Sexual Hormones: Influences on the Electrophysiology of the Brain

Papers by
Manuel Alcaraz, C. A. Barraclough, Carlos Beyer et al.

MSS Information Corporation
655 Madison Avenue, New York, N. Y. 10021

Library of Congress Cataloging in Publication Data

Main Entry under title:

Sexual hormones.

1. Hormones, Sex,--Addresses, essays, lectures.
2. Neuroendocrinology--Addresses, essays, lectures.
3. Brain--Addresses, essays, lectures. I. Alcaraz, Manuel. [DNLM: 1. Brain--Drug effects--Collected works. 2. Electrophysiology--Collected works.
3. Sex Hormones--Pharmacodynamics--Collected works.
WK900 S518 1974]
QP376.S437 599'.01'88 74-4137
ISBN 0-8422-7214-3

TABLE OF CONTENTS

CREDITS AND ACKNOWLEDGEMENTS

Alcaraz, Manuel; Carlos Guzmán-Flores; Manuel Salas; and Carlos Beyer, "Effect of Estrogen on the Responsivity of Hypothalamic and Mesencephalic Neurons in the Female Cat," *Brain Research*, 1969, 15:429-446.

Barraclough, C.A.; and B.A. Cross, "Unit Activity in the Hypothalamus of the Cyclic Female Rat: Effect of Genital Stimuli and Progesterone," *Journal of Endocrinology*, 1963, 26:339-359.

Beyer, Carlos; V. Domingo Ramirez; David I. Whitmoyer; and Charles H. Sawyer, "Effects of Hormones on the Electrical Activity of the Brain in the Rat and Rabbit," *Experimental Neurology*, 1967, 18:313-326.

Chhina, G.S.; A.S. Chakrabarty; K. Kaur; and B.K. Anand, "Electroencephalographic Responses Produced by Genital Stimulation and Hormone Administration in Sexually Immature Rhesus Monkeys," *Physiology and Behavior*, 1968, 3:579-584.

Komisaruk, Barry R.; Peter G. McDonald; David I. Whitmoyer; and Charles H. Sawyer, "Effects of Progesterone and Sensory Stimulation on EEG and Neuronal Activity in the Rat," *Experimental Neurology*, 1967, 19:494-507.

Lincoln, D.W., "Effects of Progesterone on the Electrical Activity of the Forebrain," *Journal of Endocrinology*, 1969, 45:585-596.

Lincoln, D.W., "Unit Activity in the Hypothalamus, Septum and Preoptic Area of the Rat: Characteristics of Spontaneous Activity and the Effect of Oestrogen," *Journal of Endocrinology*, 1967, 37:177-189.

Lincoln, D.W.; and B.A. Cross, "Effect of Oestrogen on the Responsiveness of Neurones in the Hypothalamus, Septum and Preoptic Area of Rats with Light-Induced Persistent Oestrus," *Journal of Endocrinology*, 1967, 37:191-203.

Logothetis, John; and Richard Harner, "Electrocortical Activation by Estrogens," *Archives of Neurology*, 1960, 3:290-297.

Oshima, Kiyoshi; and Aubrey Gorbman, "The Time Course of Effects of Sex Hormones on Electrically-Evoked Potentials in the Frog Forebrain," *Acta Endocrinologica*, 1969, 62:537-545.

Oshima, Kiyoshi; and Aubrey Gorbman, "Effects of Sex Hormones on Photically Evoked Potentials in Frog Brain," *General Comparative Endocrinology*, 1969, 12:397-404.

Pfaff, D.W.; and Estelle Gregory, "Correlation between Pre-Optic Area Unit Activity and the Cortical Electroencephalogram: Difference between Normal and Castrated Male Rats," *Electroencephalography and Clinical Neurophysiology*, 1971b, 31:223-230.

Pfaff, D.W.; and E. Gregory, "Olfactory Coding in Olfactory Bulb and Medial Forebrain Bundle of Normal and Castrated Male Rats," *Journal of Neurophysiology*, 1971a, 34:208-216.

Pfaff, Donald W.; and Carl Pfaffmann, "Olfactory and Hormonal Influences on the Basal Forebrain of the Male Rat," *Brain Research*, 1969. 15:137-156.

Terasawa, Ei; and Charles H. Sawyer, "Diurnal Variation in the Effects of Progesterone on Multiple Unit Activity in the Rat Hypothalamus," *Experimental Neurology*, 1970, 27:359-374.

Vogel, W.; D.M. Broverman; E.L. Klaiber; G. Abraham; and F.L. Cone, "Effects of Testosterone Infusions upon EEGs of Normal Male Adults," *Electroencephalography and Clinical Neurophysiology*, 1971, 31:400-403.

Woolley, Dorothy; and Paola S. Timiras, "The Gonad-Brain Relationship: Effects of Female Sex Hormones on Electroshock Convulsion in the Rat," *Endocrinology*, 1962b, 70:196-209.

PREFACE

The dictatorial effect of sexual hormones on mating behavior has long been known from the ancient knowledge that mating behavior can be abolished by castration. Later studies have shown that a small lesion in certain regions of the brain can mimic the effect of castration, and that implantation of a minute amount of sexual hormone into such regions can restore sexual behavior in the castrated animal. These studies and the demonstrations of the selective uptake and retention of sexual hormones by certain brain structures have convinced investigators that sexual hormones control respective behavior by directly altering brain function. Such a notion has now been extended to include non-sexual hormones (eg. ACTH) which have recently been shown to be capable of affecting such behavior as avoidance. Thus, from the studies on hormone-behavior relationships, the study of hormonal influence on brain function has become an established research field.

Electrophysiological study is one of the most employed methods in studying hormonal influence on brain function. Generally, it is done by comparing the electrophysiological measurements of brain function of the animals at different hormonal states. The brain function is usually measured either as the activity of a large portion of the brain with electroencephalographic recording, or as the activity of a certain neuron(s) with single or multiple unit recording. Studies of this kind have shown that both the activities of individual neurons as well as the brain as a whole can be affected by hormones. In addition, such studies provide information about the site(s) of hormonal influence in brain, the latency and the mode of hormonal action. This information is not only valuable in itself for understanding the hormonal influence on brain function, but can also lend some clues to further biochemical and pharmacological studies on the mechanism of hormonal action on nervous tissues.

However, there are problems and limitations in this field of study. A particular problem is the specificity of the hormonal influence. Studies on male sexual hormone, progesterone, and non-sexual hormones are still insufficient to clarify the specificity. Consider, for example estrogen, which attracted most intensive study in this field. Although most of the unit recording experiments indicate that there is a specific hormonal action, some of the electroencephalographic studies seem to indicate otherwise. The electrophysiological study in this field, like all other electrophysiological studies in general, has its restrictions, but it can be supplemented with other techniques. This potential application is still in the developing stage; once fully developed, our understanding will be greatly enhanced.

Lee-Ming Kow
March, 1974

Sexual Hormones

EFFECT OF ESTROGEN ON THE RESPONSIVITY OF HYPOTHALAMIC AND MESENCEPHALIC NEURONS IN THE FEMALE CAT

MANUEL ALCARAZ, CARLOS GUZMÁN-FLORES, MANUEL SALAS AND CARLOS BEYER

INTRODUCTION

Evidence exists that mating behavior is produced by the direct action of sex steroids on the brain[6,13,14]. The intimate mechanism through which estrogen elicits mating in the female is not known, but it is commonly believed that it involves changes in hypothalamic excitability[2,16]. We considered it interesting to test this hypothesis by studying the responsivity of anterior and medial hypothalamic neurons to diverse stimuli in both estrous and anestrous cats. Additional observations were made in neuronal pools of the mesencephalic reticular formation whose excitability has been shown by Kawakami and Sawyer[10] to be influenced by gonadal steroids.

METHODS

Twenty-five female cats were ovariectomized under barbiturate anesthesia. Four to 8 weeks after ovariectomy the subjects were allotted to the following two groups: (1) anestrous cats, which received a daily injection of 0.5 ml sesame oil, for 4–6 days and (2) estrous cats, which were daily injected for 4–6 days with estradiol benzoate (20 μg, estradiol benzoate, Syntex, in 0.5 ml of sesame oil). Subjects were tested daily by perineal tapping for lordosis and treading. Only subjects clearly in estrus were included in group 2.

Surgery was performed under ether. A metal cannula was placed in the trachea, and the saphenous vein was cannulated with a blunt needle for intravenous injections. Blood pressure was monitored from a polyethylene tube introduced into the right femoral artery. The subjects were placed in a stereotaxic frame (Kopf), and two small holes were drilled through the bone.

Metal cannulas (28 gauge) were stereotaxically guided through the holes and fixed with dental cement to the skull when the tip was located either in the ventral thalamic region or the mesencephalic tectum. EEG was recorded from stainless steel screws fixed by dental cement in the skull over the frontal and parietal cortex.

Multi-unit activity was recorded from the cut tip of an insulated nichrome wire (tip approximately 60 μ). The electrode was driven through one of the implanted cannulas with a microdrive manipulator (Alvar). By means of a voltage gate, neuronal spikes of a chosen height were selected from the start of the experiment. The selected spikes were used to trigger a pulse generator. The pulses of the generator activated a pen of the Grass polygraph producing a record of the neuronal firing frequency. The technique employed to record and integrate multineuronal activity has been described in detail elsewhere[5]. This technique permits the recording of the activity of a relatively small number of neurons (neuronal pool).

At the end of surgery, ether anesthesia was discontinued, pressure points and wound margins were infiltrated with novocaine, and flaxedil was administered. Artificial respiration was started. At least 4 h were allowed to pass before recording was initiated. Flaxedil was administered whenever the subjects started to show muscular activity, and novocaine infiltration was routinely performed every 3 h. Multi-unit activity was recorded from the medial and anterior hypothalamus (F 11 to 13; L 0.5 to 1; H –1 to –5 of the Jasper and Ajmone Marsan atlas[8]). In the mesencephalon, the electrodes were aimed at the region limited by the following planes: F 3 to 5; L 3; H 0 to –3.

The electrodes were advanced in small steps, and the unit activity recorded in each site was monitored for several minutes allowing for stabilization of discharge before the application of any stimulus. Neuronal pools with an erratic, unpredictable type of discharge were usually excluded from testing. Usually, two tracks were explored in each subject.

Thirty-second records of 'spontaneous' activity were taken and recorded in an Ampex tape recorder (Model SP 300) before every stimulation. The responsivity of each pool to the following stimuli was tested: tactile (lightly touching the back of the

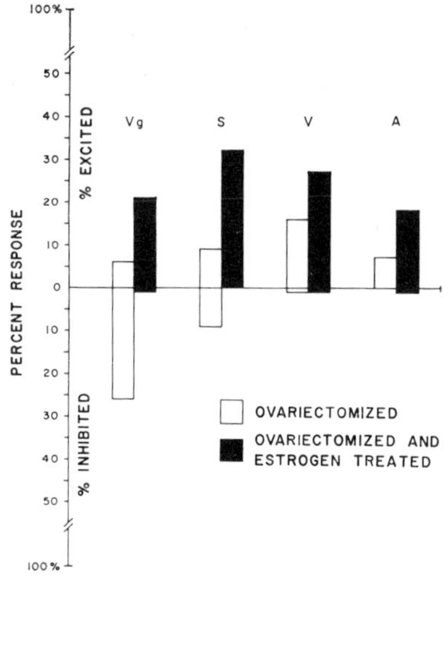

Fig. 1. Histogram showing the percentages of hypothalamic neuronal pools in ovariectomized (anestrous) and ovariectomized estrogen-treated (estrous) cats responding with acceleration or deceleration to the following stimuli: vaginal probing (Vg), tactile (S), visual (V), and acoustic (A).

subject), visual (5/sec flashes), auditory (clapping hands, beating a tin drum outside the recording room) and vaginal stimulation (probing the vagina with a glass rod lubricated with mineral oil). Standard stimulation periods lasted 30 sec. Unit activity was continuously recorded on tape during stimulation. Several minutes were allowed between stimulation periods.

Thirty-second control of stimulation records were divided into ten 3-sec samples, and the number of pulses occurring in each sample was counted with a pulse counter. The mean frequency discharge and its standard deviation were calculated for every control and experimental period. A pool was considered responsive when as a result of stimulation it increased or decreased its mean discharge frequency beyond the value of the previous control mean $\pm$ 2 standard deviations.

At completion of the observations the subjects were killed with an overdose of pentobarbital. The brain was perfused with 10% formalin through the carotid arteries. Placement of the electrodes was histologically determined.

RESULTS

General features

The EEG of most of the subjects was characterized by low voltage, fast activity interspersed with trains of slow high amplitude waves. Prolonged periods of spindle sleep were occasionally noted in some subjects when undisturbed. No clear relation was found between EEG activity and the discharge of most hypothalamic pools analyzed. Conversely, the activity of some mesencephalic neuronal pools was related to the state of vigilance of the subject. Generally, spontaneous blood pressure fluctuations did not affect either hypothalamic or mesencephalic unit activity.

Hypothalamic activity

Anestrous cats. A total of 213 hypothalamic pools was tested in 9 ovariectomized cats. With the above-mentioned criterion only 94 out of 213 pools (44%) responded either with excitation or inhibition to the diverse stimuli employed. As shown in Fig. 1, excitatory responses predominated after the application of visual and auditory stimuli. An equal number of pools showed excitatory and inhibitory responses to tactile stimulation, while vaginal probing, when effective, generally resulted in a slowing of unit firing. Fig. 2 shows a typical inhibitory response to vaginal stimulation in an anestrous cat.

Estrous cat. 156 pools were tested in 6 ovariectomized estrogen-treated subjects. Fifty-five percent (84 pools) responded to some type of stimulation. The proportion of responsive neuronal pools in estrous subjects was not significantly different from that found in ovariectomized anestrous animals (χ^2 test). However, a clear shift to excitatory responses was found after vaginal and somatic stimulation (Figs. 1 and 3). Inhibitory responses were rarely noted in estrogen-treated subjects.

No clear correlation was found between the neuronal responses and either

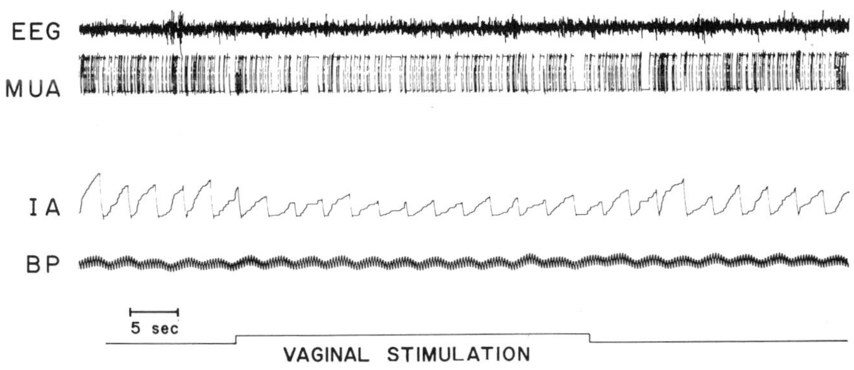

Fig. 2. Effect of vaginal probing on the multi-unit activity of the ventromedial hypothalamic nucleus in an anestrous cat. The slowing in the unitary discharge was not correlated with EEG or blood pressure changes. Abbreviations: MUA, multi-unit activity of the ventromedial hypothalamus; IA, integrated unit activity; BP, blood pressure.

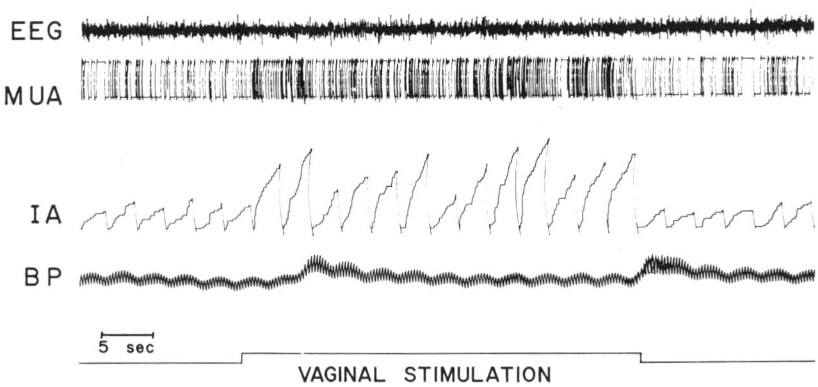

Fig. 3. Acceleration of ventromedial hypothalamic units by vaginal probing in an estrous cat. Note that the unitary response precedes the rise in blood pressure. Abbreviations as in Fig. 2.

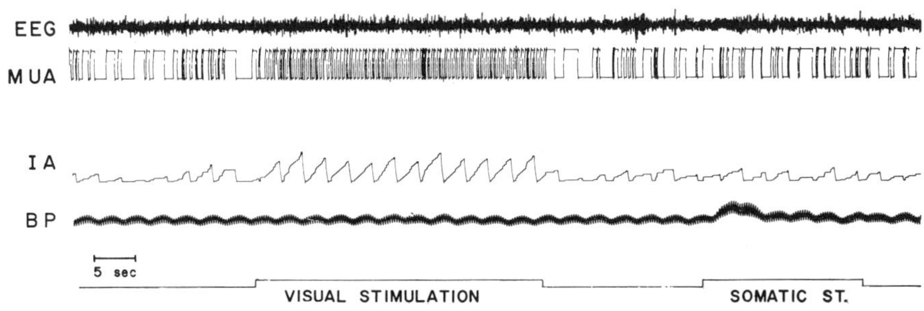

Fig. 4. Record showing the differential effect of visual and tactile stimulation on hypothalamic unit activity and blood pressure.

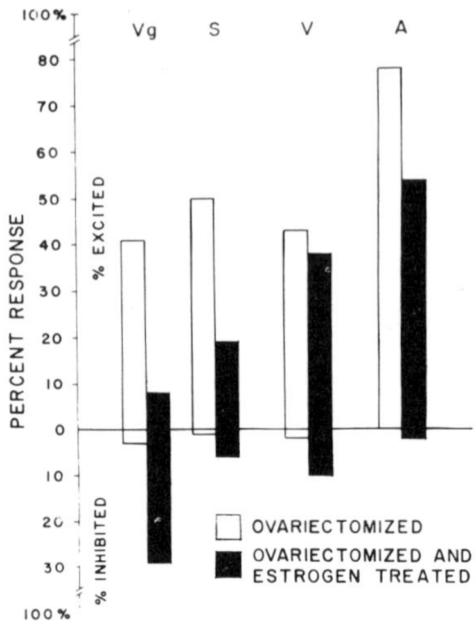

Fig. 5. Histogram showing the percentages of mesencephalic neuronal pools in ovariectomized (anestrous) and ovariectomized estrogen-treated (estrous) subjects that responded to the diverse stimuli employed. Abbreviations as in Fig. 1.

blood pressure or EEG changes. Fig. 4 shows a clear response to light flashes without any blood pressure alterations, whereas tactile stimulation which elicited a rise in blood pressure did not significantly alter unit discharge.

The effect of vaginal stimulation on blood pressure was somewhat inconsistent, though this procedure usually caused blood pressure rises in both estrous and anestrous subjects. Yet the direction and magnitude of the neuronal response to vaginal probing was independent of the change in blood pressure. Frequently the responses overlasted the period of stimulation. This was particularly clear for vaginal stimulation in which the effects occasionally persisted for several minutes after the cessation of the stimulus.

Mesencephalon

Anestrous cats. Most of the mesencephalic pools (86%) tested in 5 anestrous subjects responded at least to one type of stimulation. Excitatory responses clearly predominated over inhibitory ones in all stimulus modalities (Fig. 5). Vaginal stimulation rarely decelerated the discharge of mesencephalic pools in anestrous subjects.

Estrous cats. Estrogen treatment produced a slight but non-significant reduction in the proportion of responsive pools (80% responded in estrous subjects against 86% in anestrous subjects). Yet a shift towards inhibitory responses, particularly striking during vaginal stimulation, was observed (Fig. 5).

DISCUSSION

Kawakami and Sawyer[10] found that the administration of gonadal steroids to ovariectomized rabbits lowers the threshold elicitation of both EEG arousal and the

EEG after reaction by cerebral stimulation. This and similar studies (see Sawyer[16]) strongly suggest that the effects of gonadal hormones on brain functions are produced by altering the excitability of some neural circuits.

The critical site of action of estrogen on the brain is unknown. Recently, Lincoln and Cross[12], working on the rat under urethane, reported differential effects of estrogen on the responsivity of hypothalamic and septal neurons. Estrogen enhanced the proportion of inhibitory responses to pain, cold and cervical stimulation in the anterior hypothalamus, whereas in the septum the number of inhibitory responses was reduced. The above-mentioned effects were generally related to EEG changes, an observation suggesting that they were the result of generalized changes in brain excitability. More recently, Kawakami and Saito[9] studied in both ovariectomized and estrogen-treated cats the responsivity of neurons from a wide hypothalamic region to vaginal stimulation. Acceleration in the firing rate of anterior hypothalamic neurons following vaginal stimulation was noted, though the authors did not state the endocrine condition of their animals. On the other hand, vaginal stimulation decreased the firing rate of ventromedial neurons in anestrous cats, whereas it augmented it in estrous animals. Our results fully agree with the changes observed in the ventromedial hypothalamic nucleus by the Japanese workers. On the other hand, opposite effects to those obtained in the rat by Lincoln and Cross[12] were observed by ourselves in the anterior hypothalamus. Moreover, in our experiments hypothalamic unitary responses were independent of EEG and changes in blood pressure. This contrasts with results obtained in the rat under urethane by several workers[1,11,12] who found that a large proportion of hypothalamic neurons or neuronal pools vary their activity in parallel with EEG or blood pressure fluctuations. The discrepancy between our results and those obtained in the rat must be due either to species differences or to the different experimental conditions in which the animals were tested.

Our results show that estrogen can also alter the responsivity of mesencephalic reticular neurons to peripheral stimulation. Opposite effects to those observed in the hypothalamus were usually obtained. This suggests an inverse relationship between the activity of the mesencephalic reticular formation and the anterior hypothalamus. Our results, however, do not allow us to assert whether there exists a causal relationship between the activity of the mesencephalon and the anterior hypothalamus. Reciprocal interaction between the firing of mesencephalic and posterior hypothalamic neurons has been found by Slusher *et al.*[17] after intracerebral administration of hydrocortisone.

Our experiments do not permit us to differentiate direct from indirect actions of estrogen on hypothalamic or mesencephalic neurons. Estrogen can affect either the excitability of the recorded neurons themselves or the physiological conditions and excitability of the elements involved in the transmission of afferent impulses to the brain stem, *i.e.* receptors, internuncial neurons. It is interesting that estrogen treatment did not significantly alter the overall proportion of responsive neuronal pools, a finding suggesting that no marked change in the excitability of the recorded neurons occurred. This suggests that transmission along some of the pathways leading to the brain stem might be facilitated or inhibited by estrogen. In this connection it is important to recall that afferent transmission to the brain stem is affected by the blood level of some adrenal corticoids[3,4,7].

Vaginal stimulation is known to elicit the mating pattern in estrous cats. Moreover, it is known that the integrity of the anterior hypothalamus is essential for the manifestation of estrus in the female cat[15]. Hence it is tempting to speculate that the increase in firing rate of hypothalamic neurons that normally followed vaginal stimulation in estrous cats was an electric correlate of mating behavior. However, there is no evidence indicating that the mating pattern in the cat or any other species is produced by an increase in the firing frequency of hypothalamic or other neurons. Moreover, the physiological meaning of changes in frequency discharge is far from clear (see Beyer and Sawyer[2]). Therefore, the significance of our results for brain functioning must await further elucidation.

SUMMARY

The responsivity of hypothalamic and mesencephalic neurons to somatic, visual, acoustic and vaginal stimulation was studied in ovariectomized (anestrous) and estrogen-treated ovariectomized conscious cats (estrous) immobilized with Flaxedil. Comparison between the results obtained in the two groups revealed that in the anterior and medial hypothalamus estrogen facilitated the appearance of excitatory responses to all the types of stimulus used, whereas it reduced the number of inhibitory responses to vaginal stimulation. Excitatory responses to all sensory modalities clearly predominated over inhibitory ones in the mesencephalic reticular formation of anestrous cats. By contrast, a marked increase in the proportion of inhibitory responses, particularly to vaginal stimulation, was observed in estrous subjects. Our results suggest that estrogen affects differentially the responsivity of hypothalamic and mesencephalic neurons to peripheral stimulation.

REFERENCES

1 Beyer, C., Ramírez, V. D., Whitmoyer, D. I., and Sawyer, G. H., Effects of hormones on the electrical activity of the brain in the rat and rabbit, *Exp. Neurol.*, 18 (1967) 313–326.

2 Beyer, C., and Sawyer, C. H., Hypothalamic unit activity related to control of the pituitary gland. In L. Martini and F. Ganong (Eds.), *Frontiers in Neuroendocrinology*, Oxford University Press, Oxford, 1969, pp. 255–287.

3 Chambers, W. F., Freedman, S. L., and Sawyer, C. H., The effect of adrenal steroids on evoked reticular responses, *Exp. Neurol.*, 8 (1963) 458–469.

4 Feldman, S., Electrophysiological alterations in adrenalectomy, *Arch. Neurol. (Chic.)*, 7 (1962) 106–116.

5 Guzmán-Flores, C., and Alcaraz, M., A technique for recording and integrating unit activity, *Bol. Inst. Estud. méd. biol. (Méx.)*, 1969, in press.

6 Harris, G. W., and Michael, R. P., The activation of sexual behaviour by hypothalamic implants of estrogen, *J. Physiol. (Lond.)*, 171 (1964) 275–301.

7 Hoagland, H., Studies of brain metabolism and electrical activity in relation to adrenocortical physiology, *Recent Progr. Hormone Res.*, 10 (1954) 29–63.

8 Jasper, H. H., and Ajmone Marsan, C., *A Stereotaxic Atlas of the Diencephalon of the Cat*, Nat. Res. Council of Canada, Ottawa, 1954.

9 Kawakami, M., and Saito, H., Unit activity in the hypothalamus of the cat: Effect of genital stimuli, luteinizing hormone and oxytocin, *Jap. J. Physiol.*, 17 (1965) 466–486.
10 Kawakami, M., and Sawyer, C. H., Neuroendocrine correlates of changes in brain activity threshold by sex steroids and pituitary hormones, *Endocrinology*, 65 (1959) 652–668.
11 Komisaruk, B. R., McDonald, P. G., Whitmoyer, D. I., and Sawyer, C. H., Effect of progesterone and sensory stimulation on EEG and neuronal activity in the rat, *Exp. Neurol.*, 19 (1967) 494–507.
12 Lincoln, D. W., and Cross, B. A., Effect of oestrogen on the responsiveness of neurons in the hypothalamus, septum and preoptic area of rats with light-induced persistent oestrus, *J. Endocr.*, 37 (1967) 191–203.
13 Lisk, R. D., Diencephalic placement of estradiol and sexual receptivity in the female rat, *Amer. J. Physiol.*, 203 (1962) 493–496.
14 Palka, Y. S., and Sawyer, C. H., The effect of hypothalamic implants of ovarian steroids on oestrous behaviour in rabbits, *J. Physiol. (Lond.)*, 185 (1966) 251–269.
15 Robinson, B. L., and Sawyer, C. H., The loci of sex behavioural and gonadotrophic centers in the female cat hypothalamus, *Physiologist*, 1 (1957) 72 (abstract).
16 Sawyer, C. H., Effect of hormonal steroids on certain mechanisms in the adult brain. In L. Martini, F. Fraschini and M. Motta (Eds.), *Proceedings of the Second International Congress on Hormonal Steroids*. Int. Congr. Series No. 132, Excerpta Medica, Amsterdam, 1967, pp. 123–134.
17 Slusher, M. A., Hyde, J. E., and Laufer, M., Effect of intracerebral hydrocortisone on unit activity of diencephalon and midbrain in cats, *J. Neurophysiol.*, 29 (1966) 157–169.

UNIT ACTIVITY IN THE HYPOTHALAMUS OF THE CYCLIC FEMALE RAT: EFFECT OF GENITAL STIMULI AND PROGESTERONE

C. A. BARRACLOUGH AND B. A. CROSS

SUMMARY

Unit activity in the hypothalamus and other diencephalic regions was recorded with stereotaxically oriented steel microelectrodes in adult female rats under light urethane anaesthesia.

Spontaneous firing rates of neurones varied from < 1/10 sec. to > 50/sec., but the majority fired at 1–10/sec. Some variations in the pattern of firing are described.

Acceleration of firing rate was most readily induced by pain stimuli (64 % of neurones) and then by cold (60 %), probing the cervix (47 %), smell (20 %), light (5 %) and noise (3 %) in that order. A minority of neurones were inhibited by the stimuli.

Many neurones responded to several different stimuli, most commonly by accelerating to cervical probing, cold and pain. Inhibitory convergence was also observed, e.g. blockade of the response to cervical probing by an olfactory stimulus, and inhibition by cervical probing of the response to cold or pain.

The proportion of neurones excited by smell in prooestrous rats was more than double that in oestrous or dioestrous rats. Oestrous rats had relatively more neurones which were unresponsive or inhibited by the test stimuli.

Slow intravenous injection of 400 μg. progesterone induced a selective depression of the response of lateral hypothalamic neurones to cervical probing. The effect was maximal at about 30 min. and full recovery occurred in 1 hr.

The possible significance of these observations is discussed with particular reference to the neural control of luteotrophin secretion.

INTRODUCTION

Unit recording from the hypothalamus has proved a useful method of furthering understanding of certain neuro-endocrine mechanisms. The postulated osmoreceptor role of supraoptic and preoptic neurones in regulating antidiuretic hormone release from the neurohypophysis has been studied in this way in rabbits (Cross & Green, 1959) and cats (Brooks, Ushiyama & Lange, 1962) and the participation of lateral and posterior hypothalamic neurones in the adrenomedullary discharge initiated by hypercapnia has also been investigated in rabbits (Cross & Silver, 1963). Incidental observations have been reported which might bear on anterior pituitary function, e.g. the finding that ambient light intensity can affect the discharge rate of certain supraoptic neurones (Cross & Green, 1959), but so far there have been no unit studies directed specifically to the elucidation of the neural mechanisms regulating secretion of adenohypophysial hormones.

The cyclic female rat seemed to us a suitable subject for such a study for several reasons. Animals at any desired stage of the oestrous cycle can be chosen by examining vaginal smears. Mechanical stimulation of the cervix of oestrous females with a glass rod is known to induce pseudopregnancy through the secretion of luteotrophic hormone from the adenohypophysis. Stereotaxic procedures have been in routine use and excellent stereotaxic atlases of the rat brain are available. Our central objective therefore was to gather information on the responses of hypothalamic neurones to genital stimulation which might reflect, in part at least, the neural mechanism initiating the secretion of luteotrophin.

MATERIALS AND METHODS

Animals

Forty-eight female albino rats, 210–320 g. in body weight, were used. They were all bred in the laboratory from the same Wistar strain, maintained on rat pellets and water *ad lib.* and kept at a room temperature of 68° F. For 1 week or more before operations daily vaginal smears were taken.

Operative procedure

The rats were anaesthetized with urethane injected i.p. as a 20 % aqueous solution in a dose of 1·5 g./kg. After shaving the head and exposing the external auditory meatus they were secured in the stereotaxic instrument in an earthed metal wire cage to shield against electrical interference. A small burr hole was drilled in the skull slightly to the right or left of the bregma suture and the dura mater carefully incised and reflected. During the subsequent period of the experiment no further surgical manipulation of the animal was required, and often unit recording was continued for 6–8 hr. with minimal or no supplemental doses of anaesthetic. For the whole of this period the rats were kept warm by means of an overhead infra-red lamp. For experiments involving i.v. injection of hormones a preliminary operation was performed to cannulate the femoral vein with thin polythene tubing. Slow injections of normal saline, progesterone dissolved in propylene glycol (8 mg./ml.) or propylene glycol were made from a 1·0 ml. tuberculin syringe graduated in 0·01 ml.

Unit recording

Stainless steel microelectrodes were made from straight intestinal suture needles electropolished by a.c. at 5–10 V, first in concentrated HCl and finally in a mixture of 21 parts H_3PO_4, 17 parts H_2SO_4 and 12 parts distilled water. The resulting tips were approximately 1–3 μ in terminal diameter. The electrodes were dipped in lacquer (E–33–N, Insl–X Company Inc., Ossining, New York), turned up and allowed to dry and harden for at least 24 hr. before use. The tip resistance of the microelectrodes was 0·5–5 MΩ. They were mounted in the electrode carrier and a.c.-coupled to the input stage which was a Tectronix type 123 preamplifier with a gain of 100, an input impedance of 10 MΩ and a passband of 3 cyc./sec. to 25 kc. The recording was single-ended with the earthed input connected to one of the metal ear plugs. The Tectronix preamplifier was plugged directly into the input socket of one channel of a dual beam oscilloscope (Nagard type D.T. 103).

In all experiments, loudspeaker monitoring of unit activity was employed, for which purpose the amplified signals from the Y plates of the cathode-ray oscilloscope were capacity-coupled to an audio-amplifier. By means of a simple co-axial distribution box these amplified signals could also be fed to a monitoring oscilloscope, and a dekatron fast counter and timing unit (Labgear Ltd. types D4131 and D4102). Permanent records of all important test procedures were made on magnetic tape using a two-channel tape recorder (EMI model 76). Unit activity was recorded on one channel and a spoken commentary on the other to facilitate later analysis of the records. To obtain a visual reproduction of the unit discharges the appropriate tape record was sometimes played back into the oscilloscope with the sweep generator turned off and the vertical deflexions photographed on moving film, but usually the unit discharges were written out on paper by means of a Grass Polygraph. For the latter purpose the unit channel output from the tape recorder was made to trigger a square wave pulse generator (Nagard type 5002) connected in turn to one channel of the polygraph, so that each neurone spike caused a deflexion of the pen. For fast-firing units it was preferable to write out only every tenth spike by using the output of the first decade of the dekatron counter as the triggering stimulus (Fig. 3).

Locating microelectrode sites

The rat stereotaxic atlas of de Groot (1959) was used to orientate the microelectrodes in the diencephalon. An accurate micrometer reading for the horizontal plane of the surface of the cerebral cortex was first obtained by slowly lowering the microelectrode with the micro-manipulator until the characteristically abrupt change in the noise level was heard on the loudspeaker. After depressing the electrode a little deeper into the cortex the hole in the skull was sealed by applying warm agar solution which quickly solidified around the microelectrode. Note was kept of the depth from cortex surface of each unit studied and also of the horizontal co-ordinates and final depth of all electrode tracks. Small Prussian blue spots were made at strategic sites in electrode tracks to aid later histological reconstruction. An anodal d.c. current of $< 5\ \mu$A. was passed through the steel microelectrode for a few seconds to deposit iron in the tissue. The rats were killed by i.v. 'Nembutal' and after removing them from the stereotaxic instrument the heads were perfused via the heart with a weak solution of potassium ferrocyanide in normal saline to develop the Prussian blue reaction and then fixed by perfusion of 20 ml. 10% formol saline. Finally the brains were carefully removed from the cranial cavity and stored in 10% formol saline. Frozen sections were cut transversely at 50 μ using the method of Marshall (1940) and mounted serially. The sections were stained with cresyl violet or neutral red, the latter to give greater contrast for the Prussian blue spots. The upper portions of the electrode tracks in the plane of section were readily identified, but the finely tapered tips often left little trace in the sections, so that the Prussian blue spots were of great help. Shrinkage was not more than $\frac{1}{8}$th and the site of all recorded neurones could be estimated by their distance either from cortex or a Prussian blue spot or both.

Characteristics and distribution of recorded neurones

From the first experiment the rat proved to be a rewarding subject for the study of unit activity in the forebrain. As the microelectrode tip penetrated the cerebral cortex action potentials were readily picked out, and an abundance of units could

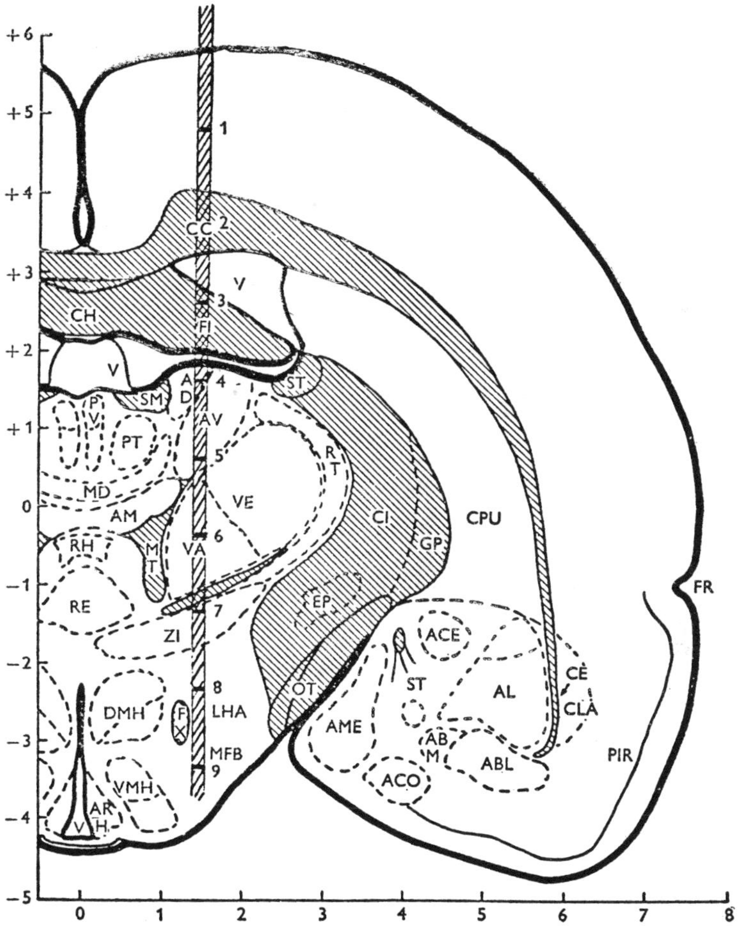

Fig. 1. Diagram showing the path most commonly traversed by the electrodes as a hatched band superimposed on a diagram of the A 5·4 plane of the Rat Brain Atlas of de Groot (1959).

generally be found in the cortex and deeper in the thalamus. They were usually large and distinct with signal-to-noise ratios as great as 40:1. As previously observed in the rabbit (Cross & Green, 1959; Cross & Silver, 1963), stable units became scarcer as the electrode passed into the hypothalamus, but in many cases it was possible to study 4–6 hypothalamic units over a distance of 1·5 mm. in one passage through the hypothalamus (see Fig. 1).

Fig. 2 illustrates the waveform of four units recorded in one microelectrode track. Typically, the action potentials were about 0·75 mV. in amplitude and 1·5 msec. in duration. All the units studied were positive/negative and most showed evidence of a prespike potential. Occasionally, as in cell F in Fig. 2, the prespike potential occurred without an accompanying main spike potential. Minor variations were

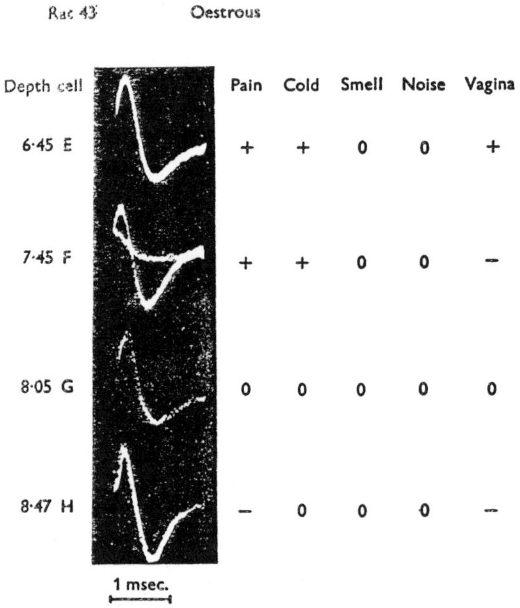

Fig. 2. Photographs of superimposed oscilloscope sweeps to show the waveform (upward deflexion positive) of four neurones recorded successively in a single microelectrode track. The action potentials triggered the sweeps internally and the initial part of the waveform from the stationary spot was therefore missed. The figure-of-eight appearance of cell F was due to the fact that the prespike potential sometimes fired separately (see text). Responses of neurones to five test stimuli are shown to right of their waveforms: acceleration of firing rate indicated as +, slowing as – and no change as 0. Cell H, located with the help of a Prussian blue spot, was in the dorsal premammillary nucleus, cells F and G in the posterior hypothalamic area and E in the ventromedial thalamic nucleus.

apparent in the waveform of different units, but in individual units the waveform persisted unchanged for long periods. The particular waveform observed seemed to depend largely upon the location of the microelectrode tip in relation to the neurone. By carefully advancing the microelectrode with the fine adjustment of the micromanipulator, we were sometimes able to record from the same unit for a distance of 100 μ or more. In these instances a change in the relative prominence of the prespike and main spike potentials was commonly observed. The type of unit waveform described above we regarded as the action potential recorded from the vicinity of a nerve cell body. Small negative spikes of less than 1 msec. duration sometimes appeared transiently in the corpus callosum and other areas of white matter as well as occasionally in nuclear regions. They were interpreted as impulses from nerve fibres and were disregarded for the purposes of this investigation.

As a general procedure the microelectrodes were oriented through the brain in a sagittal plane about 1·3 mm. from the midline near the bregma, so as to bring the tip of the electrode into the lateral area of the hypothalamus at about 7·5 mm. from the surface of the cortex (Fig. 1). More medial and more anterior regions of the hypothalamus appeared, in initial explorations, to yield few neurones suitable for study.

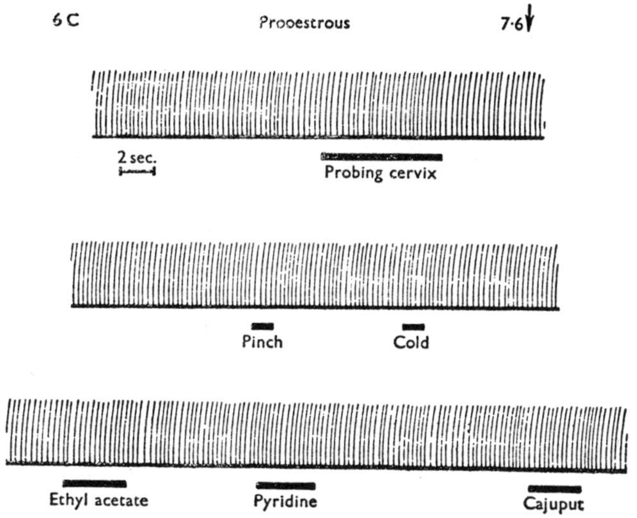

Fig. 3. Fast-firing thalamic neurone, probably in the reticular nucleus. Note regularity of firing rate and lack of response to test stimuli. Polygraph records prepared from magnetic tape of experiment to show every *tenth* spike (see methods). In this and all remaining figures duration of stimuli indicated by solid bars under unit records. Stage of oestrous cycle, rat no. and serial letter of neurone, together with its depth from cortex surface, shown at top of each figure.

Our usual procedure was to examine first the spontaneous activity and responsiveness of a few neurones in the thalamus before making a more exhaustive examination of the patterns of activity displayed by hypothalamic neurones. From examination of the electrode tracks in histological sections of the brains it was evident that neurones were recorded in many thalamic nuclei including the anterodorsal, anteroventral, reticular, ventralis anterior, mediodorsal and ventromedial. However, since the Prussian blue marker spots were all placed in the hypothalamus, identification of the sites of thalamic units could not be made with the same degree of precision. About one-third of the neurones were found to be situated in the hypothalamus, mostly in the lateral area. The rest were in the thalamus or zona incerta.

Usually before commencing tests of the responsiveness of a neurone to various stimuli, its spontaneous firing frequency was determined over 10 sec. intervals with the dekatron fast counter. Firing rates varied very considerably from less than one impulse/10 sec. to over 50 impulses/sec. However, more than half the neurones counted had firing frequencies in the range 1–10/sec. There was a tendency for hypothalamic neurones to exhibit a more regular rate of firing than thalamic neurones. Some neurones were found, notably in the region of the zona incerta, which fired at a steady fast rate, e.g. 40/sec. for upwards of an hour (Fig. 3). Usually the firing pattern was much less constant than this, even in the hypothalamus. Two variants often observed were intermittent bursts of impulses apparently unconnected with any external stimulation, or alternatively a train of fairly evenly spaced spikes interspersed by groups of two or three action potentials in very rapid succession, giving a characteristic 'beep' sound on the monitoring loudspeaker. When these 'beeps' were replayed from the magnetic tape to the polygraph, the pen was unable to follow the individual signals and produced instead a summated signal. The resulting records thus provided a clear graphical representation of the incidence of such activity (Figs. 4, 10 and 11). Single neurones were studied for periods varying from a few minutes to over 2 hr., the average duration being about 20 min. During the longer periods of observation we sometimes found a change in the pattern of firing, e.g. a fast-firing neurone which was unresponsive to various sensory stimuli would slow down and then become excitable to previously negative stimuli. Such bimodal neurones were usually situated above the hypothalamus and the shift in activity would be from a steady firing rate of 10–50/sec. to a slow irregular pattern of firing frequently with a tendency to 'beep'.

Effect of visual, acoustic and olfactory stimuli

Table 1 shows that only a small percentage of neurones gave any response to noise or light. One sound-sensitive neurone located in the dorsomedial hypothalamic nucleus was inhibited not only by the shrill blast of the whistle used routinely as an acoustic stimulus, but also by the very much less intense stimulus provided by lightly snapping the fingers. Another neurone inhibited by noise was found in the lateral hypothalamic area. Of six neurones whose firing rate was accelerated by acoustic stimuli three were situated in the lateral hypothalamic area and three in the thalamus.

Illumination of the eyes was effected by means of a small pocket flashlamp. This stimulus rarely evoked any apparent change in firing rate. Only five neurones showed a reproducible response and in these it took the form of an accelerated firing during the period of ocular illumination. Two of the neurones were located in the lateral hypothalamic area, one in the zona incerta and two in the thalamus. Finding so few neurones responsive to light we discontinued this stimulus in our testing procedures after twenty-eight experiments.

For studying responsiveness to olfactory stimuli we first tried a variety of odorous chemicals, i.e. ethyl acetate, pyridine, clove oil, terpineol and oil of cajuput. These were fairly quickly reduced to two—ethyl acetate and oil of cajuput and in many experiments only the latter was used. A piece of surgical gauze damped with the chemical was placed about half a centimetre from the animal's nostrils and left in position for 5–30 sec., i.e. long enough to ensure that inhalation of the odour had occurred. In some experiments the rat stopped breathing momentarily as a result of this procedure and quite often an increased rate of respiration was observed.

Three-quarters of the neurones tested gave no response to olfactory stimuli (Figs. 3–5), though in many cases an altered respiration showed that the odour had been inhaled. Of the forty-seven neurones that did show a response forty were accelerated and the others slowed. Twenty-seven of the excited neurones were distributed in the lateral and perifornical area of the hypothalamus and the rest in various thalamic nuclei including the anteroventral, reticular, mediodorsal and ventralis anterior. Four hypothalamic neurones, all situated in the lateral hypothalamic area, were inhibited by the odour of cajuput oil or ethyl acetate. An indication of differential sensitivity to various odours was seen in some neurones, e.g.

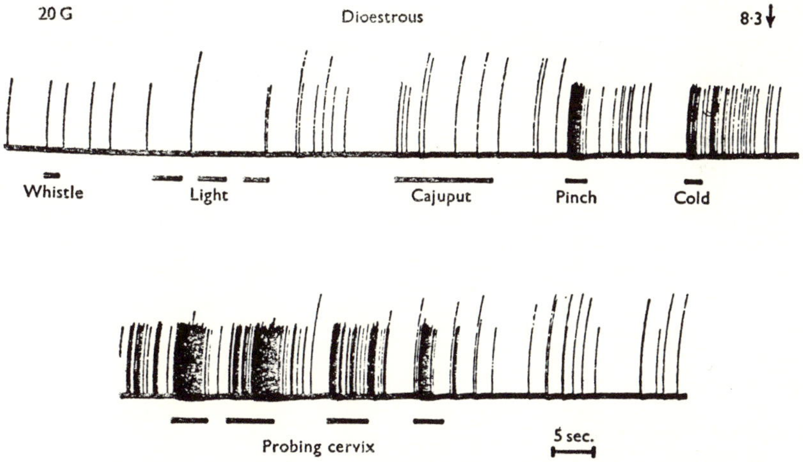

Fig. 4. Lateral hypothalamic neurone unaffected by acoustic, light and olfactory stimuli but responsive to pain, cold and cervical probing (see also Fig. 10). The taller deflexions or 'beeps' represent the summated response of the polygraph pen to two spikes arriving very close together (< 10 msec. apart).

acceleration to cajuput oil but not ethyl acetate, but opposite effects, i.e. slowing to one odour and accelerating to another were never observed.

It is of interest that all the neurones from which olfactory responses were elicited also responded to other sensory modalities, usually pain, cold or vaginal stimulation (see below). It seemed likely, therefore, that so far as the neurones in the lateral hypothalamic area were concerned a convergence of afferent impulses occurred from spinal pathways and the medial forebrain bundle.

An interesting inhibitory phenomenon resulting from olfactory stimuli was seen in one lateral hypothalamic neurone. A slight diminution in firing frequency occurred during exposure to the odour of either cajuput oil or ethyl acetate; but a much more striking effect was the blockade of the excitatory response to cold and genital stimulation (see below). Recovery from this inhibitory influence followed within 15 sec. of removing the odorous agents (Fig. 8).

Effect of pain and cold stimuli

Both these sensory stimuli were applied to the tail of the rats. A manual pinch constituted the pain stimulus, and local cooling was produced by spraying the tail for 1 sec. with ethyl chloride. Both stimuli gave reproducible responses in most neurones tested and nearly two-thirds of them exhibited a clear acceleration of firing rate (Table 1 and Figs. 4 and 7). About a tenth of the neurones were inhibited in varying degrees (Fig. 5). As both stimuli involved a tactile component we looked for evidence of responsiveness to this modality but found only three neurones which were excited by touching or stroking the tail.

Table 1. *Summary of responses obtained in* **306** *recorded neurones*

(Percentages are calculated to nearest whole number.)

Stimulus	No. rats	No. cells	% excited	% inhibited	% unchanged
Noise	46	203	3	2	95
Light	26	94	5	0	95
Smell	45	197	20	4	76
Pain	48	282	64	12	24
Cold	47	267	60	9	31
Probe cervix	48	256	47	13	40

A pronounced after-discharge was a common feature of the response to pain, as illustrated in Fig. 11. A similar long-lasting increase in firing rate frequently occurred also following cold (Fig. 7), though in this case the true duration of the cooling effect was less readily controlled. In responsive neurones with a marked 'beeping' tendency both pain and cold had the effect of diminishing the incidence of 'beeps' during the period of accelerated firing, with a recurrence of the 'beeps' after the waning of the response. In such cases there was clearly a change in the pattern of firing as well as in the frequency (Fig. 4). Moreover, some of the bimodal neurones referred to in the first section would only respond to pain or cold during the slow-firing phase commonly associated with 'beeping', and were unaltered by application of the stimuli during the phase of fast regular firing. A related phenomenon occurred in one thalamic neurone which responded to none of the test stimuli except glass-rod stimulation of the cervix (see below). This slowed the firing rate of the neurone from about 20/sec. to less than 1/sec. When thus slowed by cervical probing the neurone could be accelerated by pain stimuli. It would seem that excitatory connexions from pain or cold pathways were present for all these neurones, but they were unable to respond because their firing rates were already maximal or near maximal.

As previously noted inhibitory effects of pain and cold on the frequency of discharge of neurones were much less common. A good example, however, is seen in Fig. 5 which illustrates the response of a lateral hypothalamic neurone to cold and pain. This neurone was also slowed by cervical stimulation. Such parallelism was not by any means the normal rule. In one thalamic neurone the after-discharge resulting from cervical excitation was actually suppressed by cold and pain stimuli though the initial burst of spikes was not blocked. In this case the effects of pain and cold were the same and both were antagonistic to the genital response. Cold and pain usually elicited comparable responses, but a dozen neurones were found in which different effects were observed to follow stimulation of these sensory modalities. Four neurones were inhibited by pain and accelerated by cold. Two were in the thalamus and two in the hypothalamus. The reverse situation, acceleration to pain and inhibition to cold stimuli, was noted in two experiments, both neurones being situated in the lateral hypothalamic area. In addition, six neurones, four in the hypothalamus, one in the zona incerta and one in the mediodorsal thalamic nucleus, responded to only one of the two stimuli, either by an acceleration or by slowing.

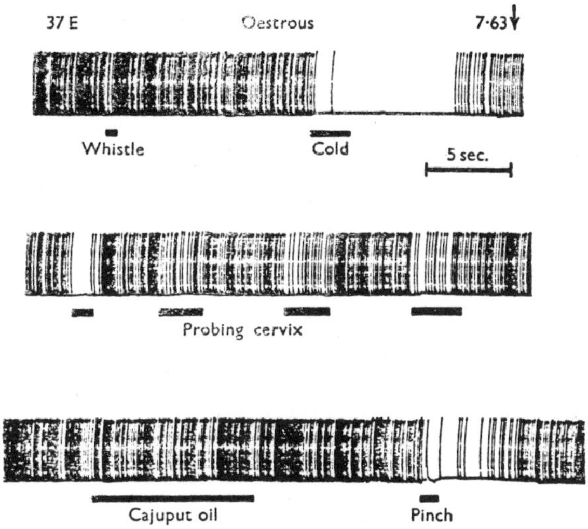

Fig. 5. Lateral hypothalamic neurone showing inhibitory responses to cold, pain and cervical probing and no response to acoustic and olfactory stimuli.

Effect of genital stimuli

A tapered glass rod with rounded end was used for mechanical stimulation of vulva, vagina or cervix. The rod was lubricated with liquid paraffin before insertion into the reproductive tract. The most effective stimulus consisted in probing deep into the vagina so as to bring the tip of the glass rod into firm contact with the os cervicis. Nearly half the 256 neurones tested in this way responded by a clear acceleration of firing rate. A much smaller proportion of neurones showed a diminution or arrest of firing activity. Thus the general effect of genital stimulation was intermediate between that of pain or cold on the one hand and olfactory stimulation on the other (Table 1).

Responsiveness to genital stimulation was shown in equal degree by neurones in the thalamus and hypothalamus. Nor was there any apparent segregation of neurones showing inhibition from those which were excited. Neurones displaying both types of response were found in the lateral hypothalamic area, zona incerta and the ventral nucleus of the thalamus. Fig. 6 illustrates the contrasted behaviour of two neurones in the lateral hypothalamic area, the first of which was less than half a millimetre above the other. Many other examples were seen of different responses to genital stimuli in nearby neurones (Fig. 2).

After-discharge was less commonly observed to follow genital stimuli than pain or cold. More often the frequency of firing would wane during a sustained contact of the glass rod with the cervix, suggesting a process of sensory adaptation. This sort of change in excitability was particularly evident following stimulation of the vulva or vagina, and it was therefore difficult to obtain reproducible responses from these parts of the female tract. A burst of impulses might follow the initial insertion of the glass rod into the vagina, but thereafter movement of the rod in the vagina usually produced little change in the activity of the recorded neurones. On the other hand,

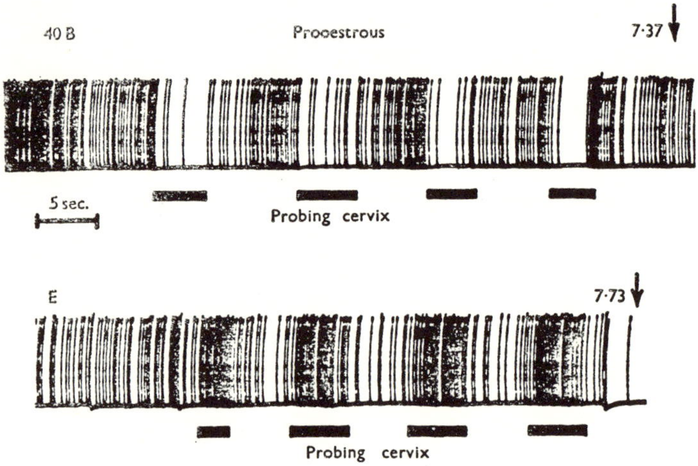

Fig. 6. Two lateral hypothalamic neurones showing contrasting responses to cervical probing. 40B, inhibited, was situated 0·46 mm. above 40E which was accelerated by the stimuli.

the response to probing the cervix could be elicited repeatedly (Figs. 4, 6, 8 and 9). In some experiments we compared the intensity of the response in individual neurones to different forms of genital manipulation. As a rule cervical probing gave the biggest effect, followed by stimulation of the vagina and vulva in that order. Often no response at all could be evoked by the latter two types of stimulation. We encountered only one neurone which responded in opposite ways to the different kinds of genital stimulus. This was a neurone in the anteroventral nucleus of the thalamus which was inhibited by cervical probing but excited by stimulation of the vulva.

We were particularly interested to discover if any neurones would show a response to genital stimulation only. Three neurones came near to satisfying this degree of specificity. The first, a lateral hypothalamic neurone, gave no response when tested with light, whistles, pain, cold and the odour of cajuput oil but acceleration of the firing rate was repeatedly induced by probing the cervix. Of special interest was the striking response produced in this neurone by gently stroking the loin, e.g. a site which normally receives tactile stimulation from the male during coitus. A comparable tactile stimulus delivered to the hind paw had no effect. The second neurone, also in the lateral hypothalamic area, was observed in an oestrous rat. This was a very slow-firing neurone which could not be accelerated by any of the test stimuli except probing the cervix, which provoked bursts of impulses at rates of 3–4/sec. from a background activity of less than one impulse/10 sec. The response was highly reproducible, but in this animal stroking the loin had no effect on the neurone. The third neurone to respond only to genital stimulation was found in a dioestrous rat, high in the thalamus, probably in the mediodorsal nucleus.

The majority of neurones which responded to genital stimuli also exhibited a sensitivity to more than one other stimulus modality. Commonest were neurones

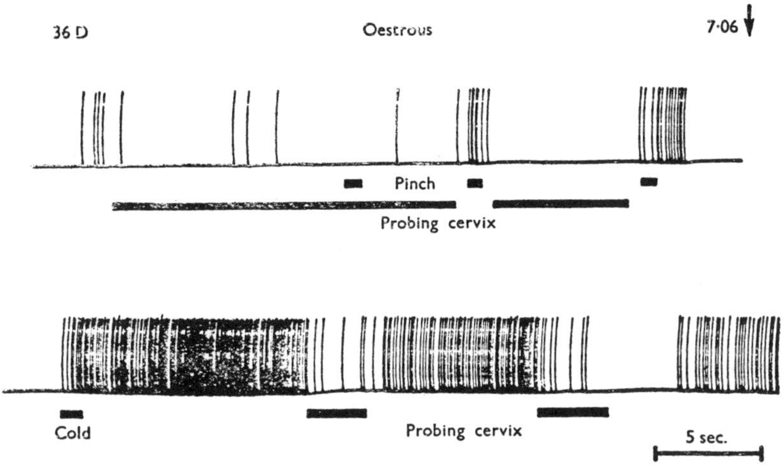

Fig. 7. Neurone in zona incerta showing interaction of convergent sensory stimuli. Upper record shows inhibitory effect of cervical probing on response to a pain stimulus, and lower record illustrates a similar inhibitory influence of cervical probing on the after-discharge following a cold stimulus.

which were excited alike by cervical probing, pain and cold (Figs. 2 and 4). Ninety-four neurones showed this pattern of responsiveness. The cervical stimulus was clearly distinct from pain, however, for some neurones responded to probing the cervix and remained unaffected by pain stimuli, and others were found which responded in the opposite sense to the two stimuli, e.g. being inhibited by cervical probing and accelerated by pain (Fig. 2). Several thalamic neurones, for example, could be induced to alternate between slow firing with 'beeps' under the influence of genital stimuli and fast regular firing under the influence of pain stimuli. Presumably these phenomena reflected a high degree of convergence in the afferent pathways deriving from the spinothalamic tracts. A similar, though less pronounced, convergence was also present in the pathways transmitting the genital, olfactory, visual and auditory stimuli, since individual neurones were found responding to combinations of these sensory modalities.

In some experiments we were able to observe a well-defined interaction between convergent sensory stimuli. Fig. 7 shows one such experiment. A slow-firing neurone in the zona incerta could be excited by pain or cold, but whenever the cervix was probed with the glass rod the response to these stimuli was suppressed. A similar effect was seen in a lateral hypothalamic neurone of another rat. An inhibitory effect of olfactory stimuli on the response of a lateral hypothalamic neurone to probing the cervix is shown in Fig. 8. This neurone was accelerated by pain, cold and cervical stimulation and slowed by the odour of ethyl acetate and cajuput oil. During the time these odours were presented to the rat the response of the neurone to cervical probing, pain and cold was attenuated or absent, but within seconds of removing the odours they could once again be elicited in full intensity. Unfortunately we were unable to duplicate this effect in other experiments.

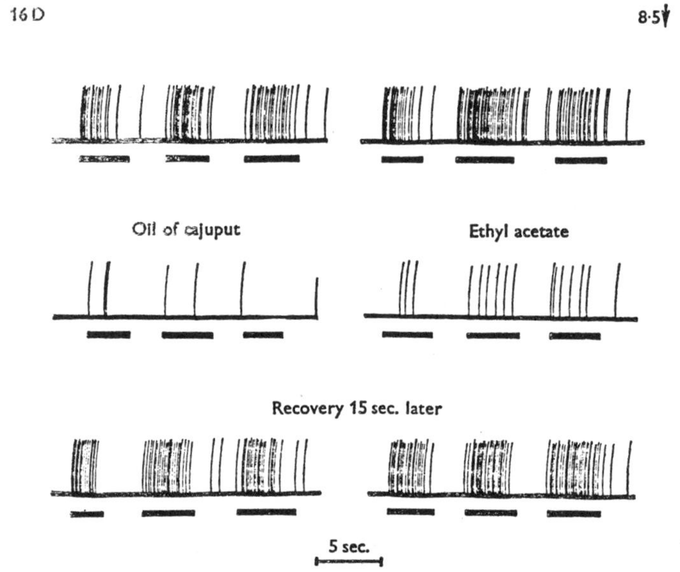

Fig. 8. Lateral hypothalamic neurone showing blockade of response to cervical probing by simultaneous exposure to odour either of cajuput oil or of ethyl acetate.

Effect of ovarian activity

The high degree of reproducibility in the responses described in the previous sections encouraged us to look for influences of ovarian hormones on the patterns of responsiveness. As vaginal smears were taken from the rats before recording, and usually for a week previous to that, the stage of the cycle could be confidently assessed. Most of the rats selected were in oestrus as we were primarily interested in unit responses to genital stimuli which mimic coitus and might therefore be related to the initiation of pseudopregnancy. Our experiments were not specially designed to reveal differences of excitability of diencephalic neurones at the various stages of the oestrous cycle. Nevertheless, we did examine rats in prooestrus and dioestrus, and a few which had been ovariectomized a week earlier. The observations made on these groups of animals yielded suggestive evidence of cyclical changes in neurone responsiveness as will now be described.

Several interesting points emerge from inspection of the data summarized in Table 2. With regard to smell, the highest level of responsiveness to olfactory stimuli occurred in rats in prooestrus. In this group the percentage of neurones excited was more than three times the corresponding value during oestrus, and more than twice that in dioestrus. Moreover, none of the neurones in prooestrous rats was inhibited by odours, whereas a significant minority of neurones in oestrous and dioestrous rats showed inhibitory effects. For pain and cold, however, it was the

Table 2. *Responses of neurones to pain, cold, smell and cervical probing in three stages of the oestrous cycle*

(Percentages are calculated to nearest whole number.)

		Stimulus							
		Pain				Cold			
Stage of cycle	No. of rats	No. cells	% +	% −	% 0	No. cells	% +	% −	% 0
Prooestrus	9	51	72	8	20	48	69	6	25
Oestrus	21	124	61	15	24	118	53	14	33
Dioestrus	11	57	65	5	30	51	66	6	28

		Stimulus							
		Smell				Probe cervix			
Stage of cycle	No. of rats	No. cells	% +	% −	% 0	No. cells	% +	% −	% 0
Prooestrus	9	39	41	0	59	45	53	16	31
Oestrus	21	102	12	5	83	113	39	17	44
Dioestrus	11	50	16	4	80	51	55	6	39

oestrous pattern of responsiveness which stood in contrast to that of prooestrus and dioestrus. Thus the percentage of neurones in oestrous rats which showed inhibition to these stimuli was two or three times the figure obtaining in the other two stages of the cycle, and conversely the percentage of neurones excited by pain and cold during oestrus was less than during prooestrus and dioestrus. A different relationship again is seen in the responsiveness to cervical probing. Here the percentage of inhibited neurones was greater in both prooestrus and oestrus than in dioestrus, but the oestrous females had the lowest percentage of excited neurones. If we take the figures in Table 2 as a whole it appears that during oestrus there was a trend towards a reduction of excitability, as indicated by more unresponsive neurones and fewer neurones accelerated by the test stimuli. A greater frequency of inhibitory responses was an associated feature in the unit activity of oestrous rats.

We experienced some difficulty in finding stable units in ovariectomized rats and at first thought the loss of ovarian hormones might adversely affect the activity of the neurones. However, in three spayed rats we collected a total of twenty neurones whose responses to the various test stimuli were similar to those previously described. Three neurones were unresponsive to all test stimuli and two responded only to olfactory stimuli. Nine neurones were excited by pain, cold and cervical probing, and two were inhibited by these three stimuli. With so small a sample we could discern no alteration in the pattern of responsiveness as compared with cyclic rats, but it was clear that ovarian hormones were not indispensable for the response of hypothalamic neurones to genital stimulation.

Effect of intravenous progesterone

A more direct approach to the problem of hormone influences on unitary responses was attempted in acute experiments by testing hypothalamic neurones at various intervals before and/or after slow i.v. injections of progesterone dissolved in propylene glycol. In the first of these experiments 400 μg. progesterone was given after the sixth successive neurone had responded in the same way, i.e. by accelerating to

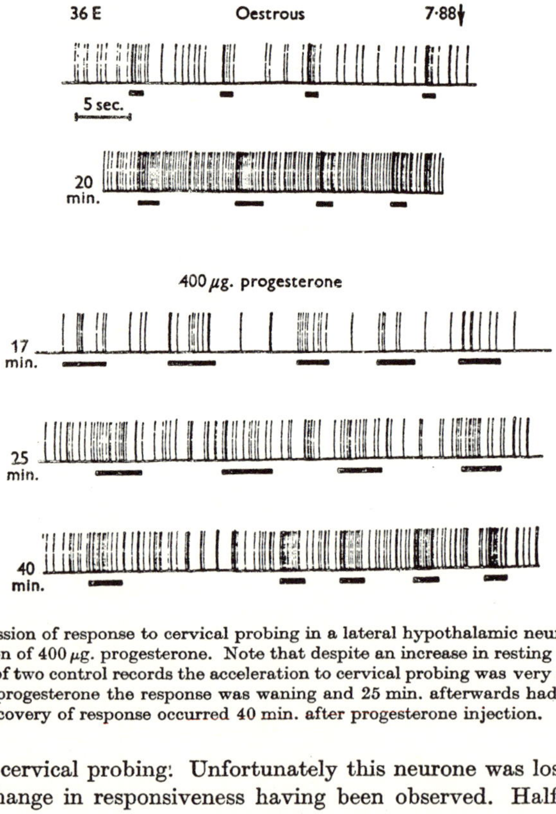

Fig. 9. Depression of response to cervical probing in a lateral hypothalamic neurone produced by i.v. injection of 400 μg. progesterone. Note that despite an increase in resting discharge rate in the second of two control records the acceleration to cervical probing was very distinct, while 17 min. after progesterone the response was waning and 25 min. afterwards had virtually disappeared. Recovery of response occurred 40 min. after progesterone injection.

pain, cold and cervical probing. Unfortunately this neurone was lost 10 min. later without any change in responsiveness having been observed. Half an hour after giving the progesterone another neurone was found which gave a similar response to pain and cold but for the first time no response to cervical stimulation. Then we repeated the progesterone tests on a third neurone with the results illustrated in Figs. 4 and 10. The response of the neurone to cervical probing showed a progressive reduction to a minimal level at 30 min. followed by recovery to the pre-injection level after 1 hr. During this same period the response to pain and cold was apparently unchanged.

A comparable diminution in the responsiveness of hypothalamic neurones to genital stimuli was seen in nine other experiments following injection of progesterone (Figs. 9, 11). The smallest dose which produced an effect was 40 μg. progesterone, and this reduced the response at 12 min. but allowed full recovery in 21 min. 400 μg.

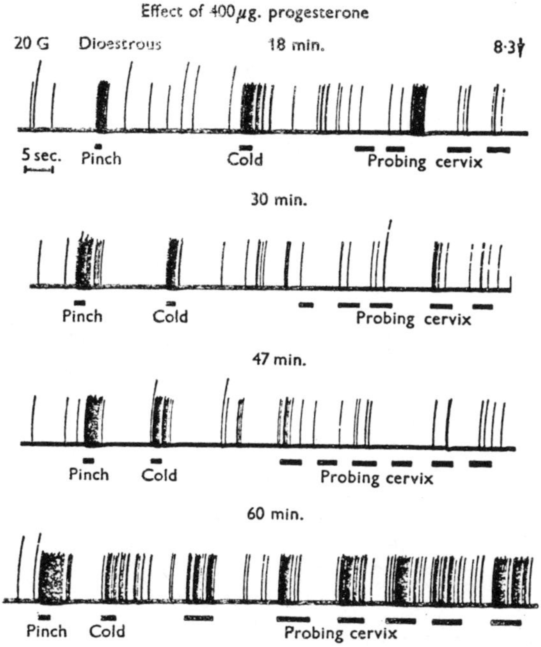

Fig. 10. Showing effect of 400 μg. progesterone (i.v.) on response to pain, cold and cervical probing. This (lateral hypothalamic) neurone is the same as that illustrated in Fig. 5. Note poor responsiveness to cervical probing (but not pain or cold) at 18, 30 and 47 min. and full recovery at 60 min.

was the usual dose given and in all cases the maximum depression of the response to cervical probing was reached between 15 and 40 min. and recovery was complete 1 hr. after the injection. As indicated in Figs. 10 and 11 the progesterone appeared to exert a selective action on the response to genital stimuli, i.e. pain and cold still accelerated the neurones to a comparable extent.

In one experiment a lateral hypothalamic neurone was tested over a period of $2\frac{1}{2}$ hr., during which time injection of 400 μg. progesterone on two occasions produced the selective depression of the response to cervical probing just described. When finally a dose of 800 μg. was given, however, there was a loss of responsiveness to all previously effective stimuli, i.e. pain and cold as well as cervical probing. In a further experiment doses of 400 and 800 μg. progesterone depressed the response to the genital stimulus without affecting cold or pain. It would seem therefore that in optimal dosage a reproducible depression of responsiveness to genital stimuli could be produced by progesterone, but that high doses in some circumstances could bring about a general lowering of responsiveness to all stimuli.

Intravenous injection of equivalent volumes of propylene glycol, i.e. 0·05–0·1 ml. had no effect on the responses of the neurones. The lack of involvement of the vehicle in the production of the effect described above was also indicated by the failure of a dose of 32 μg. progesterone to change the response of one neurone and by a similar negative result when 400 μg. progesterone was tried in an ovariectomized rat. Most

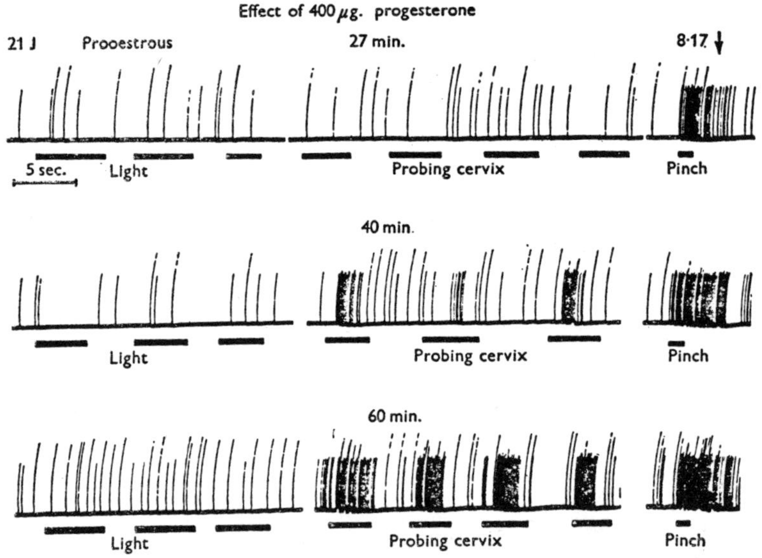

Fig. 11. Stages in recovery of responsiveness to cervical probing in a lateral hypothalamic neurone to show selective action of progesterone. Note uniformly negative response to light stimuli recorded 27, 40 and 60 min. after 400 μg. progesterone, and positive response at these times to pain stimuli. Response to cervical probing completely lost at 27 min., recovering at 40 min. and fully restored at 60 min.

of the neurones studied were in the lateral hypothalamic area and they were chosen for their responsiveness to pain, cold and genital stimuli. It was of interest that one fast unresponsive neurone in the zona incerta was completely unaffected by injection of 400 μg. progesterone, and fired continuously at a rate of 26/sec. for more than 45 min. after the injection. In view of the known anaesthetic action of large doses of progesterone we injected 400 and 800 μg. progesterone i.v. in four conscious female rats. At this dose level there was no anaesthesia, nor even torpor. The rats appeared behaviourally normal.

DISCUSSION

These experiments were planned as a reconnaissance into an unexplored field of rat neuro-endocrinology. A great deal has been accomplished in this species with techniques of neuro-pharmacological blockade, electrical stimulation and ablation, and we now have a broad picture of the regulation of the sexual cycle and the role of the hypothalamus therein (for review see Everett, 1961). Sooner or later, however, it will be necessary to provide an explanation of the neural mechanism of these cyclical events in terms of the patterning of activity of single neurones. In this context our results constitute a modest but encouraging beginning, for they have shown the feasibility of unit recording in the rat hypothalamus and yielded data which may lead eventually to a new conception of the shifting balance of neuronal activity which determines gonadotrophic activity of the pituitary and perhaps behavioural responsiveness as well.

So far studies of unit activity in the hypothalamus have been few, and confined to the rabbit and cat. None has been specifically concerned with sexual function or the control of adenohypophysial secretion. There has been general agreement on certain features of the behaviour of single units in the hypothalamus in the species studied, despite differing anaesthetics and operative conditions. The reports agree that most units tend to discharge at relatively steady rates and that few fire at frequencies much greater than 20/sec. Though individual neurones can be found which seem to respond in a fairly specific fashion to changes in the humoral environment, e.g. osmotic pressure (Cross & Green, 1959; Brooks *et al.* 1962), oxygen or carbon dioxide tension (Cross & Silver, 1963) and temperature (Nakayama, Eisenman & Hardy, 1961), many neurones show evidence of activation by several afferent nervous modalities. The present study shows these findings also hold for the rat. The high degree of sensory convergence which we have observed in this species is consistent with the notion that the brain stem reticular activating system extends rostrally into the hypothalamus (Bernhaut, Gellhorn & Rasmussen, 1953; French, Verzeano & Magoun, 1953), though it is uncertain if thalamic relays were involved in any of the responses we obtained in the hypothalamus. To be sure many thalamic neurones responded to one or more of our test stimuli, but none was in the classical relay nuclei, and it is probable that they were responding as part of a non-specific thalamic arousal system.

Turning now to the particular effects of genital stimulation we may note the striking quality of the response of many neurones in the hypothalamus, subthalamus and thalamus (Figs. 4, 6, 8 and 11). The sum of all these unit responses to an elementary stimulus, i.e. touching the cervix with a glass probe, must constitute a rich pattern of neuronal discharges: how much more vivid the pattern provoked by the genital stimulation in natural coitus. Our sample of hypothalamic unit responses was largely restricted to the lateral and perifornical areas, and gives little idea of the spatial organization of the neuronal effects within the hypothalamus. We should like to know, for example, the reaction of cells in the anterior, ventromedial and arcuate areas which may be nearer the final neural link to the pituitary gland (Donovan & Van der Werff ten Bosch, 1959; Barraclough & Gorski, 1961). However, Barraclough (1959, 1960) found that a sharply differentiated electrical ('EEG') response to stimulation of the cervix in late prooestrous or oestrous rats could be recorded only in the lateral preoptic and lateral hypothalamic areas. There is also the work of Porter, Cavanaugh, Critchlow & Sawyer (1957) in oestrous cats which revealed a characteristic sequence of electrical changes in the lateral hypothalamus induced by mechanical stimulation of the cervix. The precise relation of such effects to our unit responses is in doubt, but taken together all these results strongly suggest that neuronal systems located in the lateral hypothalamic area participate in the sequence of events initiated by coitus and culminating in specific alterations in gonadotrophic secretion by the adenohypophysis.

If we proceed on the supposition that the responses we have observed in neurones in the lateral hypothalamus are in some way causally connected to the induction of pseudopregnancy some interesting relationships appear. There is the notorious lack of specificity in the adequate stimulus for pseudopregnancy. The latter condition may result from coitus, mechanical or electrical stimulation of the cervix, suckling or mechanical stimulation of the nipples, and electrical stimulation of the brain (Everett, 1961). A rough parallel with this situation may be seen in the tendency of lateral hypothalamic neurones to respond in a similar way to a variety of stimuli (Figs. 4, 5). Very few neurones responded exclusively to genital stimulation.

Then there is the question of the relation of the olfactory block of the unit response to cervical probing (Fig. 8) and the olfactory block to pregnancy observed in mice (Bruce, 1960; Bruce & Parrott, 1960) and which is attributable to interference with the secretion of luteotrophin (Bruce & Parkes, 1960). Here it should be said at once that apart from the species difference, and the 'Bruce effect' has not yet been confirmed for the rat, the block we have observed appears altogether too crude a mechanism to account for the highly specific sensory and temporal properties of the pregnancy block phenomenon. In the latter the inhibitory influence, i.e. any male mouse odour differing from that of the successful mate, occurs much later than the coital stimulus that initiated luteotrophin secretion. In our experiment two contrasted odours were effective, neither of which remotely resembled that of a male rat. They blocked the response to pain and cold as well as to cervical probing, and were effective only when applied at the same time as these stimuli. Though no strict parallel can be drawn for the two phenomena it is at least clear that olfactory connexions to lateral hypothalamic neurones can modulate their response to genital stimuli. In this regard the apparent increase of responsiveness to olfactory stimuli in prooestrous rats (Table 2) could be of considerable biological significance, for if a reflection of increased olfactory acuity it might be a necessary prelude to the 'imprinting' of the odour of the mate as required by the 'Bruce effect'. It is established that fluctuations of olfactory acuity occur in the human menstrual cycle (Elsberg, Brewer & Levy, 1935), so a comparable phenomenon in the rat is not improbable.

This brings us to the general problem of the relation of hypothalamic activity to the various stages of the oestrous cycle. Our observations suggest that the neurones may exhibit variations in responsiveness which probably reflect the differing hormonal status in prooestrus, oestrus and dioestrus. Perhaps the most surprising finding was that the level of responsiveness was lowest in oestrous rats (Table 2), though a higher proportion of neurones were inhibited by genital stimuli, pain or cold than in dioestrous rats. This might indicate that, contrary to expectation, oestrogen actually enhances the inhibitory connexions to the lateral hypothalamic neurones. Extending this line of argument we might find in that inhibitory action a partial explanation of why maximal secretion of luteotrophin from the adenohypophysis occurs when the gland is removed entirely from the influence of the hypothalamus, e.g. grafted in the renal capsule (Everett, 1954, 1956; Nikitovitch-Winer & Everett, 1958) or even in tissue culture (Meites, Kahn & Nicoll, 1961). It could also account for the luteotrophic effect of oestrogen in rats (Selye, Collip & Thomson, 1935; Merckel & Nelson, 1940), which is mediated by the pituitary gland.

Progesterone is believed to be secreted in appreciable amounts only after mating and the induction of luteotrophin secretion. Hence to see if the dramatic effect of injected progesterone on the response of lateral hypothalamic neurones to cervical probing (Figs. 9–11) approximates to a naturally occurring condition it will be necessary to study unit activity in pseudopregnant rats. Despite the rapid clearance of progesterone from the blood (see Short, 1961) which may account for the short duration of the selective depressant effect, the peak concentrations achieved probably greatly exceeded the normal level of endogenous hormone. It would be reasonable to expect therefore that the effect we observed represents at best an exaggerated form of physiological process. There are many questions about this phenomenon for which answers are not presently available. We do not yet know if inhibitory effects are depressed as well as excitatory effects, or how oestrogens modify the effect, or even the site of action of progesterone. It is tempting to postulate a direct action of the hormone on hypothalamic neurones, though a mechanism involving afferent synaptic relays or even a change of threshold in the receptors of the cervix might be no less probable. Plainly much remains for further investigation. It would seem, however, that the progesterone effect we have observed is the first example to be reported of a sex hormone influencing unit activity or responsiveness. In recent years there have been several papers indicating an effect of progesterone on electrical activity of the brain, but none has been at the level of single units. Kawakami & Sawyer (1959) working with rabbits described changes in the 'EEG' arousal threshold involving the brain stem reticular formation and in the 'after-reaction' threshold involving the rhinencephalon and hypothalamus evoked by injection of sex steroids and pituitary hormones. In the rat Barraclough (1959) reported differences in the electrical response to cervix stimulation in untreated ovariectomized females and those given oestrogen with or without progesterone; while Woolley & Timiras (1962) have described alterations in seizure thresholds to electroshock in rats treated with female sex hormones. We may hope that effective exploitation of the techniques of unit recording and analysis may soon begin to reveal something of the mechanisms underlying such neuro-endocrine phenomena.

We wish to thank Mr Derek Thurlbourn and Miss Ann Vipers for technical assistance, and Miss Valerie Pink for care of the animals. The work was supported by a Contract, AF 61(052)–301, with the Air Force Office of Scientific Research, O.A.R., through the European Office, Aerospace Research, U.S.A.F., and also by a U.S. Public Health Service Grant, No. B2958.

REFERENCES

Barraclough, C. A. (1959). Localised alterations in electrical activity of the hypothalamus associated with stimulation of the vaginal cervix in estrous rats. *XXI Internat. Physiol.-Congr. Buenos Aires.* (Abst. Comm.), p. 28.

Barraclough, C. A. (1960). Hypothalamic activation associated with stimulation of the vaginal cervix of proestrus rats. *Anat. Rec.* **136**, 159.

Barraclough, C. A. & Gorski, R. A. (1961). Evidence that the hypothalamus is responsible for androgen-induced sterility in the female rat. *Endocrinology*, **68**, 68.

Bernhaut, M., Gellhorn, E. & Rasmussen, A. T. (1953). Experimental contributions to problem of consciousness. *J. Neurophysiol.* **16**, 21.

Brooks, C. McC., Ushiyama, J. & Lange, G. (1962). Reactions of neurons in or near the supraoptic nuclei. *Amer. J. Physiol.* **202**, 487.

Bruce, H. M. (1960). A block to pregnancy in the mouse caused by proximity of strange males. *J. Reprod. Fertil.* **1**, 96.

Bruce, H. M. & Parkes, A. S. (1960). Hormonal factors in exteroceptive block to pregnancy in mice. *J. Endocrin.* **20**, xxix.

Bruce, H. M. & Parrott, D. M. V. (1960). Role of olfactory sense in pregnancy block by strange males. *Science*, **131**, 1526.

Cross, B. A. & Green, J. D. (1959). Activity of single neurones in the hypothalamus: Effect of osmotic and other stimuli. *J. Physiol.* **148**, 554.

Cross, B. A. & Silver, I. A. (1963). Unit activity in the hypothalamus and the sympathetic response to hypoxia and hypercapnia. *Exptl. Neurol.* (in the Press).

Donovan, B. T. & Van der Werff ten Bosch, J. J. (1959). The hypothalamus and sexual maturation in the rat. *J. Physiol.* **147**, 78.

Elsberg, C. A., Brewer, E. D. & Levy, I. (1935). Concerning conditions which may temporarily alter normal olfactory acuity. *Bull. neurol. Inst. N.Y.* **4**, 31.

Everett, J. W. (1954). Luteotrophic function of autografts of the rat hypophysis. *Endocrinology*, **54**, 685.

Everett, J. W. (1956). Functional corpora lutea maintained for months by autografts of rat hypophyses. *Endocrinology*, **58**, 786.

Everett, J. W. (1961). The mammalian female reproductive cycle and its controlling mechanisms. In *Sex and internal secretions*, 3rd ed. (ed. W. C. Young), vol. I, p. 497. London: Baillière, Tindall and Cox.

French, J. D., Verzeano, M. & Magoun, H. W. (1953). An extra-lemniscal sensory system in the brain. *Arch. Neurol. Psychiat., Chicago*, **69**, 505.

Groot, J. de (1959). The rat forebrain in stereotaxic coordinates. *Verh. Akad. Wet. Amst.* (b), **52**, no. 4.

Kawakami, M. & Sawyer, C. H. (1959). Neuroendocrine correlates of changes in brain activity thresholds by sex steroids and pituitary hormones. *Endocrinology*, **65**, 652.

Marshall, W. H. (1940). An application of the frozen section technic for cutting serial sections through the brain. *Stain Tech.* **151**, **133**.

Meites, J., Kahn, R. H. & Nicoll, C. S. (1961). Prolactin production by rat pituitary *in vitro*. *Proc. Soc. exp. Biol., N.Y.*, **108**, 440.

Merckel, C. & Nelson, W. O. (1940). The relation of the estrogenic hormone to the formation and maintenance of corpora lutea in mature and immature rats. *Anat. Rec.* **76**, 391.

Nakayama, T., Eisenman, J. S. & Hardy, J. D. (1961). Single unit activity of anterior hypothalamus during local heating. *Science*, **134**, 1.

Nikitovitch-Winer, M. & Everett, J. W. (1958). Comparative study of luteotropin secretion by hypophysial autotransplants in the rat. Effects of site and stages of estrus cycle. *Endocrinology*, **62**, 522.

Porter, R. W., Cavanaugh, E. B., Critchlow, B. V. & Sawyer, C. W. (1957). Localised changes in electrical activity of the hypothalamus in estrous cats following vaginal stimulation. *Amer. J. Physiol.* **189**, 145.

Selye, H., Collip, J. B. & Thomson, D. L. (1935). Effect of oestrin on ovaries and adrenals. *Proc. Soc. exp. Biol., N.Y.*, **32**, 1377.

Short, R. V. (1961). Progesterone. In *Hormones in blood* (eds. C. H. Gray and A. D. Bacharach), p. 379. London: Academic Press.

Woolley, D. E. & Timiras, P. S. (1962). The gonad–brain relationship: effects of female sex hormones on electroshock convulsions in the rat. *Endocrinology*, **70**, 196.

Effects of Hormones on the Electrical Activity of the Brain in the Rat and Rabbit

CARLOS BEYER, V. DOMINGO RAMIREZ, DAVID I. WHITMOYER, AND CHARLES H. SAWYER[1]

A study has been made of the effects of various hormones on the electrical activity (EEG and background activity) of the brain in the rat and rabbit. In the rat under weak urethane or ether anesthesia the intravenous injection of vasopressin epinephrine or progesterone induced EEG synchronization and a concomitant decrease in diencephalic background activity. These electrical changes were invariably associated with a rise in blood pressure and were probably the result of activation of baroceptors. In rabbits under urethane, injections of these hormones also elevated the blood pressure but in this species the rise was associated with EEG activation and an increase in background activity. These effects were apparently due to direct excitation of the reticular activating system by the sudden rise in blood pressure.

Introduction

The electrical activity of the brain can be modified by the action of hormones. Changes in both the electroencephalogram (EEG) and unit activity have been reported by a number of workers (11, 14, 32) following the administration of various hormones. The mechanisms through which hormones alter cerebral activity are not completely understood. A direct action on neurons has been postulated frequently (2, 9, 17, 20, 21, 30, 31). The possibility of an indirect effect on the brain has also been suggested (1, 7, 12, 29) particularly for hormones that exert widespread actions in the organism, e.g., the catecholamines. In the present work we have studied the effects of a variety of hormones on EEG activity and on the discharge of discrete populations of cortical and subcortical neurons. Preliminary results led us to analyze the involvement of certain visceral mechanisms in the hormone-induced changes in electrical activity in the brain.

Materials and Methods

Thirty-four Sprague-Dawley female rats (210-290 g) and ten New Zealand White female rabbits (3.5-5.0 kg) were used. Some of the rabbits were ovariectomized. In the rats vaginal smears were taken daily.

Various anesthetics were used in the rat experiments: urethane (1 g/kg in a 20% aqueous solution, ip), Methohexital (Brevital sodium, 30-40 mg/kg), pentobarbital (33 mg/kg) and ether. All the rabbits were anesthetized with urethane (1 g/kg in a 20% aqueous solution, ip). Routinely, in both species a polyethylene cannula was introduced into the trachea, and one jugular vein was cannulated to facilitate intravenous injections. In most

[1] The authors thank Miss Virginia Tompkins, Miss Cora Rucker and Miss Arlene Koithan for technical assistance, and Mr. Rudolph Sabbot for photographing the illustrations. The work was supported in part by grants from the National Institutes of Health (NB 01162) and the Ford Foundation.

cases the carotid artery on the same side was cannulated for recording blood pressure. The animal was placed in a stereotaxic apparatus and several screws (three to five) were fixed in the skull to record EEG and to ground the preparation. A small part of the dorsal surface of the brain was exposed and the dura reflected. A warm agar solution was applied to prevent dessication and movements of the brain. In some rats ether anesthesia was discontinued at the completion of surgery, and the skin was infiltrated with xylocaine at the wound margins and pressure points of the stereotaxic holder. Most of the animals were immobilized with Flaxedil and artificially respired. In three rats the carotid sinuses were denervated according to the technique of Farris and Griffith (16). During the experiment a lamp was employed to keep the animal warm.

Localized activity of a small region of the brain was recorded with large microelectrodes made from Clay Adams pins No. 00, insulated with epoxy resin except at the tip, which was tapered to a diameter of 30-60 μ. The electrode was oriented according to the rat atlas of de Groot (15) and the rabbit atlas of Sawyer *et al.* (33). A hydraulic micromanipulator was used to drive the electrode in an exploration which focused on diencephalic areas. The technique for recording multiple unit activity (background activity) was basically that described by Weber and Buchwald (35). As shown in Fig. 1, the multiple unit activity data channel consisted of a Grass P6 preamplifier, audio monitor, high pass filter, Tektronix 502 oscilloscope modified for vertical signal output and an R-C integrator. A four channel Offner type R dynograph was employed to record integrated background activity, blood pressure, respiration, and a selected channel of cortical EEG. The EEG from other cortical loci and the EKG were simultaneously recorded with a multichannel Grass model IV EEG instrument.

The pharmacological agents and hormones employed in these experiments were epinephrine (Adrenalin, Parke Davis), nor-epinephrine (Levophed, Winthrop), vasopressin (Pitressin, Parke Davis), acetyl-β-methylcholine (Mecholyl, Merck), oxytocin (Pitocin, Parke Davis; and Syntocinon, Sandoz), ergotamine (Gynergen, Sandoz) and progesterone. Fresh solutions of all these substances with the exception of progesterone were prepared daily. Progesterone was dissolved in propylene glycol (2 mg/ml). In nearly all cases the drugs were injected intravenously within 30 sec. Injections of progesterone were given more slowly (2-3 min). In a few experiments amyl

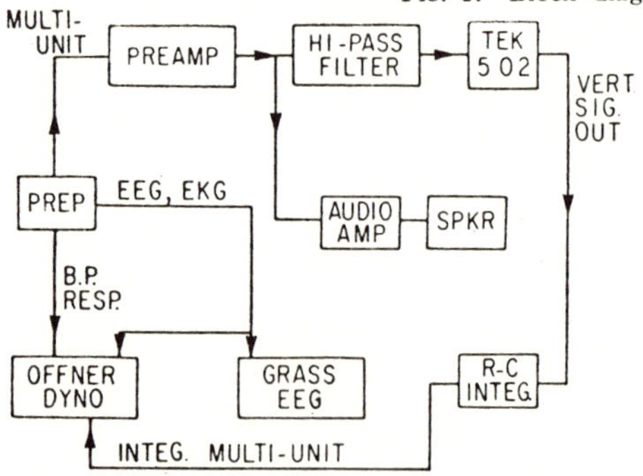

Fig. 1. Block diagram of recording system.

nitrate vapor was applied to lower the blood pressure rapidly. Ovariectomized rabbits were primed with estrogen (estradiol benzoate 0.1 mg for 2 days).

Results

A brief description of the multiple unit activity patterns in rat and rabbit brains will be given since, to our knowledge no study of this type has been made in these species. The magnitude of the background activity varied with the region of the brain and the state of the animal. Urethane anesthesia impaired the multiple unit activity very little whereas pentobarbital even in subanesthetic doses (10-20 mg/kg) suppressed it almost completely. The cerebral cortex, the dorsomedial thalamus and the ventral thalamus consistently showed intense background activity. The hypothalamus registered background activity generally lower than that of the thalamus, but within the hypothalamus such regions as the dorsomedial, ventromedial and paraventricular nuclei revealed background activity relatively higher than the low activity characteristic of the base of the tuber.

Shifts in background activity, observed in most of the structures explored, were generally associated with EEG changes. A drop in the level of background activity frequently coincided with the appearance of spindling in the EEG. This relationship was particularly clear in certain regions of the diencephalon (Fig. 2) but not in the tuber. In the cerebral cortex surges of background activity were related to EEG slow waves, though drops in background level were also found during spindling. The surges in background activity during spindling were produced by the synchronous discharge of many neurons generating large spikes. Correlations of background

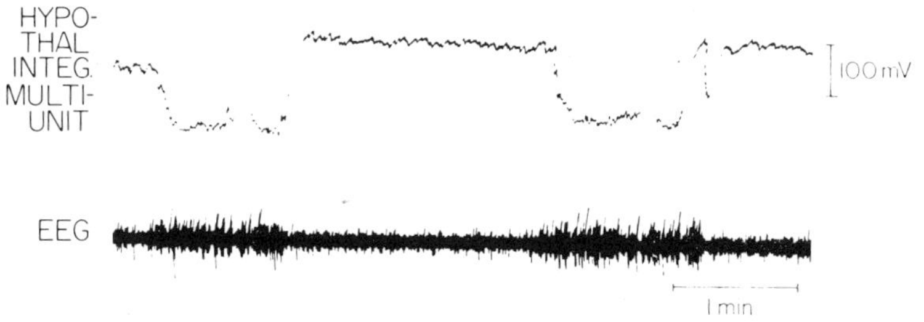

Fig. 2. Rat under urethane. Relation between EEG activity of the cerebral cortex and background activity of the ventromedial nucleus of the hypothalamus. Note the decrease in background activity during EEG spindling.

activity and EEG were observed in both anesthetized (ether and urethane) and unanesthetized animals.

Changes in background activity and EEG were observed to coincide with fluctuations in blood pressure and respiratory rate. Although these parallel changes were seen in all types of preparation, they were clearest in animals under urethane anesthesia. Under these conditions the EEG is composed of periods of spindling interspersed with fast activity rhythms. A decrease in respiratory rate was commonly observed during EEG spindling and low background activity. Spontaneous or induced drops in blood pressure were usually associated with an increase in background activity and EEG

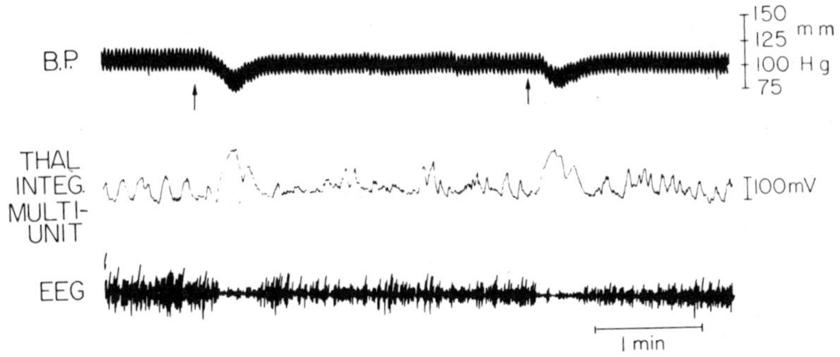

FIG. 3. Rat under light ether anesthesia. Simultaneous recording of blood pressure, thalamic background activity and electrocorticogram. At arrows the rat's tail was pressed gently. Note the close relationship between fall in blood pressure and changes in cerebral electrical activity.

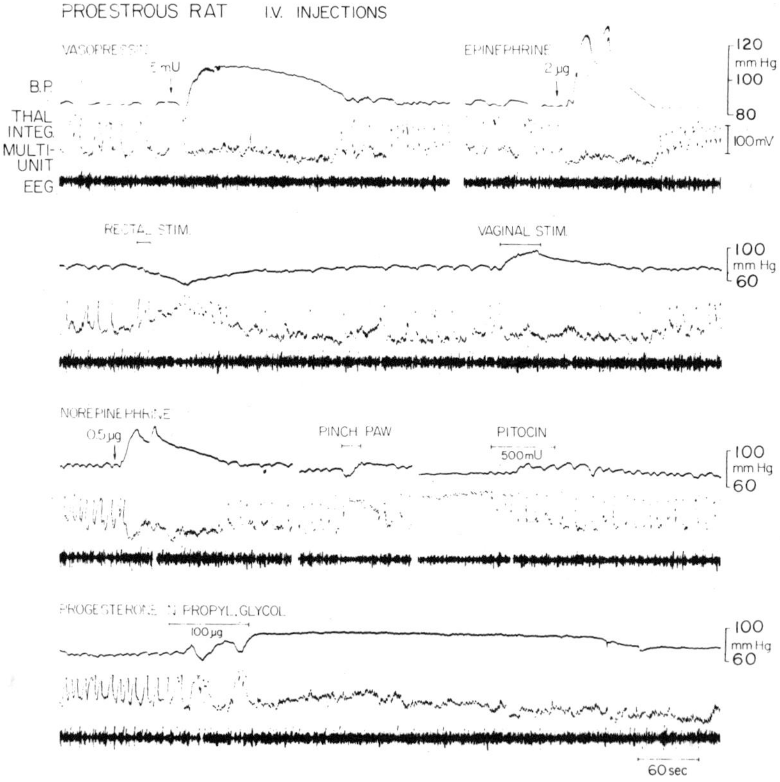

FIG. 4. Rat under urethane. Effects of various experimental treatments on blood pressure, background activity and cortical EEG. Note that all of the procedures that induced a rise in blood pressure (injections of vasopressin, epinephrine, norepinephrine, pitocin, progesterone and vaginal stimulation) also evoked a decrease in background activity and EEG spindling. Conversely, those eliciting a fall in blood pressure resulted in EEG arousal and increase in background activity.

"arousal" (Figs. 3 and 4), whereas rises in blood pressure were related to decreases in background activity and EEG synchronization.

Background activity changes could be induced by extrinsic stimulation (tactile, thermic, rectal probing, etc.), which usually induced a rise in background activity, EEG and behavioral arousal, acceleration of respiration and a fall in blood pressure. This background activity response was found in both telencephalic and diencephalic structures, though some regions (e.g., the tuber) were generally unresponsive. Rhythmic stimulation of the rat's vaginal cervix with a glass rod frequently elicited a decrease in diencephalic background activity and EEG spindling (Fig. 4), changes associated with a rise in blood pressure. This type of response to vaginal stimulation was commonly observed in proestrous rats but not during early diestrus.

Effects of Vasopressin and Oxytocin. In doses ranging from 2 to 50 milliunits, vasopressin induced synchronization of the EEG and a decrease in diencephalic background activity in most rats under urethane or light ether anesthesia (Figs. 4 and 5). As can be seen in Fig. 5, there was a relation

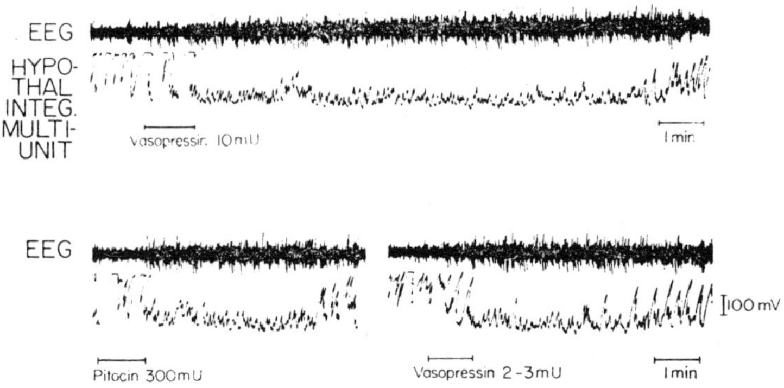

FIG. 5. Rat under urethane. Effects of neurohypophyseal hormones. In the upper tracing, 10 milliunits of vasopressin elicited a decrease in background activity and EEG synchronization that lasted for 10 min. Note that the effect of injecting 300 milliunits of pitocin (lower tracing) is comparable in magnitude and duration with that obtained by administering only 3 milliunits of vasopressin.

between the amount of vasopressin injected and the duration of the changes in electrical activity of the brain. The dose of vasopressin required to elicit these alterations varied from animal to animal and throughout the experiment in the same rat. As a rule larger amounts of vasopressin were required to induce EEG synchronization and depression of background activity in rats showing an activated EEG pattern (low voltage, fast activity). In similar or even smaller doses than those required to elicit changes in the electrical activity of the brain, vasopressin inhibited muscular activity (jaw and limb movements, shivering, etc.) in rats that were not under Flaxedil.

Natural oxytocin (Pitocin) also induced synchronization of the EEG and a drop in background activity (Fig. 5), but usually larger amounts were required (100-500 milliunits). Synthetic oxytocin (Syntocinon) was found to be ineffective in most cases.

In the nonanesthetized rat under Flaxedil showing low voltage, fast EEG rhythms, the administration of vasopressin (5-100 milliunits) did not elicit clear-cut changes in electrical activity. Vasopressin induced EEG synchronization and a decrease in background activity only when the rat showed a somewhat drowsy EEG pattern. The injection of large amounts of vasopressin (100-500 milliunits) to highly aroused rats actually increased the background activity in some cases.

The simultaneous recording of blood pressure revealed some interesting facts. It was found that the EEG and background activity shifts never preceded the vasopressin-induced rise in blood pressure. Moreover no changes in EEG or background activity were seen when vasopressin failed to raise the blood pressure. In some experiments the changes in electrical activity occurred almost simultaneously with the rising phase of the blood pressure curve (Fig. 4) whereas in others the electrical changes had a longer latency (Fig. 6). It was generally found that the re-establishment of an alert EEG coincided with the return of the blood pressure to its previous level (Figs. 4 and 6).

In three rats under urethane in which the carotid and aortic baroceptor areas had been surgically denervated, vasopressin injections failed to induce EEG synchronization or depression of the background activity.

In the rabbit under urethane, the alterations in the electrical activity of the brain induced by vasopressin differed markedly from those obtained in the rat. With doses of vasopressin adequate to raise the blood pressure (200-2000 milliunits) the initial response was an activation of the EEG and a dramatic rise in background activity (Fig. 7). The EEG activation was particularly clear in the limbic cortex, in which a 4 to 6 per sec sinusoidal rhythm was established. The activation period varied in its duration; however, it was clearly associated with the elevation in blood pressure (Fig. 7). In many cases the activation phase was followed by spindling. The administration of pentobarbital (20 mg/kg) blocked the activating effect of vasopressin.

A slowing of heart rate followed the injection of a hypertensive dose of vasopressin. Bradycardia was usually maximal during the rising phase of the blood pressure curve, but it persisted for a long time, suggesting a sustained effect on vasomotor centers. However, there was no clear temporal relationship between the cerebral electrical changes and the alterations in heart rate.

Effects of Catecholamines. Epinephrine and nor-epinephrine were administered to rats under urethane in doses from 0.5 to 5 µg. Those doses induced synchronization of the EEG and a fall in background activity in the diencephalon. As can be seen in Fig. 4 these effects coincided with the rise in blood pressure elicited by the hormones. EEG arousal and increases in background activity were rarely observed following administration of catecholamines to rats under urethane.

However, in rabbits anesthetized with urethane the injection of epinephrine or nor-epinephrine in amounts ranging from 0.5 to 5 µg/kg usually produced a clear increase in background activity associated with EEG and behavioral

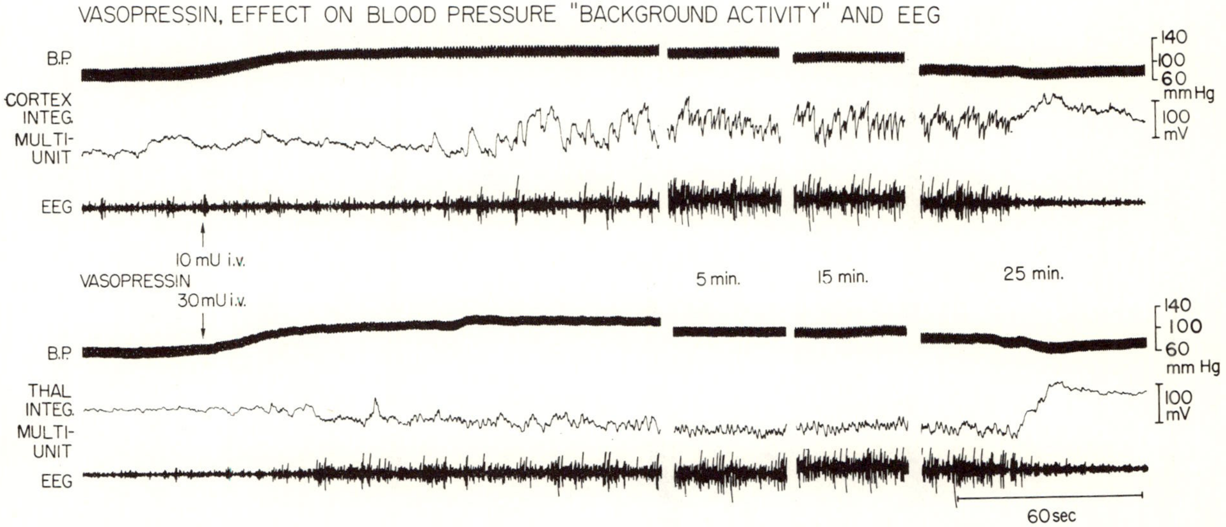

FIG. 6. Rat under urethane. At arrows, injection of vasopressin was started. Note that the rise in blood pressure precedes the changes in electrical activity of the brain. In the upper tracing it can be seen that surges of cortical background activity are associated with EEG spindling whereas a drop in background activity is the principle change in diencephalic background activity during spindling (lower tracing). Note that abrupt rises in background activity coincide with the sudden return of blood pressure to its previous level.

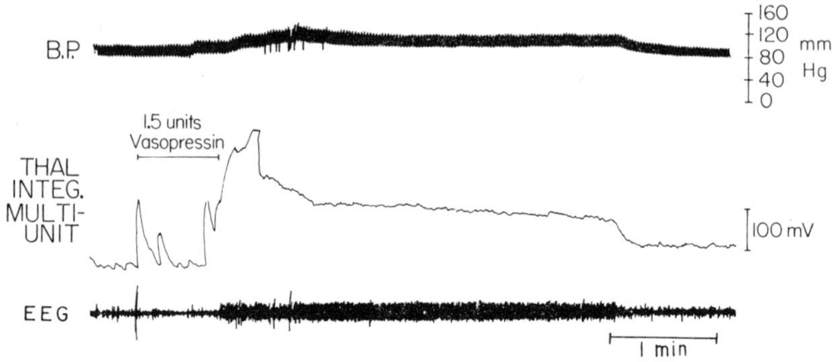

FIG. 7. Rabbit under urethane. Bar indicates vasopressin injection (1500 milliunits). Note the marked increase in background activity that is closely related to the rise in blood pressure. The EEG activity, recorded from the limbic cortex, shows a high amplitude synchronous theta rhythm which in nonimmobilized preparations was associated with behavioral arousal.

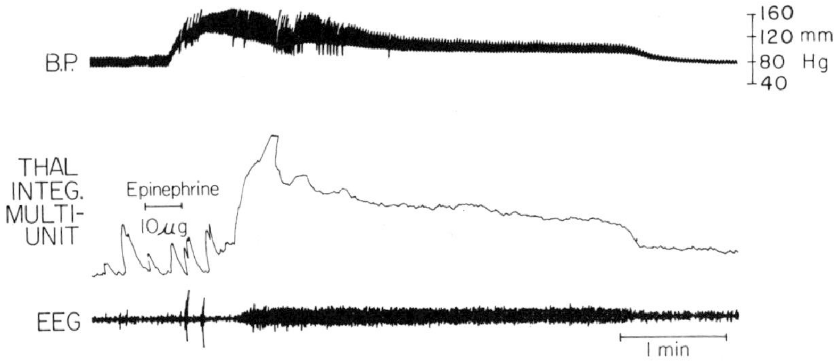

FIG. 8. Rabbit under urethane. The bar indicates time of epinephrine injection. Note the striking activation of background activity and EEG (high amplitude theta rhythm) that were clearly related to the rise in blood pressure (see Fig. 6).

arousal. These changes followed a rise in blood pressure (Fig. 8). The epinephrine-induced EEG arousal and increase in background activity were temporarily blocked by the administration of ergotamine (500 μg/kg). This drug also blocked the blood pressure response to catecholamines.

Effects of Progesterone. Progesterone (100-200 μg iv, in propylene glycol) was slowly injected in several anesthetized and unanesthetized rats. In cases in which the EEG was not highly activated at the time of injection, progesterone administration was followed by EEG spindling and a decrease in diencephalic background activity. As can be seen in Fig. 4, electrical changes were clearly correlated with a rise in blood pressure that lasted for several minutes. The rise in blood pressure was preceded in most cases by a fall of brief duration that was apparently due to the propylene glycol. No consistent effects of progesterone on the electrical activity of the brain was observed in the rabbit experiments.

Discussion

Various effects on cerebral activity have been reported following administration of the hormones employed in the present study. For example, epinephrine has been found to induce either behavioral and EEG arousal (7, 9, 12, 27, 28, 31) or EEG synchronization and a sleeplike condition (22-24, 29). Both increases and decreases in the rate of discharge of cerebral neurons have been noted following epinephrine injections (4, 5, 10). Contradictory results have also been obtained with vasopressin administration. Thus, Capon (12) found vasopressin elicited EEG arousal in the rabbit. However, Kawakami and Sawyer (20) noted that in the female rabbit vasopressin can produce a characteristic sleeplike pattern, the EEG afterreaction. This response includes a phase of paradoxical sleep which is always preceded by a phase of EEG synchronization. The induction of spindle sleep in the rabbit by vasopressin has also been reported by Faure (17).

Our results indicate that the animal's state of vigilance at the time of hormone administration largely determines the direction of the alterations in EEG and background activity. Thus, EEG synchronization was induced by small doses of vasopressin or epinephrine in rats showing a drowsy EEG pattern, whereas in the fully awake animal the injection of these hormones, even in large doses, rarely induced similar electrical changes.

The mechanisms through which the catecholamines induce EEG alterations have been debated. Some workers (9, 31) have proposed that epinephrine acts directly on the neurons of the reticular activating system. Other investigators (1, 5, 7, 12) have suggested that the EEG arousal is a result of the rise in blood pressure induced by the catecholamines.

Our findings indicate that the immediate effects on electrical activity of the brain induced by either epinephrine or vasopressin are the result of changes in blood pressure. This is supported by the findings that any agent (hormones, peripheral stimulation, rapid injections of saline, etc.) that increased the blood pressure produced activation phenomena in the rabbit, whereas they produced the opposite effects (EEG synchronization and decrease in diencephalic background activity) in the rat. Moreover, when administration of hormones did not alter the blood pressure, no EEG or background activity changes were observed in either of the species studied.

Although both activation of cerebral electrical activity in the rabbit and its deactivation in the rat were due primarily to rises in blood pressure, the mechanisms involved in the two responses appear to be different. Koch (22) found that sudden distension of the carotid bodies in wakeful dogs induced a sleeplike condition. Bonvallet, Dell and Hiebel (8, 9) working also with dogs observed that increased pressure on the isolated carotid sinus produced EEG synchronization. Signs of decreased excitability of the central nervous system such as inhibition of movements and suppression of convulsions (18, 19, 23) have been reported following a pressure rise in the baroceptor areas. This mechanism appears to be responsible for the EEG synchronization and depression in background activity that follows administration of vasopressin or epinephrine in the rat. This idea is supported by the finding that EEG changes were not induced by vasopressin injections in rats in which the baroceptor areas had been presumably denervated. On the other hand, the activation of electrical activity that follows administration of epinephrine or vasopressin in the rabbit appears to be due to a direct action of the elevated blood pressure on brain neurons. This explanation is based on the remarkable temporal relationship between the rise in blood pressure and the activation phase. Moreover, there have been recorded EEG arousal and changes in neuron firing by augmenting blood pressure in the cat (4-6, 26).

It is of interest that progesterone in relatively small doses in the rat produced spindling and a drop in background activity with a short latency. This effect was clearly associated with a rise in blood pressure. The hypertensive action of progesterone in the rat has been reported only recently (13). Progesterone was also found to induce an EEG pattern of sleep in the rat by Kobayashi *et al.* (21). However, the amounts of progesterone injected by the Japanese workers were much larger than those used in our experiments and therefore probably involved other mechanisms. It is important to recall that progesterone and other steroids in large doses can induce deep anesthesia (34) in all probability acting directly on nervous tissue. The primary rise in blood pressure induced by progesterone in our experiments may represent a central effect of the hormone.

We can only speculate about the neural structures involved in the production of electrical changes described in this paper. Our observations failed to demonstrate differential alterations in the electrical activity of restricted regions of the brain following administration of the hormones. It was found that the background activity shifts evoked by hormones were nonspecific and that they were related to changes in brain excitability of a more general nature. It can be suggested, however, that the hormonally induced blood pressure changes activate or deactivate electrical activity of the brain by acting on two neural mechanisms: (a) the reticular activating system located in the mesencephalic tegmentum and caudal hypothalamus and (b) the EEG synchronizing mechanism located in the lower part of the brain stem, i.e., medulla and lower pons (3). The capacity of a sudden rise in blood pressure to stimulate neurons of the reticular activating system has been demonstrated by the experiments of Baust and his co-workers (4-7). On the other hand it is known that EEG synchronizing structures are susceptible to influences originating in the baroceptor areas, and therefore rises in blood pressure such as those obtained by injecting hypertensive hormones may activate this mechanism. In this connection it is important to recall that stimulation of the area of the tractus solitarius has been found to elicit EEG synchronization in cats which showed a drowsy EEG (25).

In conclusion, the data reported in this paper indicate that short-latency changes in the electrical activity of the brain following the administration of certain hormones are primarily attributable to peripheral rather than central effects. These findings do not, however, exclude the possibility of a direct action of these hormones on the brain. Our results emphasize the importance of polygraphic recording when studying the action of hormones on the electrical activity of the brain.

References

1. Albe-Fessard, D., and O. Hesse. 1953. Le facteur de pression arterielle dans l'accroissement adrenalinique de l'activite corticale chez le lapin. *J. Physiol.*

Paris **45**: 16-20.

2. Barraclough, C. A., and B. A. Cross. 1963. Unit activity in the hypothalamus of the cyclic female rat: effect of genital stimuli and progesterone. *J. Endocrinol.* **26**: 339-359.
3. Batini, C., F. Magni, M. Palestini, G. F. Rossi, and A. Zanchetti. 1959. Neural mechanisms underlying the enduring EEG and behavioral activation in the midpontine pretrigeminal cat. *Arch. Ital. Biol.* **97**: 13-25.
4. Baust, W., and P. Katz. 1961. Untersuchungen zur Tonisierung enzelner Neurone im hinteren Hypothalamus. *Arch. Ges. Physiol.* **272**: 575-590.
5. Baust, W., and H. Niemczyk. 1963. Studies on the adrenaline-sensitive component of the mesencephalic reticular formation. *J. Neurophysiol.* **26**: 692-704.
6. Baust, W., H. Niemczyk, H. Schaefer, and J. Vieth. 1962. Über ein pressosensibles Areal im hinteren Hypothalamus der Katze. *Arch. Ges. Physiol.* **274**: 374-384.
7. Baust, W., H. Niemczyk, and J. Vieth. 1963. The action of blood pressure on the ascending reticular activating system with special reference to adrenaline-induced EEG arousal. *Electroencephalog. Clin. Neurophysiol.* **15**: 63-72.
8. Bonvallet, M., P. Dell, and G. Hiebel. 1953. Sinus carotidien et activité électrique cérébrale. *Compt. Rend. Soc. Biol.* **147**: 1166-1169.
9. Bonvallet, M., P. Dell, and G. Hiebel. 1954. Tonus sympathique et activité électrique corticale. *Electroencephalog. Clin. Neurophysiol.* **6**: 119-144.
10. Bradley, P. B., and A. Mollica. 1958. The effect of adrenaline and acetylcholine on single unit activity in the reticular formation of the decerebrate cat. *Arch. Ital. Biol.* **96**: 168-186.
11. Campbell, H. J., and J. T. Eayrs. 1965. Influence of hormones on the central nervous system. *Brit. Med. Bull.* **21**: 81-86.
12. Capon, A. 1960. Analyse de l'effet d'éveil exercé par l'adrenaline et d'autres amines sympathicomimétriques sur électrocorticogramme du lapin non narcotisé. *Arch. Intern. Pharmacodyn.* **127**: 141-162.
13. Cession, G., A. Cession-Fossion, and R. Limet. 1966. Action de la progestérone sur trois agents endogènes à action hypertensive. *Compt. Rend. Soc. Biol.* **159**: 1864-1866.
14. Cross, B. A., and I. A. Silver. 1966. Electrophysiological studies on the hypothalamus. *Brit. Med. Bull.* **22**: 254-260.
15. de Groot, J. 1959. The rat forebrain in stereotaxic coordinates. *Verhandel. Koninkl. Ned. Akad. Wetenschap (b)*, **52**, *No. 4.*
16. Farris, E. J., and J. Q. Griffith. 1942. "The Rat in Laboratory Investigation," 2nd ed., pp. 441-442. Lippincott, Philadelphia, Pennsylvania.
17. Faure, J. M. A. 1965. Hormones in relation to sleep-wakefulness mechanisms, pp. 606-611. *In* "Proceedings of the Second International Congress of Endocrinology," Part 1. Excerpta Medica Int. Congr. Ser. #83.
18. Gellhorn, E. 1943. "Autonomic Regulations. Their Significance for Physiology, Psychology and Neuropsychiatry." Interscience, New York.
19. Gellhorn, E., and L. Yesinick. 1942. The significance of carotid sinus reflexes for the effects of anoxia and carbon dioxide on convulsions. *Am. J. Physiol.* **137**: 404-408.
20. Kawakami, M., and C. H. Sawyer. 1959. Induction of behavioral and electroencephalographic changes in the rabbit by hormone administration or brain stimulation. *Endocrinology* **65**: 631-643.
21. Kobayashi, T., T. Kobayashi, S. Takezawa, K. Oshima, and H. Kawamura. 1962. Electrophysiological studies on the feed-back mechanism of progesterone. *Endocrinol. Japon.* **9**: 302-320.
22. Koch, E. 1932. Die Irradiation der pressoreceptorischen Kreislaufreflexe. *Klin. Wochschr.* **11**: 225-227.
23. Kreindler, A. 1946. Recherches experimentales sur les relations entre le sinus carotidien et la systeme nerveux central. *Bul. Sec. Scient. Acad. Roumaine* **28**: 448-481.

24. Longo, V. G. 1962. "Electroencephalographic Atlas for Pharmacological Research. Effects of Drugs on the Electrical Activity of the Rabbit Brain," pp. 46–48. Elsevier, Amsterdam.

25. Magnes, J., G. Moruzzi, and O. Pompeiano. 1961. Synchronization of the EEG produced by low-frequency electrical stimulation of the region of the solitary tract. *Arch. Ital. Biol.* **99**: 33-67.

26. Mantegazzini, P., K. Poeck, and G. Santibañez. 1959. The action of adrenaline and nor-adrenaline on the cortical electrical activity of the "encéphale isolé" cat. *Arch. Ital. Biol.* **97**: 222-242.

27. Marley, E. 1966. Behavioural and electrophysiological effects of catecholamines. *Pharmacol. Rev.* **18**: 753-768.

28. Marley, E., and B. J. Key. 1963. Maturation of the electrocorticogram and behaviour in the kitten and guinea pig and the effect of some sympathomimetic amines. *Electroencephalog. Clin. Neurophysiol.* **15**: 620-636.

29. Nakao, H., H. M. Ballin, and E. Gellhorn. 1956. The role of the sino-aortic receptors in the action of adrenaline, nor-adrenaline and acetylcholine on the cerebral cortex. *Electroencephalog. Clin. Neurophysiol.* **8**: 413-420.

30. Ramirez, V. D., B. R. Komisaruk, D. I. Whitmoyer, and C. H. Sawyer. 1967. Effects of hormones and vaginal stimulation on the EEG and hypothalamic units in the rat. *Am. J. Physiol.* (in press).

31. Rothballer, A. B. 1956. Studies on the adrenaline-sensitive component of the reticular activating system. *Electroencephalog. Clin. Neurophysiol.* **8**: 603-621.

32. Sawyer, C. H. 1967. Effects of hormonal steroids on certain mechanisms in the adult brain, pp. 763-775 Excerpta Medica Int. Congr. Ser. #132. *In* Proceedings of the 2nd International Congress on Hormonal Steroids, Milan, Italy.

33. Sawyer, C. H., J. W. Everett, and J. D. Green. 1954. The rabbit diencephalon in stereotaxic coordinates. *J. Comp. Neurol.* **101**: 801-824.

34. Selye, H. 1941. Studies concerning the anesthetic action of steroid hormones. *J. Pharmacol. Exptl. Therap.* **73**: 127-141.

35. Weber, D. S., and J. S. Buchwald. 1965. A technique for recording and integrating multiple unit activity simultaneously with the EEG in chronic animals. *Electroencephalog. Clin. Neuro* [illegible]: 190-192.

ELECTROENCEPHALOGRAPHIC RESPONSES PRODUCED BY GENITAL STIMULATION AND HORMONE ADMINISTRATION IN SEXUALLY IMMATURE RHESUS MONKEYS

G. S. Chhina, A. S. Chakrabarty, K. Kaur and B. K. Anand

CENTRAL NERVOUS system regulates reproductive activity through a coordinated control over the secretion of sex hormones and sex behavior [2]. The neural mechanisms for regulation of gonadotropin secretion, as well as regulation and determination of sex behavior, are possibly located in the hypothalamus. The observations of Lisk [14], and Sawyer and Kawakami [20] support the presence of well localised areas in the hypothalamus which regulate each of these functions.

It is still not very clear where, and if so how far, the hypothalamic control of gonadotropin activity is linked with the automatic self-regulation of gonadotropic hormones. Present evidence indicates that the gonadal hormones feed back into the hypothalamic region [21], and probably only excessive amounts of these may have any direct effect on the pituitary gland. This feed back of sex hormones possibly takes place into the anterior hypothalamic region as auto-transplantation of small fragments of ovarian tissue [9], or injection of estrogen [11], or implantation of fine needles containing estradiol [7, 14] into anterior hypothalamus leads to inhibition of gonadotropin secretion. There is also feed back of information into the hypothalamic region via sensory afferents originating from the reproductive organs, as Porter *et al.* [17] showed that in the estrous cat responding to coitus or vaginal stimulation by producing after-reaction, bursts of high voltage activity appear in the EEG records localised to the anterior lateral hypothalamus. Barraclough [3] also obtained hypothalamic activation in rats on vaginal stimulation, and Chhina [5], and Chakarbarty *et al.* [4] observed EEG changes in cats and monkeys in response to genital stimulation.

These studies were carried out in sexually mature animals in which both the gonadal hormones, and the sensory afferents from the reproductive organs together feed back into the central nervous regions regulating reproductive activity. In these it is not possible to study the integrative role played by the feed back of gonadal hormones and the sensory afferents in influencing the nervous regulatory activity.

The present experiments were, therefore, undertaken to study the effect of sensory afferents from the reproductive organs on nervous activity in sexually immature monkeys and to further observe if injections of gonadal hormones would influence this mechanism.

METHODS

Fifteen sexually immature rhesus monkeys (13 male and 2 female), weighing between 1.5–2.5 kg, were used for this study. Sexually immature status of the animals was judged from their weight and sex behavior.

In all these monkeys bipolar insulated stainless steel electrodes, with their tips scraped for about 1 mm, were stereotaxically implanted in different regions of the hypothalamus and limbic system using the technique of Anand [1]. The outer ends of these electrodes were connected to a socket which was secured to the skull with dental cement and screws.

After the animals had recovered from the effects of surgical trauma, the electrical activity of the different regions of the brain was recorded through these electrodes on a 3 channel Grass EEG machine. The monkeys were not anaesthetised and were made to sit in a special chair for this purpose while recording the EEG activity. Penile stimulation by rubbing with a cotton pad was carried out in male monkeys and vaginal stimulation with the help of a lubricated glass rod carried out in female monkeys. As control measures similar stimulations of nipples and skin over abdomen and back, as well as pinching different parts of the body, were carried out. The behavioral responses of the animals to genital stimulation were also noted.

After repeating these manoeuvres for a few days in the sexually immature animals, daily intramuscular injections of gonadal hormones were started. Male monkeys were given testosterone propionate (Perandren, Ciba) in daily doses of 0.4 mg/kg body weight; while female monkeys were injected diethylstilboestrol dipropionate (Clinestrol, Glaxo) in daily doses of 0.25 mg. EEG recordings were carried out everyday after the injection of gonadal hormone and changes produced by penile or vaginal stimulations observed. These were repeated for a period of 2–3 weeks.

After completion of experimental procedures, electrode sites were marked by passing a direct current of 15 mA for 30 sec to produce small iron deposits at the electrode tips. The animals were sacrificed and their brains perfused with 10% formaline solution containing 1% potassium ferrocyanide. This produced a Prussian blue reaction with the iron deposits, resulting in blue spots at the sites of electrode tips, thus making their postmortem identification quite easy.

RESULTS

Fifteen brain regions were explored with the help of 54 electrodes. The distribution of electrode sites in different brain regions is shown in Table 1.

Effects of Genital Stimulation in Immature Monkeys

Genital stimulation in the sexually immature male and female monkeys did not result in any specific response either in the hypothalamic or the limbic regions investigated (Figs. 1–4). Such manoeuvres produced a generalised desynchronisation (arousal) response in those animals which did not have EEG arousal at the time of stimulation. In those already showing EEG arousal, no further changes resulted from genital stimulation. Stimulation of other body areas produced similar responses. Behaviorally the animals did not like the genital stimulation as demonstrated by an avoidance response.

Effects of Gonadal Hormone Injections

Injections of Perandren in sexually immature male monkeys did not produce any specific EEG responses *per se*, even after these had been given for 2–3 weeks (Figs. 1, 2 and 3).

On the other hand, sexually immature female monkeys showed some EEG changes resulting from Clinestrol injections, after the hormone had been given for about a week (Fig. 5). Subsequent injections produced an increasing tendency to spontaneous spindle activity, localised in the first few days to the anterior hypothalamic regions only, but generally spreading to other regions of the brain on following days.

Effects of Genital Stimulation Following Gonadal Hormones in Males

During the first 4–5 days after starting Perandren injections penile stimulation did not produce any specific changes in the EEG. After maintaining daily injections beyond this period genital stimulation resulted in specific changes in the EEG response. These were mostly located in the rostral supraoptic hypothalamic regions, and mainly resulted in the

TABLE 1

DISTRIBUTION OF ELECTRODES IN DIFFERENT REGIONS OF THE BRAIN

	Number of Monkeys	Anterior Commissure	Preoptic Area	Supraoptic Region	Optic Chiasma and Tract	Anterior Hypothalamus	Median Eminence including Ventromedial Nucleus	Lateral Hypothalamus	Posterior Hypothalamus	Mamillary Body	Tip of Temporal Lobe	Amygdala	Hippocampus	Cerebral Peduncle	Thalamus	Cerebral Cortex
Male	13	1	4	5	2	2	5	1	2	4	1	5	2	2	1	3
Female	2	—	2	2	1	1	1	1	—	2	—	2	—	—	—	2
Total	15	1	6	7	3	3	6	2	2	6	1	7	2	2	1	5

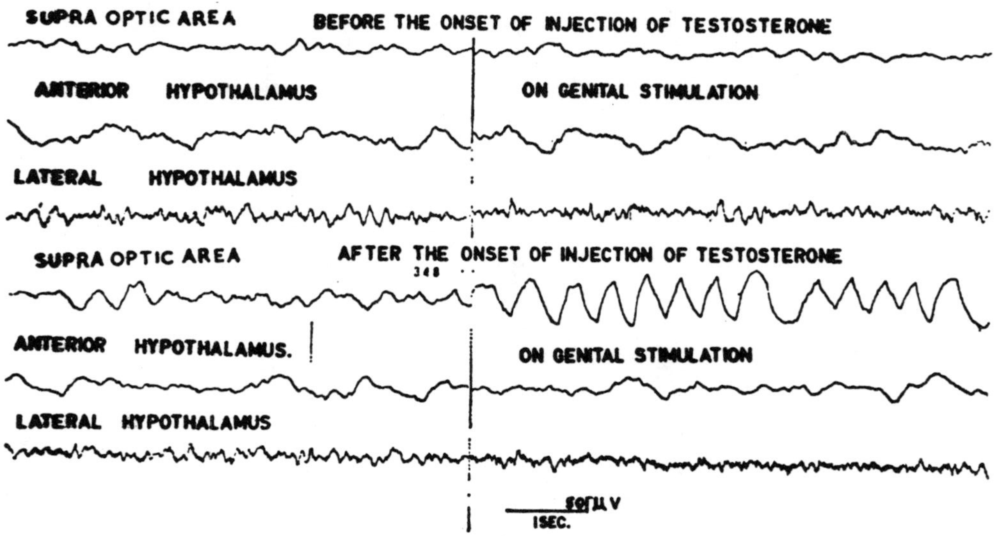

FIG. 1. Bipolar recordings from a male monkey. Before injections of testosterone, genital stimulation did not produce any changes in the EEG activity. After 5 days of testosterone injection, supraoptic area showed high voltage low frequency waves on genital stimulation, while anterior and lateral hypothalamus had no such response.

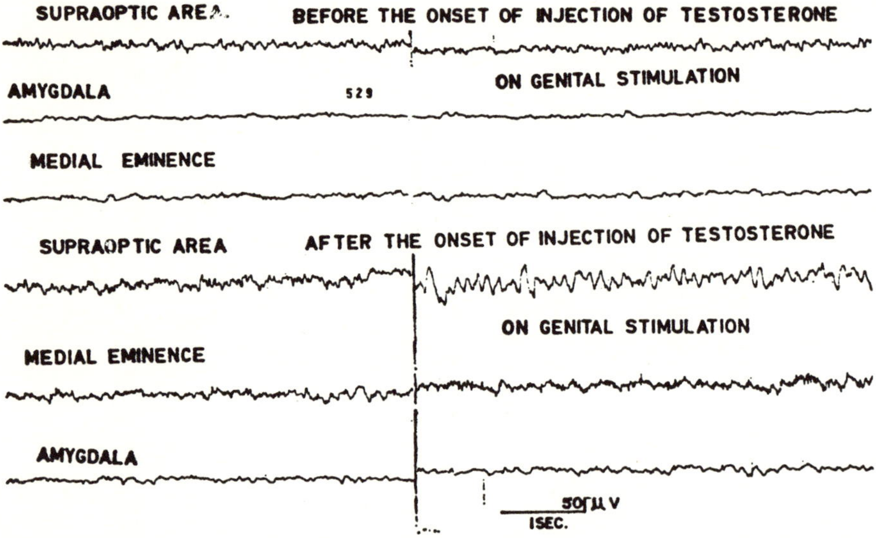

FIG. 2. Before the injections of testosterone in a male monkey genital stimulation did not produce any changes in the EEG activity. After 6 days of testosterone injection supraoptic area showed high voltage low frequency waves on genital stimulation, whereas median eminence and amygdala did not show any such response.

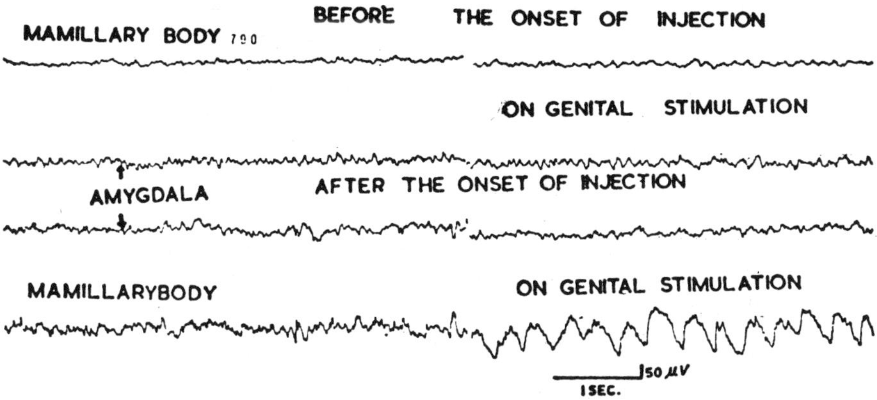

FIG. 3. Before injection of testosterone in a male monkey genital stimulation did not result in any changes in the EEG activity. After 10 days of testosterone injection, mamillary body showed high voltage low frequency waves on genital stimulation, whereas amygdala did not show any such change.

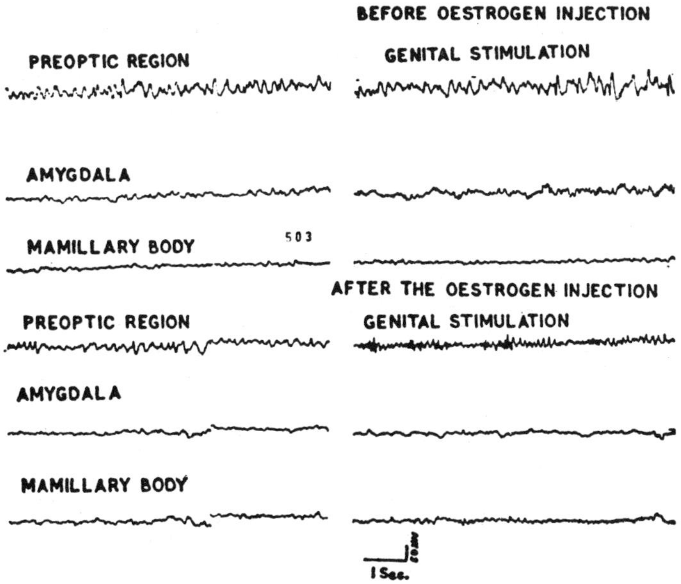

FIG. 4. Before estrogen injection in a female monkey genital stimulation did not produce any changes in EEG activity. Twenty minutes after the first estrogen injection genital stimulation resulted in high frequency spindles localised to the preoptic region, while no changes were produced in other regions.

production of high amplitude slow waves (Figs. 1 and 2). However, after a longer duration of testosterone injection these slow waves resulting from genital stimulation were also observed in the mamillary region. Such changes were not produced in any other region even after the injection had been continued for over 2–3 weeks. Furthermore, these were not elicited by stimulation of other parts of the body.

Effects of Genital Stimulation Following Gonadal Hormones in Females

Specific EEG changes on genital stimulation were produced in female monkeys even after the first injection of Clinestrol (Fig. 4). These consisted of the appearance of spindles located only in the rostral preoptic hypothalamic region. Later on, as the injections of estrogen produced spontaneous spindling in the preoptic and other regions, vaginal stimulation resulted in making this much more pronounced (Fig. 5). Even when this response gradually spread to other brain areas, it was always most prominent in the preoptic region. Such responses did not result from stimulation of other parts of the body.

Behavioral Responses

The animals, both male and female, stopped resisting attempts for genital stimulation after hormone injections had been continued for some days. They sat rather quietly through the period of stimulation and appeared to like the manoeuvre. This change in behavior appeared to coincide with the development of the EEG changes, and was noticed earlier in the females, and much later in the males.

DISCUSSION

The results of the present study provide suggestive evidence that: (a) the feed back of specific sensory information from the genital organs into the hypothalamic region occurs only in those animals which have been primed by the gonadal hormones, and (b) that in monkeys also this feed back occurs mainly into the rostral hypothalamic regions.

Previous studies [3, 6, 7, 8, 10, 12, 13, 14, 15, 16, 18, 19, 21] have demonstrated that gonadal hormones, as well as stimulation of genital organs, both result in changes in the functional activity of the hypothalamus, which brings about the regulation of reproductive activity in the animals. The present study indicates that the feed back of gonadal hormones, as well as the sensory information from the genital structures, have an integrative role to play in influencing hypothalamic activity. Without the priming effect of a certain level of gonadal hormones circulating in the blood, the sensory

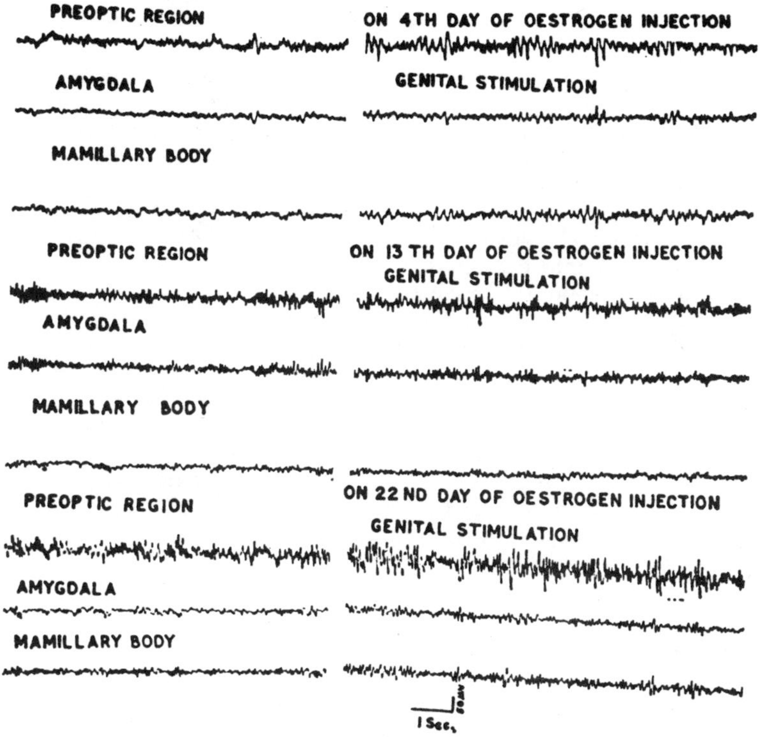

FIG. 5. EEG tracing showing responses to estrogen injection and genital stimulation on the 4th, 13th, and 22nd day of the injection in a female monkey. The spindle activity, which appeared in the preoptic area only after genital stimulation on the 4th day of injection, was later observed in other regions after estrogen injection, as well as on genital stimulation when it became more pronounced. The changes in any experimental situation were most marked in the preoptic region.

information from the genital structures is not able to bring about any specific changes in the hypothalamic activity. A certain level of concentration of gonadal hormones (at least in the female) is able to specifically influence the activity of the hypothalamic region. It is only on this previous conditioning of the hypothalamic regions that the sensory information from the genital structures can play its influencing role.

In line with the observations of other workers who have demonstrated the feed back of hormones and genital sensory information into the anterior hypothalamus in some species of animals [8, 12, 13, 14, 16], the present study confirms that even in a primate like monkey this feed back of information mostly occurs into the rostral hypothalamic regions. Previous experimental studies [6, 17, 19] have also suggested that this feed back into the anterior hypothalamus is a negative one, bringing about inhibition of certain functional activities. The EEG changes observed in the present study were either the production of high amplitude slow waves, or of spindles, both of which possibly signify depressed nervous excitability. These may be suggestive of an inhibitory feed back mechanism.

The significance of the appearance of high amplitude slow waves in the mamillary region on genital stimulation, in some of the male monkeys, is not clear. This may have something to do with the passage of sensory afferents from the genital region through this area.

REFERENCES

1. Anand, B. K. A method for permanent implantation of electrodes in the central nervous system for stimulation and recording of action potentials in conscious animals. *Indian J. Physiol. all. Sci.* **9**: 1–6, 1955.
2. Anand, B. K. Nervous regulation of reproductive behavior. *Bull. natn. Inst. Sci. India.* **27**: 20–27, 1964.
3. Barraclough, C. A. Hypothalamic activation associated with stimulation of vaginal cervix in proestrous rats. *Anat. Rec.* **136**: 159, 1960.
4. Chakrabarty, A. S., B. K. Anand and B. Singh. Effect of gonadal hormone and genital stimulation on the electrical activity of limbic system in monkeys. *Indian J. Physiol. Pharmac.* **11**: 35–36, 1967.
5. Chhina, G. S. Role of the limbic system of brain in the regulation of affective behavior. Doctorate Thesis, Punjab University, Chandigarh, India. 1960.
6. Davidson, J. M. Control of Gonadotrophin Secretion in the Male. In: *Neuroendocrinology, Vol.* 1, edited by L. Martini and W. F. Ganong. New York: Academic press, 1966, 565–611.

7. Davidson, J. M. and C. H. Sawyer. Effects of localised intracerebral implantation of oestrogen on reproductive function in the female rabbit. *Acta endocr.* **37**: 385–393, 1961.
8. Everett, J. W. Preoptic stimulative lesions and ovulation in the rat. Thresholds and LH release time in late diestrus and proestrus. In: *Major Problems in Neuroendocrinology*, edited by E. Bajuoz and G. Jasmin. Basal: S. Kargu, 1964, 346–366.
9. Flerko, B. and J. Szentagothai. Oestrogen sensitive nervous structures in the hypothalamus. *Acta endocr.* **26**: 121–127, 1957.
1C. Harris, G. W., R. P. Michael and P. P. Scott. Neurological site of action of stilboestrol in eliciting sexual behavior. In: *Ciba foundation symposium on the Neurological basis of Behavior*, Boston: Little, Brown and Co., 1958, 236–251.
11. Horowitz S. and J. J. van der Werff ten Bosch. Hypothalamic sexual precocity in female rats operated shortly after birth. *Acta endocr.* **41**: 301–313, 1962.
12. Law, O. T. and G. P. Sacket. Hypothalamic potentials in female rat evoked by hormones and by vaginal stimulation. *Neuroendocrinology.* **1**: 31–44, 1965/1966.
13. Lincoln, D. W. and B. A. Cross. Effect of oestrogen on the responsiveness of neurones in the hypothalamus, septum and preoptic area of rats with light induced persistent oestrus. *J. endocr.* **37**: 191–203, 1967.
14. Lisk, R. D. Estrogen sensitive centres in the hypothalamus of the rat. *J. exp. Zool.* **145**: 197–208, 1960.
15. Lisk, R. D. Diencephalic placement of oestradiol and sexual receptivity in the female rat. *Am. J. Physiol.* **203**: 493–496, 1962.
16. Michael, R. P. Oestrogens in the central nervous system. *Br. med. Bull.* **21**: 87–90, 1965.
17. Porter, R. W., E. B. Cavanaugh, B. V. Critchlow and C. H. Sawyer. Localised changes in electrical activity of the hypothalamus in estrous cats following vaginal stimulation. *Am. J. Physiol.* **189**: 145–151, 1957.
18. Ramirez, V. D., B. R. Komisaruk, D. I. Whitmoyer and C. H. Sawyer. Effect of hormones and vaginal stimulation on EEG and hypothalamic units in rats. *Am. J. Physiol.* **212**: 1376–1384, 1967.
19. Sawyer, C. H. and M. Kawakami. Neuroendocrine correlates of changes in brain activity thresholds by sex steroids and pituitary hormones. *Endocrinology* **65**: 652–668, 1967.
20. Sawyer, C. H. and M. Kawakami. Interactions between the central nervous system and hormones influencing ovulation. In: *Control of Ovulation*, edited by C. A. Villee, London: Pergamon Press, 1961, 79–97.
21. Smith, E. R. and J. M. Davidson. Differential responses to hypothalamic testosterone in relation to male puberty. *Am. J. Physiol.* **212**: 1385–1390, 1967.

Effects of Progesterone and Sensory Stimulation on EEG and Neuronal Activity in the Rat

BARRY R. KOMISARUK, PETER G. McDONALD,

DAVID I. WHITMOYER, AND CHARLES H. SAWYER[1]

The effects of intravenous injections of progesterone and the application of various sensory stimuli on neuronal activity in the hypothalamus, cortex, and thalamus were investigated in urethane-anesthetized rats. Multiple facets of neural activity were registered by simultaneously recording cortical EEG, single-unit firing and integrated multiple-unit activity in these brain regions. Changes in adjacent single- and multiunit activity recorded from the cerebral cortex and thalamus were closely correlated with alterations in cortical EEG, while hypothalamic activity was relatively independent of the cortical EEG. Intravenous progesterone quickly induced a sleeplike EEG which lasted between 20 and 60 min, and single- and multiunit activity changed to the patterns characteristic of sleep. During this period arousal responses to all types of sensory stimuli were partially or completely blocked. Progesterone in this preparation is thus considered to exert differential effects on neurons through a nonspecific depression of arousal. Since the activity of individual neurons is bound more or less closely to the arousal level, neurons are differentially affected by the general depression induced by progesterone.

Introduction

Recent evidence indicates that progestins exert profound effects on the nervous system, perhaps by direct action. Courtship behavior in the ring dove (14) and mating and ovulation in the rabbit (11) are inhibited by implanting crystalline progestins into particular regions of the brain.

[1] This study was supported by grants from the National Institutes of Health (NB 01162 and 1 F2 HD-14711 01 REP), Ford Foundation, and Population Council. It has received bibliographic aid from the UCLA Brain Information Service which is a part of the National Information Network of the NINDB and supported under contract PH-43-66-59. Dr. Komisaruk was a National Institute of Health Postdoctoral Fellow; his present address is Institute of Animal Behavior, Rutgers, The State University, Newark, New Jersey, 07102. Dr. McDonald was a Population Council Postdoctoral Fellow; his present address is Department of Physiology, Royal Veterinary College, London, N. W. 1, England. We are grateful to Dr. V. D. Ramirez, Dr. B. J. Meyerson, and Dr. C. Beyer for advice and assistance and to Miss Virginia Tompkins and Miss Cora Rucker for technical help. Critical comments by Dr. R. J. Barfield and Dr. B. Sachs on the manuscript are appreciated.

Behavioral and electroencephalographic sleep patterns have been induced by inserting progesterone into the preoptic region in cats (9). Progesterone injected intravenously in rats induce a sleeplike EEG (12), and profoundly inhibits excitatory responses of hypothalamic neurons to probing the vaginal cervix (2). Selective effects of progesterone on hypothalamic neurons have been postulated by Barraclough and Cross (2) and Cross and Silver (6); they reported that progesterone blocked responsiveness to probing the vaginal cervix but not to painful or thermal stimuli. This interpretation has been questioned by Ramirez *et al.* (18), however, on the basis that progesterone induces generalized inhibitory changes in brain activity, and that individual neurons as well as groups of neurons (3) simply reflect this nonspecific depression. The present experiments analyze further the question of whether progesterone has selective or generalized inhibitory effects on neurons. Our criteria for a selective effect on a neuron have been that its firing rate should be altered by the treatment in the absence of effects on adjacent groups of neurons or on the cortical EEG, all recorded simultaneously.

Materials and Methods

Mature intact female Sprague-Dawley rats, each weighing about 300 g, were used. They were anesthetized with urethane (1.2 g/kg), placed in a stereotaxic frame, and a 5-mm-long rectangular aperture was drilled through the left side of the skull extending across bregma and from the midline to about 3 mm lateral. The cortex was exposed and covered with a drop of lukewarm 3% agar. A polyethylene tracheal cannula facilitated breathing and an intravenous injection cannula was placed in a femoral vein. Blood pressure was monitored from a cannula placed usually in the right femoral artery but sometimes in the right carotid artery. The EEG was recorded from stainless steel screws fixed in the skull over the olfactory bulb, frontal and parietal cortex on the side contralateral to the aperture. Single-unit activity was recorded with electrolytically polished No. 00 stainless steel insect pins (8) which were insulated with Epoxylite. The tip diameter was 3-5 μ. The multiunit electrodes were constructed of similar insect pins, and tips abraded on fine emery cloth to a diameter of approximately 80 μ and about 60 μ of the shaft exposed. The two electrodes were joined along their lengths with DeKhotinsky's Cement. The single-unit electrode extended slightly beyond the multiunit electrode so that the distance between the tips was about 300 μ. In the brain, the single-unit electrode was placed medial to the multiunit electrode.

Single-unit activity was amplified by a Grass model P6 amplifier with cathode follower probe (gain 500, bandpass 5-10 kHz) connected to one beam of a Tektronix 502 oscilloscope. The oscilloscope was used to monitor shape and amplitude of single-unit discharges and to amplify them for presentation to a pulse height discriminator (PHD). Output from the PHD was a train of pulses (3 msec; 12 v), one for each input spike with peak amplitude lying between selected upper and lower limits. These output pulses were a-c coupled to one channel of an Offner type R Dynograph to give a single-unit firing rate record. The spike potentials of all neurons recorded were greater than 250 μv, while the noise level was approximately 100 μv. The number of neurons firing spontaneously in a given volume of the hypothalamus was notably less than in cortex or thalamus.

Almost all single-unit recordings were made in the following regions, between 0.5 and 1.0 mm lateral to midline: Cortical, between 1.5 mm anterior to and 0.5 mm posterior to bregma and between 0.5 and 3.0 mm below surface of brain; thalamic, almost all in or near nuclei reuniens and incerta; and hypothalamic, almost all in or near anterior, ventromedial, dorsal, and arcuate nuclei.

The multiunit signal channel was composed of a solid-state preamplifier, the remaining Tektronix 502 beam, a rectifier and RC integrator, and one channel of the Dynograph. Here again the oscilloscope served both as a wave-form monitor and as an amplifier, since the vertical signal output was used to drive the integrating circuit. The integrator output was d-c coupled to a Dynograph channel, giving a qualitative record of activity vs. time. The calibrations shown for this data channel reflect only the gain settings of the Dynograph.

The electrode pair showing the most distinctive cortical EEG transitions from "sleep" to "arousal" was selected and recorded on a third Dynograph channel. Blood pressure was recorded on a fourth channel by means of a Statham P23 pressure transducer. In addition EEG, EKG, respiration and the unit write-out were recorded simultaneously with a Grass model IV EEG apparatus.

To identify the recording site, electrolytic lesions were made by passing a direct current of 3 μamp for 30 sec through the single-unit electrode and 5 μamp for 30 sec through the multiunit electrode. Before staining with thionine, the brain was perfused with a solution of 3% potassium ferrocyanide and 3% potassium ferricyanide to obtain a Prussian Blue reaction.

Results

Cortical EEG under Urethane Anesthesia. Two distinctive EEG patterns were seen under urethane anesthesia, a high-amplitude slow-wave pattern closely resembling the sleeping EEG in unanesthetized rats, and a low-amplitude fast-wave pattern characteristic of arousal. We have used the terms "sleep" and "arousal" even under urethane because of observed relationships between the EEG pattern and the behavior of the rats (although it is limited) as follows. Under urethane, when high-amplitude slow waves were present, a pinch to a hind foot would almost immediately induce low-amplitude fast waves. If the pinch was strong enough, leg flexion, body twisting, vibrissa twitching, and jaw movements would occur concomitantly with the low-amplitude fast activity of the EEG. These effects were not specific to any sensory modality and were readily elicited by sufficiently strong tactile, auditory, cold, or heat stimulation. Body movements were absent during high-amplitude slow-wave periods. At our standard dose of 1.2 g urethane/kg, these periods characteristically lasted several minutes, interspersed with periods of low-amplitude fast activity also lasting several minutes. When lower doses of urethane were administered, there were longer and more numerous periods of low-amplitude fast-wave activity, during which body movements were frequently observed, and low-amplitude fast waves could be evoked more readily with mild stimulation than at higher urethane doses. The simplest characterization of all these effects is that each stimulus induced a generalized "arousal" (low-amplitude fast waves) from a condition of "sleep" (high-amplitude slow waves), urethane depressing the maximum level of arousal that could be induced. We shall therefore use the conventions of "arousal" and "sleep" in referring to low-amplitude fast waves and high-amplitude slow waves, respectively, in the urethane-anesthetized rat.

Correlation of Single- and Multiunit Activity with Cortical EEG. Single- and multiunit activity throughout the brain showed marked changes which usually correlated with transitions in the cortical EEG from sleep (high-amplitude slow waves) to arousal (low-amplitude fast waves). In thirty-one of forty-nine cases (63%), single- and multiunit activity increased on EEG arousal (Fig. 1). In ten cases unit firing rate decreased while the multiunit activity increased during EEG arousal (Fig. 2). Thus, in forty-one cases (84%), changes in single- and multiunit activity occurred simultaneously with sleep-arousal transitions of the cortical EEG. In the remaining eight (16%), single-unit firing rate remained unaltered during EEG transitions despite the fact that the multiunit activity changed; in all forty-nine cases, the multiunit activity increased upon EEG arousal.

The single-unit firing patterns seen in the cortex and thalamus were very different from those encountered in the hypothalamus. Upon arousal, over 80% of the cortical and thalamic units increased their firing rates, whereas about equal numbers of hypothalamic units increased, decreased, or showed no rate change (Table 1). The hypothalamus thus appears to be relatively independent of brain arousal levels (Fig. 3).

Characteristics of Single-Unit Activity. In the cortex, the single-unit firing rate increased significantly on EEG arousal. The variability in firing rate of these units was significantly greater during arousal than sleep (Table 2).

In the hypothalamus, since almost as many units slowed as accelerated

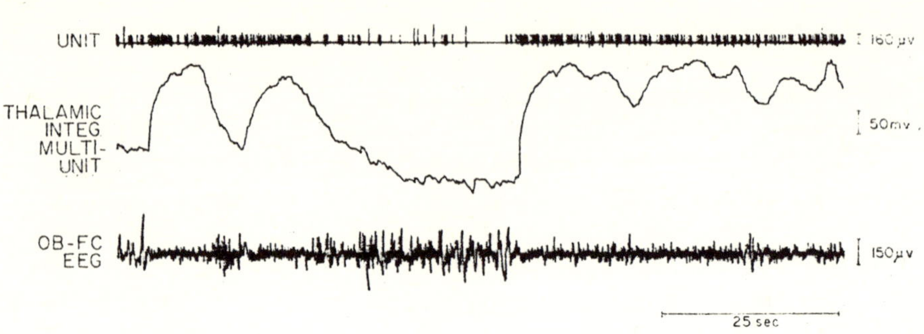

FIG. 1. Temporal correlation between changes in thalamic (neuronal) activity and the cortical EEG. Single- and multiunit activity channels show a low level of activity during the period of EEG "sleep" in the middle of the record. The sudden, spontaneous EEG arousal is accompanied by marked increases in single- and multiunit activity. The large deflections of the pen in the single-unit recording during each sleeplike period are produced by bursts of two or three spike potentials in rapid succession which the polygraph recorder cannot resolve, and which have been referred to as "beeps." See text for further explanation. Thalamic activity was recorded near zona incerta. Abbreviations in this and later figures: OB, olfactory bulb; FC, frontal cortex; PC, parietal cortex.

on arousal, there was no significant change in firing rate; however, the variability in firing rate increased significantly on arousal (Table 2). The alterations in firing rate seen in the hypothalamic units upon arousal were significantly related to their basal ("sleeping") firing rate. Hypothalamic units which speeded on arousal had the lowest basal rate; those which

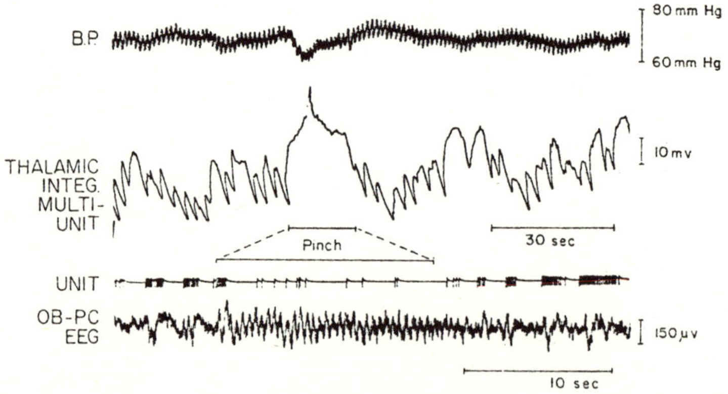

FIG. 2. Depression of thalamic single-unit activity during strong arousal, coincident with stimulation of thalamic multiunit activity and fall in blood pressure. The decrease in blood pressure upon arousal is a characteristic response in our preparation. The EEG and single-unit recordings were made on an EEG machine, simultaneously with the multiunit and blood pressure recordings made on a polygraph lacking a compatible chart-drive speed. Thalamic activity was recorded near Nucleus reuniens thalami. This thalamic unit potential was 2800 μv.

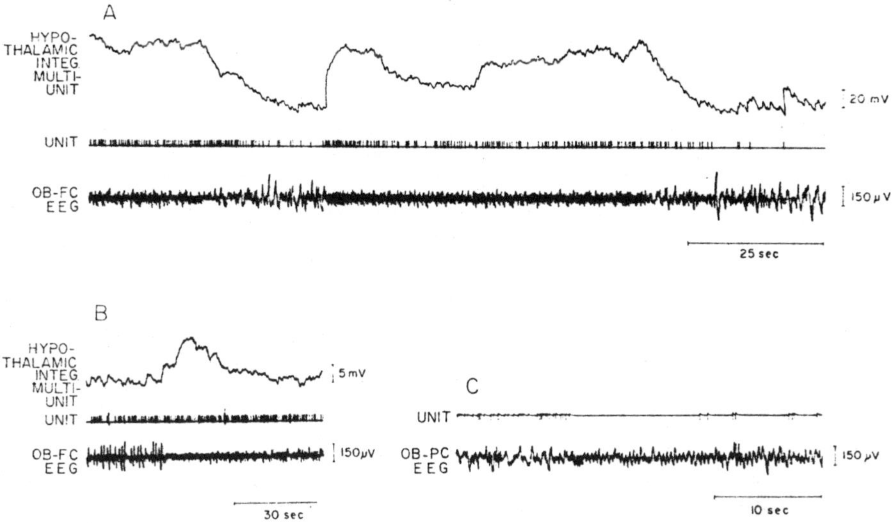

FIG. 3. Activity patterns in the hypothalamus. In (B) the unit firing rate is unchanged during spontaneous arousal although the adjacent neuronal population is activated. The high gain required in the multiunit record is indicative of the low activity found in all cases in the medial hypothalamus as compared with higher activity levels typically encountered in the cortex and thalamus. In (A) temporally parallel changes in single- and multiunit activities and cortical EEG are clearly seen. The apparently spontaneous fluctuations in arousal level were characteristically seen under urethane anesthesia in these animals. In (C) a marked depression of unit activity occurs upon "spontaneous EEG arousal" indicated by a slow (3/sec) thetalike rhythm; multiunit activity was not recorded. Unit potential and location in (A): 1400 μv, near nucleus dorsomedialis hypothalami; (B): 700 μv, dorsal anterior region of the nucleus ventromedialis hypothalami; (C): 400 μv, ventral part of the nucleus ventromedialis hypothalami.

TABLE 1

PATTERNS OF CHANGE IN SINGLE-UNIT FIRING RATE UPON EEG "AROUSAL": REGIONAL DIFFERENCES[a]

Type of firing rate change upon EEG transition from "sleep" to "arousal"	Location of single units							
	Cortex		Thalamus		Hypothalamus		Totals	
	No.	%	No.	%	No.	%	No.	%
Increase	(23)	85	(23)	82	(13)	32	(59)	61
Decrease	(4)	15	(4)	14	(12)	29	(20)	21
No change	(0)	0	(1)	4	(16)	39	(17)	18
Totals	(27)	100	(28)	100	(41)	100	(96)	100

[a] These values are based on ninety-six cases in which single-unit firing rate was determined simultaneously with EEG, and include forty-nine cases in which multiunit activity was also recorded simultaneously.

slowed on arousal had faster rates; and those which were unaffected by arousal had the fastest rates (Table 3).

TABLE 2
MAGNITUDE OF CHANGE IN SINGLE-UNIT FIRING RATE UPON EEG "AROUSAL": REGIONAL DIFFERENCES

Region of brain	No.	Firing rate (spike/sec) During EEG "sleep" Median	Inter-quartile range	Variance	During EEG "arousal" Median	Inter-quartile range	Variance
Cortex	(27)	2.4	1.2-4.4	3.4	4.6[a]	1.9-5.9	34.2[b]
Hypothalamus	(41)	2.0	0.8-4.9	23.0	2.2[c]	0.7-5.5	73.7[d]

[a] $P < 0.0001$ ($z = -3.97$) Wilcoxon matched-pairs signed-ranks test (20).
[b] $P < 0.01$ ($F = 10.0$).
[c] $P > 0.10$ ($z = -1.25$) Wilcoxon matched-pairs signed-ranks test.
[d] $P < 0.01$ ($F = 3.2$).

TABLE 3
RELATIONSHIP BETWEEN FIRING RATE AND TYPE OF CHANGE UPON EEG "AROUSAL": HYPOTHALAMIC UNITS

Type of change in rate upon transition from EEG "sleep" to "arousal"	No.	Firing rate (spike/sec) During EEG "sleep" (basal) Median	Inter-quartile range	During EEG "arousal" Median	Inter-quartile range
Speeded	(13)	0.8*a*	0.3-1.4	3.5	1.1-5.3
Slowed	(12)	1.5*b*	1.0-3.6	0.3	0.1-0.7
No definite change	(16)	4.9*c*	3.3-7.7	5.2	2.7-8.0

P *a-b* <0.10 Mann-Whitney U test (20).
P *b-c* <0.02 Mann-Whitney U test (20).
P *a-c* <0.002 Mann-Whitney U test (20).

Cortical units which speeded on arousal had significantly higher basal firing rates than hypothalamic units which speeded on arousal (Table 4).

In the thalamus, fifteen of twenty-seven units (56%) showed a distinctive pattern of activity which was seen only rarely in the cortex and hypothalamus. This pattern, described by Barraclough and Cross (2) and called "beeps," occurred almost exclusively during EEG sleep interspersed with the usual single discharges (Fig. 1). Each beep consisted of two to five spike discharges from a single unit, each discharge occurring about 2 msec after the preceding one, and being slightly lower in voltage. After each beep there was a latency of more than 200 msec before the next beep occurred. In all but one case, the unit stopped showing beeps upon EEG arousal, and the firing pattern became more regular, with single spike discharges separated by at least 50 msec. The shape and size of the spike potential was virtually the same in the single-discharge pattern as at the first spike of each beep. The units which showed this firing pattern did not differ significantly in rate during arousal from those which did not show this characteristic ($P > 0.10$; Mann-Whitney U test).

TABLE 4
BASAL FIRING RATE OF UNITS WHICH SPEED UPON EEG "AROUSAL": REGIONAL DIFFERENCES

Region of brain	No.	Firing rate (spike/sec) during EEG "sleep" Median	Inter-quartile range	Variance
Cortex	(23)	3.1	1.6-4.1	3.3
Hypothalamus	(13)	0.8[a]	0.3-1.4	6.1[b]

[a] $P < 0.02$ Mann-Whitney U test (20).
[b] There is no significant difference between the cortical and hypothalamic variances ($F = 1.9$; $P > 0.05$).

Effects of Progesterone on EEG and Single- and Multiunit Activity. Progesterone (100-300 μg in 0.05-0.15 ml propylene glycol injected intravenously) induced a profound sleeplike EEG which lasted up to 1 hour in twenty-two out of twenty-five cases. Upon injection, there was occasionally an initial EEG arousal which lasted about 1 min. Single-unit firing rate was depressed simultaneously with the onset of EEG sleep in twenty of twenty-five units studied. Each had shown a similar slowing during "spontaneous" EEG sleep prior to progesterone administration. Nine of the twenty were hypothalamic, nine thalamic, and two cortical. The five neurons which were not affected by progesterone were in the hypothalamus, and none had been altered by sleep-arousal transitions prior to progesterone administration. Thalamic units which showed beeps during spontaneous EEG sleep also showed this pattern during EEG sleep induced by progesterone administration. In seven cases, single- and multiunit activity were recorded simultaneously. A depression in multiunit activity accompanied progesterone-induced single-unit slowing and EEG sleep in each of these cases.

This single- and multiunit activity, which decreased during spontaneous and progesterone-induced EEG sleep, could be activated by any stimulus which also induced EEG arousal, such as pinching the foot or tail, probing the rectum, probing the vaginal cervix, applying ice or hot water to the foot, or jingling keys near an ear. Stimuli which failed to induce arousal also failed to affect single- or multiunit activity. Such stimuli were intense light beamed into either eye, clapping the hands or whistling, or gently stroking the fur. Under the influence of progesterone the arousing stimuli were less effective in magnitude and duration.

Figure 4 shows a typical sequence of events before and after progesterone administration. Vaginal, rectal, cold, and pinch stimuli all had strong excitatory influences on the firing rate of the single unit, the adjacent multi-

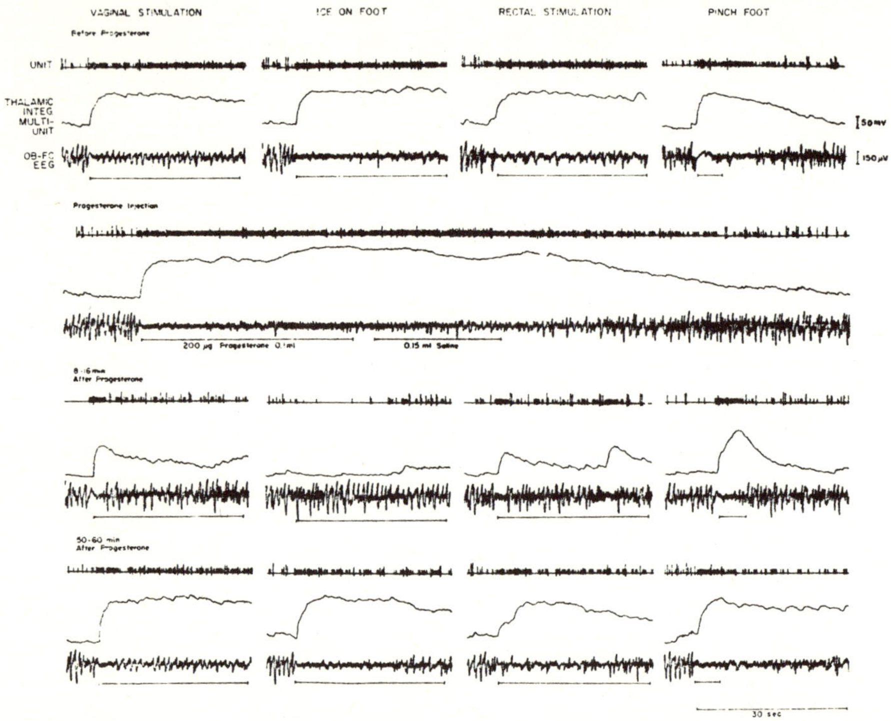

FIG. 4. Effects of progesterone on neuronal activity. After a brief arousal progesterone induces a deep sleeplike EEG accompanied by decreased basal activity of single- and multiunit recordings and decreased responsiveness to each of the afferent stimuli. Activation of neuronal activity can be predicted by the degree of arousal which the stimuli induce in the cortical EEG rather than by the modality of stimulation. The initial arousal accompanying the intravenous administration of progesterone is probably due to the toxic effect of propylene glycol. The effect of the progesterone has worn off by 1 hour after administration. Thalamic unit potential and location: 1600 μv, in the nucleus reticularis thalami.

unit population, and the cortical EEG. Upon injection of progesterone in propylene glycol there was an initial arousal. Within about 1 min, however, EEG sleep had returned and was apparently much deeper than before. Probing the vaginal cervix then had only mildly arousing effects on the EEG and single- and multiunit activity; applying ice to the foot evoked no activation whatsoever on any of these. Probing the rectum had an intermediate effect on all three, while pinching still exerted a maximal (amplitude-wise) excitatory effect. However, the response to the pinch lasted only as long as the stimulus was applied. This was in contrast to the effect before progesterone, in which the arousal continued well after the pinch was stopped. After 50 min, the responses to each of these stimuli were almost fully recovered. Note that this thalamic neuron in Fig. 4 shows the characteristic beep pattern during spontaneous sleep, shifting to a single mode of firing during arousal. During the progesterone-induced sleeplike EEG period, the unit fired exclusively in beeps except when stimuli were applied.

We often observed simultaneity between a sudden drop in arterial blood pressure and the appearance of arousal patterns in EEG, single-, and multi-unit channels. Blood pressure rose with the onset of spontaneous EEG sleep.

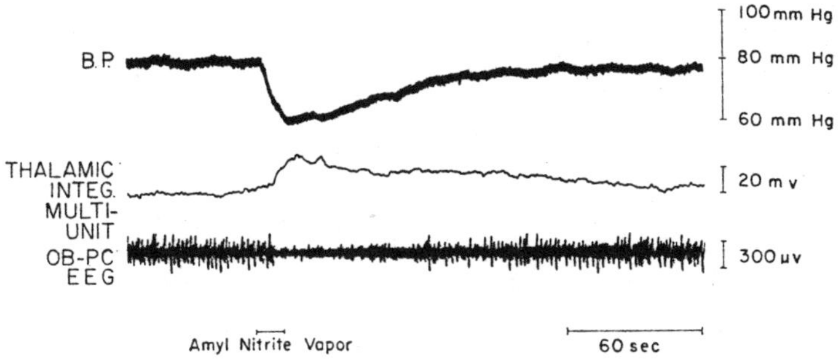

Fig. 5. Blood pressure depression induced by amyl nitrite vapor blown gently into the tracheal cannula is quickly followed by EEG "arousal" and thalamic multiunit activation.

Increasing the blood pressure by intravenous injection of saline or glucose (0.4 ml) promptly induced a sleeplike EEG which lasted for several minutes. Injection of propylene glycol (0.05-0.15 ml, followed by 0.05-0.15 ml saline) also induced a brief sleeplike condition after an initial arousal which lasted about 1 min. However, progesterone in propylene glycol (0.05-0.15 ml followed by 0.05-0.15 ml saline) induced a more prolonged increase in blood pressure and a deeper sleep, indicated by significantly ($P < 0.02$) shorter periods of arousal following the application of strong stimuli. A decrease in blood pressure was induced by gently blowing amyl nitrite vapor into the tracheal cannula. This drug quickly induces peripheral vasodilation and the precipitous fall in blood pressure was followed within seconds by a strong EEG arousal and a sharp rise in thalamic multiunit activity (Fig. 5). This progesterone effect was observed in all the phases of the estrous cycle and also in a few rats which had been ovariectomized several weeks previously.

Although an increase in blood pressure accompanied progesterone-induced EEG sleep, this blood pressure change was not necessarily the mediator for the progesterone effect. In a preliminary study, the temporal correlation between blood pressure and EEG was specifically observed. As the effect of progesterone was wearing off, a transition from EEG sleep to arousal was accompanied by a gradual fall in blood pressure in six cases, the EEG transition preceded the blood pressure fall by at least 1 min in three cases, and the EEG transition followed the blood pressure fall by several minutes in one case. In twenty-one others in which propylene glycol, glucose, or saline were administered (with a significantly shorter effect), the transition from EEG sleep to arousal accompanied the blood pressure fall in eight, preceded it in ten, and followed it in three experiments, further suggesting a correlated, rather than a causal, relationship between blood pressure and EEG activity.

Discussion

In our investigation of the effects of progesterone on neuronal activity, we were impressed by the striking temporal correlation between changes in activity of single neurons and alterations in the arousal level of the cortical EEG. Since elevated activity of the majority of the neurons we observed was closely correlated with cortical arousal, it was imperative to distinguish the effects of progesterone that might be produced indirectly by an induced change in arousal from the effects on particular neurons independent of changes in brain arousal. The close correlation between neuronal activity and level of arousal had been demonstrated by others in cortical and subcortical regions (7, 17) and is apparently not unique to our preparation under urethane (10, for review). It was therefore of great interest to observe that the hypothalamus is different from cerebral cortex and thalamus in its relative independence of the arousal level. The independent hypothalamic neurons in our study had basal firing rates significantly higher than the cortical units and the other hypothalamic neurons, while the hypothalamic neurons which speeded on arousal had significantly lower basal firing rates. The variability of firing rate was greater in arousal than sleep, and this may reflect a differentiation of function upon arousal. During EEG sleep, over-all relative inactivity of the brain would predominate, whereas in arousal some neural systems would be activated and others actively inhibited. The relative independence of the hypothalamic neurons may reflect their functions in autonomic mechanisms.

While we found ample evidence that the injection of progesterone inhibited neurons whose activity was linked to the general arousal level, we found no evidence for an effect of the steroid on independent neurons. This suggests that at least some effects of progesterone may be mediated by a general depression of arousal level and also demonstrates the importance of considering the activity of the rest of the brain when studying single neuron responses. For example, we have repeated the procedure used by Barraclough and Cross, and have confirmed almost all their findings. However, on the basis of our additional measurements, our interpretation of these findings is diametrically opposed to theirs.

Barraclough and Cross (2) found that neuronal responsiveness to stimulation of the vaginal cervix was inhibited by progesterone, and Cross and Silver (6) concluded that progesterone induces "selective depression of neuronal excitation by stimuli from the genital tract." However, we found that the neuronal response to many other stimuli as well as of the cervix is inhibited by progesterone. The effect of any stimulus on neuronal activity was predictable not so much by the specific modality as by the degree to which each stimulus aroused the brain as a whole (indicated by cortical EEG). Thus the reason that the effect of cervical probing was inhibited but the effect of pinching was not, is apparently that pinching is a stronger arousing stimulus than cervical probing. For this reason, other strongly arousing stimuli such as rectal probing and the sound of jingling keys are still effective under the effects of progesterone but other, weakly arousing, stimuli such as cervical probing and stroking the fur are no longer effective. Other findings of Barraclough and Cross can be reinterpreted to support a general inhibitory effect of progesterone. Examination of their figures show that the basal, unstimulated firing rate was lowest, and the effects of pinching were shortest-lived, when the neuron was least responsive to cervical probing. We suggest that the neurons they found to be unaffected by sensory stimulation as well as progesterone were probably unaffected by changes in arousal. They also found that while excitatory responses were suppressed by progesterone, inhibitory responses were not affected by progesterone (5). On the basis of our findings, inhibitory responses are most likely to be obtained by stimuli which induce a sleeplike EEG. Since progesterone induces EEG sleep it should not interfere with, but if anything, facilitate inhibitory responses. On the basis of our findings and a reexamination of those of Barraclough and Cross and Cross and Silver, we conclude that the selective effect which progesterone exerts on certain neurons can be accounted for by considering how closely each neuron is linked to a general arousal mechanism.

Our concept that progesterone has a general inhibitory effect on brain activity is consistent with other findings (1, 19) that this and other steroids are anesthetic if administered in dosages much higher than those used in the present experiment. However, our data do not exclude the possibility that progesterone has direct effects on hypothalamic neurons although we have seen that selective effects can be mediated by indirect mechanisms. That a general neural inhibition may release a specific behavior pattern has been demonstrated recently by Clemens and Gorski (personal communication). Mating was induced in previously unreceptive rats by spreading cortical depression. The depression produced by progesterone in our experiment may thus be involved in Lisk's (16) induction of mating in rats by dosages of progesterone within the range we used.

The question remains of the mechanism of action of progesterone; specifically, does it directly affect neurons in the brain, and if so, by what means? Progesterone raises the threshold of excitation, blocks propagated action potentials, and hyperpolarizes the cell membrane of myometrial cells in the rat, rabbit, and mouse (15). A similar mechanism might account for progesterone-induced neural inhibition. Another possible mechanism for this effect is a reflex activation of the baroceptor input: we observed a rise in blood pressure concomitant with progesterone-induced EEG sleep, and neuronal inhibition. This supports previous findings that mechanically-induced increases in carotid sinus pressure induces a behaviorally sleeplike condition in dogs (13). Beyer, *et al.* (3) observed that in rats progesterone raised blood pressure and induced sleep concomitantly with a fall in multiunit activity; denervation of the carotid sinus blocked the effects of pressor agents on EEG sleep. The pressor effect of progesterone in rats at similar dosage levels was also shown by Cession, *et al.* (4); progesterone both increased blood pressure and augmented the hypertensive effects of adrenalin, noradrenalin, and angiotensin. While progesterone may exert its effect on the EEG and neuronal activity indirectly through an increase in blood pressure, the mechanism by which progesterone increases blood pressure has not yet been demonstrated and certainly a direct effect of progesterone on the central nervous system has not been excluded. The sites of action of progesterone remain a problem for further research.

References

1. Atkinson, R. M., B. Davis, M. A. Pratt, H. M. Sharpe, and E. G. Tomich. 1965. II. Pharmacology. *J. Med. Chem.* **8**: 426-432.
2. Barraclough, C. A., and B. A. Cross. 1963. Unit activity in the hypothalamus of the cyclic female rat: effect of genital stimuli and progesterone. *J. Endocrinol.* **26**: 339-359.
3. Beyer, C., V. D. Ramirez, D. I. Whitmoyer, and C. H. Sawyer. 1967. Effects of hormones on the electrical activity of the brain in the rat and rabbit. *Exptl. Neurol.* **18**: 313-326.
4. Cession, G., A. Cession-Fossion, and R. Limet. 1966. Action de la progesterone sur trois agents endogenes à action hypertensive. *Compt. Rend.* **159**: 1864-1866.
5. Cross, B. A. 1964. Electrical recording techniques in the study of hypothalamic control of gonadotrophin secretion, pp. 513-516. *In* "Proceedings of the Second International Congress of Endocrinology." *Excerpta Med. Intern. Congr. Ser.* No. 83.
6. Cross, B. A., and I. A. Silver. 1965. Effect of luteal hormone on the behaviour of hypothalamic neurones in pseudopregnant rats. *J. Endocrinol.* **31**: 251-263.

7. Cross, B. A., and I. A. Silver. 1966. Electrophysiological studies on the hypothalamus. *Brit. Med. Bull.* **22**: 254-260.
8. Green, J. D. 1958. A simple microelectrode for recording from the central nervous system. *Nature* **182**: 962.
9. Heuser, G., G. M. Ling, and M. Kluver. 1967. Sleep induction by progesterone in the preoptic area in cats. *Electroencephalog. Clin. Neurophysiol.* **22**: 122-127.
10. Jouvet, M. 1967. Neurophysiology of the states of sleep. *Physiol. Rev.* **47**: 117-177.
11. Kanematsu, S., and C. H. Sawyer. 1965. Blockade of ovulation in rabbits by hypothalamic implants of norethindrone. *Endocrinology* **76**: 691-699.
12. Kobayashi, T., T. Kobayashi, S. Takezawa, K. Oshima, and H. Kawamura. 1962. Electrophysiological studies on the feed-back mechanism of progesterone. *Endocrinol. Japon.* **9**: 302-320.
13. Koch, E. 1932. Die Irradiation der pressoreceptorischen Kreislaufreflexe. *Klin. Wochschr.* **11**: 225-227.
14. Komisaruk, B. R. 1967. Effects of local brain implants of progesterone on reproductive behavior in ring doves. *J. Comp. Physiol. Psychol.* (in press).
15. Kuriyama, H. 1961. Recent studies on the electrophysiology of the uterus, pp. 51-71. *In* "Progesterone and the Defence Mechanisms of Pregnancy," G. E. W. Wolstenholme and M. P. Cameron [eds.]. Ciba Foundation Study Group, No. 9, Little, Brown, Boston, Massachusetts.
16. Lisk, R. D. 1960. A comparison of the effectiveness of intravenous, as opposed to subcutaneous injection of progesterone for the induction of estrous behavior in the rat. *Can. J. Biochem. Physiol.* **38**: 1381-1383.
17. Podvoll, E. M., and S. J. Goodman. 1967. Averaged neural electrical activity and arousal. *Science* **155**: 223-225.
18. Ramirez, V. D., B. R. Komisaruk, D. I. Whitmoyer, and C. H. Sawyer. 1967. Effects of hormones and vaginal stimulation on the EEG and hypothalamic units in rats. *Am. J. Physiol.* **212**: 1376-1384.
19. Selye, H. 1941. Studies concerning the anesthetic action of steroid hormones. *J. Pharmacol. Exptl. Therap.* **73**: 127-141.
20. Siegel, S. 1956. "Nonparametric Statistics for the Behavioral Sciences." McGraw-Hill, New York.

UNIT ACTIVITY IN THE HYPOTHALAMUS, SEPTUM AND PREOPTIC AREA OF THE RAT: CHARACTERISTICS OF SPONTANEOUS ACTIVITY AND THE EFFECT OF OESTROGEN

D. W. LINCOLN

SUMMARY

The frequency characteristics of the neuronal activity in the hypothalamus, septum and preoptic area of the forebrain were recorded with stereotaxically orientated steel microelectrodes in adult female rats under light urethane anaesthesia.

An exponential type of relationship was observed between the mean discharge rate of units and the frequency with which they were encountered in all areas. Thus, 40–60 % of units had firing rates of less than 1 spike/sec. and only 1·0–15 % had rates exceeding 6/sec. However, units with a mean discharge rate of 2–4/sec. contributed most to the total spike activity. The form of the interspike interval distributions was found to vary with mean firing rate, and the variability of the interspike interval decreased as the firing rate of the unit increased.

The levels of 'spontaneous' activity in the anterior hypothalamic, preoptic and septal areas of rats with light-induced persistent oestrus were lower than those observed after ovariectomy. The administration of 10 μg. oestradiol benzoate/day to the ovariectomized animals depressed the levels of activity towards those observed in the persistently oestrous animals. Reciprocal effects were observed in the lateral hypothalamic area, i.e. decreased activity in the ovariectomized rats.

The results are discussed in relation to unit recording procedures and the feedback effects of oestrogen.

INTRODUCTION

The hypothalamic, preoptic and septal areas of the forebrain are involved in many neuro-endocrine and homeostatic mechanisms. Each function can be presumed to be mediated, directly or indirectly, by changes in the pattern of action potential activity. In these areas, and in most other parts of the brain, neurones display a continuous level of action potential activity ('spontaneous' activity), and from this activity functional changes have to be deciphered. The characteristics of the activity in these forebrain areas are particularly important, since many changes may be of long duration and may not be observed in acute experiments, e.g. the feedback effects of ovarian hormones. Moreover, most unit recording techniques are dependent on this activity for the detection of units, and therefore any sample of units will be governed by the frequency characteristics of the 'spontaneous' activity. To date there have been few quantitative studies on the frequency characteristics of cell firing in these regions of the brain.

Reference has been made in many cell recording studies to the range of firing rates. In the posterior hypothalamus of cats under pentobarbitone anaesthesia, rates of 0·01–3·19/sec. were observed by Dafny, Bental & Feldman (1965), while Nakayama, Eisenman & Hardy (1961) reported a range for the anterior hypothalamus of this species, under urethane, of 3·7–27/sec. Cross & Silver (1963) and Barraclough & Cross (1963), in studies of hypothalamic neurones in rabbits and rats respectively, under urethane, recognized a wider range of firing rates, though most of the units that were studied had mean rates of 1–10/sec. Cross & Green (1959), in their original work on hypothalamic unit activity in the rabbit, found that a high proportion of units fired at slow rates, and this phenomenon has been confirmed in a number of more recent studies (for references, see Cross & Silver, 1966).

The first aim of this paper is to describe the frequency characteristics of the 'spontaneous' action potential activity displayed by single neurones and neurone populations in the septal, preoptic and hypothalamic areas of the rat forebrain. The second aim is to examine the effect of exogenous and endogenous oestrogen on the characteristics of this activity. There is considerable evidence that oestrogen influences activity in these areas. Oestrogen implants in the arcuate nucleus of the rat produce atrophy of the reproductive tract (Lisk, 1960), while similar implants in the medial preoptic and anterior hypothalamic areas may induce oestrous behaviour in spayed animals (Lisk, 1962). Studies involving stimulation of the hypothalamus and other limbic forebrain areas have shown that oestrogen influences the threshold for EEG arousal and for the induction of 'paradoxical' sleep (Kawakami & Sawyer, 1959, 1962). Finally, observations by Cross & Findlay (see Cross, 1964) have indicated a changed responsiveness of lateral hypothalamic neurones after systemic oestrogen treatment.

MATERIALS AND METHODS

Animals and pretreatment. The experiments were performed on adult female rats, of a Wistar strain with an oestrous cycle of 4 days, and weighing 210–230 g. They were maintained on rat pellets and water *ad libitum*. The environmental temperature was kept at 20° and the photoperiod controlled by artificial illumination (14 hr. light–10 hr. darkness).

Batches of 20 animals were selected at intervals of 14 days and vaginal smears taken for 5 consecutive days. The cyclic rats were transferred to continuous illumination and daily vaginal smearing recommenced after 10 days. A persistent 'light' oestrus was shown by most of these animals. The time taken to establish persistent oestrus was considerably shortened by not taking vaginal smears during the first 10 days of exposure to continuous illumination.

Animals which had shown at least 10 consecutive days of vaginal oestrus, within 35 days of exposure to continuous illumination, were divided into three groups and treated in the following way: (1) *Persistent-oestrus group*: these rats received no further treatment and unit recordings were made forthwith. (2) *Spayed group*: these animals were bilaterally ovariectomized and unit recordings were made 3 days later. (3) *Spayed oestrogen-treated group*: these animals were bilaterally ovariectomized and received 5 μg. oestradiol benzoate ('Oestroform', B.D.H.) i.m., twice daily for 3 days. Unit recordings were made 3 days after ovariectomy.

Ovariectomy was performed under ether anaesthesia and the first oestradiol injection was given immediately after this operation.

Unit recordings were made from 15 animals in each group.

Recording equipment. Microelectrodes were prepared from stainless-steel insect pins, electro-etched and polished by a technique similar to that described by Cross & Silver (1963). The polishing solution was modified by the addition of 20% (v/v) of conc. hydrochloric acid. The electrodes were insulated with a lacquer (E-33-N, Insl-X Company Inc., Ossining, New York) and stored in an oven at 40°. The final tip diameters were 1 μ or less.

For recording, the microelectrodes were mounted in a micromanipulator and the apparatus enclosed in an earthed metal cage. The electrode was capacity-coupled to a low level pre-amplifier (Tectronix, type 123, input impedance 10 MΩ, passband 3–25,000 cyc./sec.), and this was connected to the input of an amplifier on one channel of a dual-beam oscilloscope (Telequipment, amplifier type 33C). The amplified signals from the Y-plates of the oscilloscope were capacity-coupled via a co-axial distribution box to an audio-amplifier and loudspeaker, a monitoring oscilloscope, a dekatron counter and timing unit (Labgear Ltd., types D 4131 and D 4102) and to the external trigger of a square-wave pulse generator (Nagard, type 5002). Triggered 2 msec. square waves were fed from the pulse generator to the driver amplifier of one channel of a polygraph (Devices, type M-4) to produce a permanent record of action potential activity.

An electrocorticogram was recorded during the latter half of the experiments by means of a steel needle inserted into the frontal cortex and connected to an a.c. pre-amplifier (Devices, type A.C. 7) of the polygraph.

Operative procedures and recording technique. The animals were lightly anaesthetized with urethane, injected i.p. as a 25% (w/v) aqueous solution at a dose level of 1·2 g./kg. The head of the animal was secured in a stereotaxic instrument, and the scalp incised under local anaesthesia. Four small holes were drilled in the skull with a flat-ended burr, at points determined in relation to the mid-line and bregma suture. The small cap of bone left overlying the dura was removed and the dura carefully incised immediately before the microelectrode was inserted. The exposed skull was then covered with a warm agar solution.

A heating coil, positioned outside the earthed cage, kept the animals warm during these operations. A constant level of illumination, at an intensity approximately equal to that under which the animals were previously housed, was applied to the eyes by means of a glass-fibre optical system.

Two microelectrode tracks were made in each animal, one on either side of the mid-line. One track was orientated to pass through the lateral septal and anterior hypothalamic-preoptic areas and the other to pass through the thalamus and lateral hypothalamic area. The order in which the tracks were made was randomized. The stereotaxic atlas of de Groot (1959) was used to orientate the electrodes.

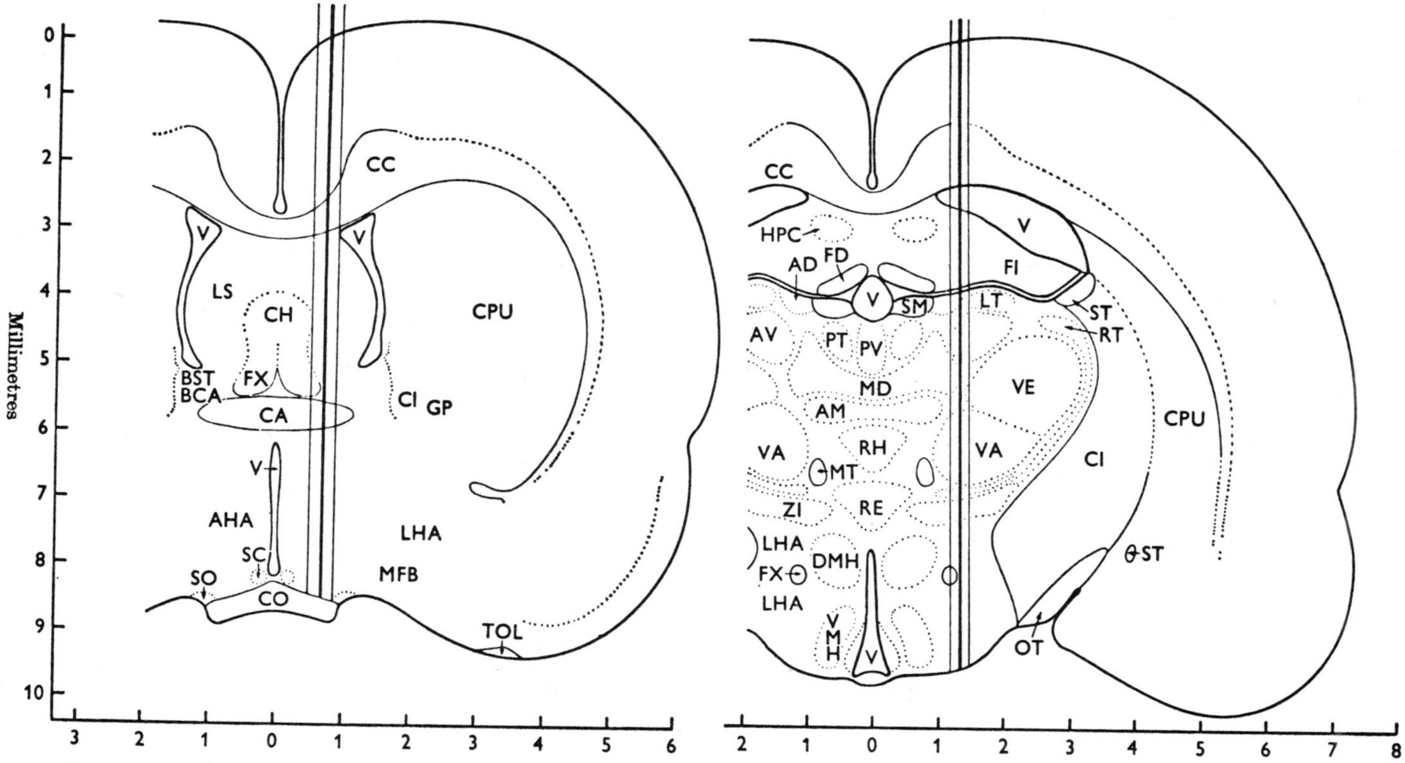

Fig. 1. Diagrams showing the paths of the two electrode tracks. The lateral standard deviations are shown by the outer lines. The lettering corresponds to that used in the Rat Brain Atlas of de Groot (1959), e.g. AHA, area anterior hypothalami; LS, nucleus lateralis septi; LHA, area lateralis hypothalami.

Assessment of firing rate. The 'spontaneous' firing rate of each unit was assessed by counting the number of action potentials during five separated 10 sec. intervals or, for slower units (< 1·5 spikes/sec.), during two separated 60 sec. intervals. Several minutes were allowed to elapse after the detection of a unit to check the stability of the recording. During these periods the EEG, recorded from the frontal cortex, normally consisted of large-amplitude slow waves.

Histological procedures. The techniques used to establish the precise ordinates of each track, and subsequently the position of individual units, were the same as those described by Barraclough & Cross (1963).

RESULTS

Location of recorded neurones

The mean ordinates of the two microelectrode tracks, together with their lateral deviations, are shown in Fig. 1. The deviations in the sagittal plane were slightly greater in the lower part of each track; thus both medial preoptic and anterior hypothalamic units were sampled. The units were grouped according to their location and Table 1 gives the number of units studied in each area.

Table 1. *Distribution of neurones studied*

Location	Number of neurones	
Medial preoptic area	136	322
Anterior hypothalamic area	186	
Lateral septal area		308
Lateral hypothalamic area		307
Thalamic area		
N. anteroventralis	122	335
N. ventralis thalami pars anterior	122	
Others	91	

Specifications of recorded activity

As the microelectrodes were moved down through areas of grey matter, numerous units were observed exhibiting 'spontaneous' action potential activity. The signal-to-noise ratios (S:N) of the extracellular waveforms were usually greater than 10:1, and frequently the signal strength was of several mv. The waveforms were similar to those observed in other studies (Cross & Green, 1959; Barraclough & Cross, 1963). Slight variations were evident from one area to another, e.g. units in the preoptic and anterior hypothalamic areas displayed waveforms with consistently larger positive to negative ratios than units elsewhere.

Entirely positive spikes, with a characteristically fast rise-time, were frequently observed in the optic chiasma and occasionally in other areas. These recordings were attributed to fibre activity since a transition was observed from the recognized fibre activity which consists of small negative spikes of short duration. All fibre activity and all recordings made when there was evidence that the microelectrode was influencing the behaviour of a unit were excluded from this investigation.

Spatial distribution of neurones

The number of units that were observed per mm. of microelectrode track varied from one area to another. In the thalamic nuclei, examined on the more caudal and lateral track, there were usually 6–8 units/mm. Consequently, the mean distance between recording positions was 110–160 μ but, by carefully advancing the microelectrode, it was possible to maintain stable recordings for 50–80 μ, and sometimes

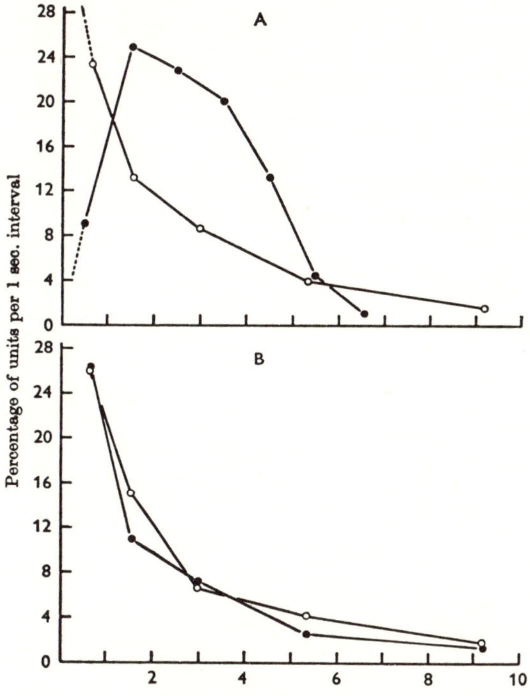

Fig. 2. Relation of the mean firing rate of units to the frequency of their occurrence (unit rate distributions). The figures given after each area refer to the number of units sampled. Note the exponential character of the curves for units in the hypothalamic, preoptic and septal areas. A: ○—○, Anterior hypothalamic/preoptic area (n = 322); ●—●, thalamic area (n = 226). B: ○—○, Lateral septal area (n = 308); ●—●, lateral hypothalamic area (n = 307).

further, before the unit was killed or passed out of recording range. Surprisingly, the monitoring of more than one unit at a time was a very infrequent occurrence. Multiple-unit recordings were easily recognized since the recordings invariably differed in their S:N ratios, waveforms and action potential rates. The number of units observed in the anterior and lateral hypothalamic areas was 2–5/mm., and slightly more in the lateral septal area.

Analysis of 'spontaneous' firing rates

For the purpose of this analysis the results of the three hormonal treatments were combined.

In the hypothalamic, preoptic, and septal areas 40–60 % of the units that were encountered fired at less than 1 spike/sec., though the range of firing rates was considerable (0 to > 50/sec.). The relationship between the number of units and their mean firing rates was of an exponential type (Fig. 2). Units firing at less than 0·3

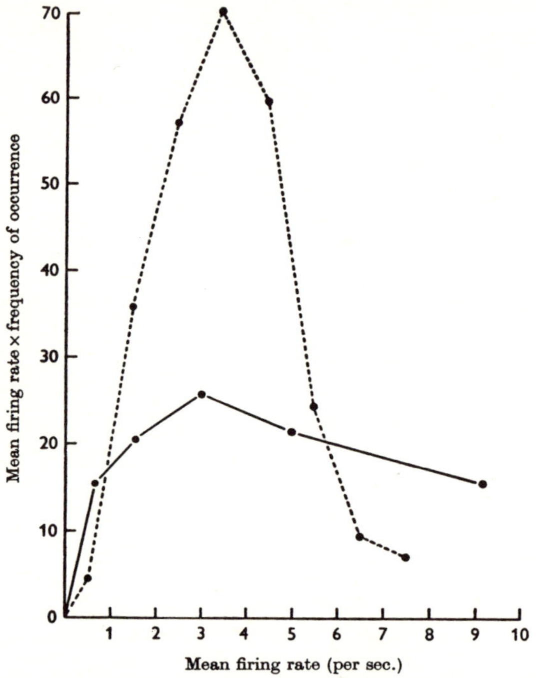

Fig. 3. Diagram showing the contribution made by units at various 'spontaneous' firing rates to the total spike activity of the anterior hypothalamic-preoptic area (●—●) and the thalamus (n. anteroventralis thalami and n. ventralis thalami pars anterior) (●---●). The areas beneath the curves for the two regions are comparable.

spikes/sec. are not included in Fig. 2 because there is a strongly subjective element in taking a comparable sample of these slow-firing units, and their number is likely to have been underestimated. However, more units were observed with firing rates of less than 0·3/sec. than with rates between 0·3–1·0/sec. By contrast, there were almost no quiescent thalamic units.

The 'exponential' distributions were similar in form, though there were minor differences. For example, in the lateral hypothalamic area there were more units with mean firing rates of less than 1 spike/sec. and fewer with rates between 1 and 2·5/sec.

than in the anterior hypothalamic area. However, these small differences have very marked effects on the total spike activity displayed by these areas.

When the mean firing rate was related to the frequency with which these mean rates were encountered, a relationship was obtained between mean spike rate and the total spike activity of the neurone population (Fig. 3). First, Fig. 3 illustrates that units in the anterior hypothalamic and thalamic areas firing at rates of 2–4/sec. contribute most to the total activity. Similar peaks were observed in the lateral hypothalamic and septal areas. Secondly, the contribution of the large number of slow firing units to the total activity is very small. Thus, 41·5 % of all anterior hypothalamic units fired at rates of less than 1 spike/sec. but only contributed 4·2 % to

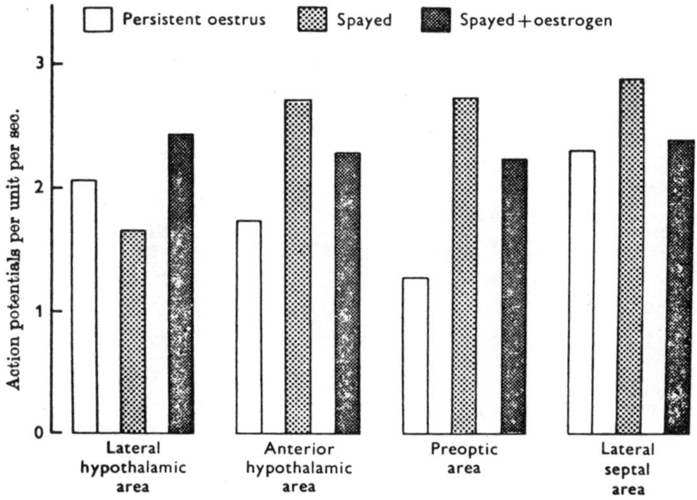

Fig. 4. Effect of oestrogen on the levels of spike activity in various forebrain areas. The histograms represent the mean spike rates of units firing between 0 and 15 spikes/sec. Note the reciprocal effects in the lateral hypothalamic area.

the total action potential activity. The corresponding figures for the lateral hypothalamic area were 55·0 % and 9·1 %, for the lateral septal area 42·8 % and 6·9 % and for the thalamic area 9·3 % and 1·7 %. Thirdly, there was considerably more action potential activity in the thalamic area than in any of the other areas examined; this difference is likely to have been underestimated since many slow-firing units, so common in the hypothalamic and septal area, may have been overlooked.

Effect of hormonal status on the level of spike activity

The unit rate distributions were similar for each hormonal treatment. However, small differences between these distributions resulted in very considerable differences in the levels of total spike activity (Fig. 4). The spayed group was consistently different from the persistent-oestrus and spayed oestrogen-treated groups. In the preoptic area the spayed groups showed 112 % more activity (number of action potentials/unit/sec.) than the group with persistent-oestrus and 22 % more than the spayed oestrogen-treated group. The corresponding figures for the anterior hypothalamic area were 57 % and 22 % and for the lateral septal area 24 % and 20 %. By contrast, the differences in the lateral hypothalamic area were in the opposite direction.

The differences in total spike activity were mainly the result of differences in the number of units with firing rates of 7–15 spikes/sec. (Table 2).

Table 2. *Relation of firing rate and unit numbers to the total spike activity values of each hormonal treatment: data for the anterior hypothalamic-preoptic area*

Rate interval (spikes/sec.) r	% of units n	Contribution to the total spike activity nr	% of total activity
Persistent-oestrus group			
0–6·8	94·7	185	94
6·8–18·0	1·3	12	6
Spayed group			
0–6·8	77·8	110	33
6·8–18·0	19·7	211	67
Spayed oestrogen-treated group			
0–6·8	88·5	145	64
6·8–18·0	7·2	82	36

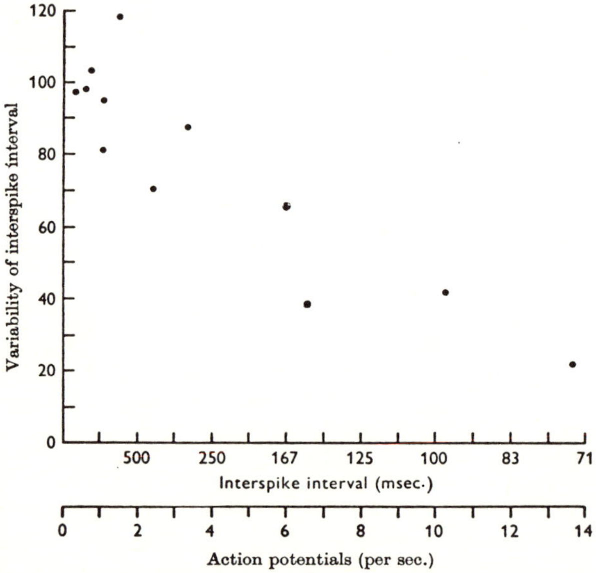

Fig. 5. Relation of mean firing rate to the variability of the interspike interval. The points were determined from the analysis of 100 interspike intervals from each of 12 different anterior hypothalamic units. The variability (ordinate) expresses the standard deviation of the interspike intervals as a percentage of the mean interval.

Analysis of interspike intervals

The mean firing rate of a unit is a measure which may conceal valuable information, e.g. changes in the temporal pattern of spike activity. It is quite possible that changes in the pattern of spike discharge, without change in mean frequency, could result from the action of a circulating hormone or signal the release of a neurohumoral transmitter. An exhaustive survey of interspike interval distributions has not been possible with the technique used in this investigation. However, sample distributions were collected for different mean firing rates and different areas, by recording with

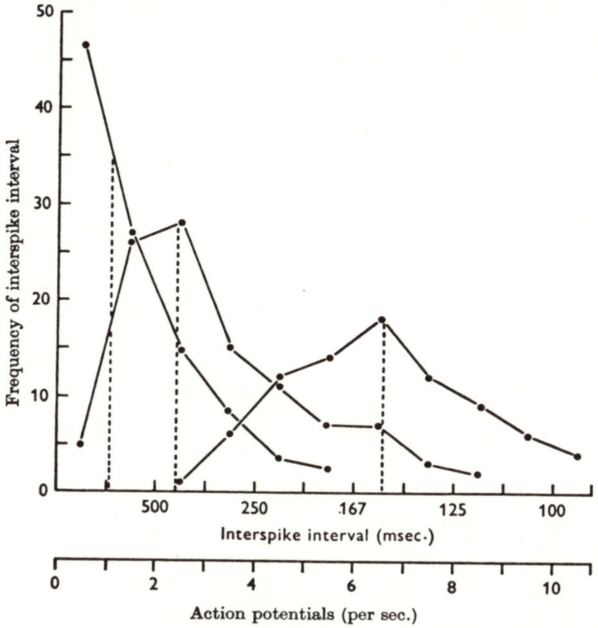

Fig. 6. Interspike interval distributions of three anterior hypothalamic units. Each distribution was calculated from 100 interspike intervals. The mean intervals are shown by the vertical dashed lines.

the polygraph paper run at fast speed (10 cm./sec.). It was not possible to detect any differences between the hypothalamic, preoptic and septal areas, but in all areas the variability of the interspike interval was greatest at slow firing rates (Fig. 5) and the form of the interspike interval distribution varied with firing rate (Fig. 6).

DISCUSSION

The exponential type of relationship between the mean discharge rate of units and the frequency of their occurrence in hypothalamic, preoptic and septal areas is clearly different from that suggested or implied by most unit studies. On the other hand, the characteristics of the interspike interval distributions are in agreement with those reported by Oomura, Kimura, Iki & Kuniyoshi (1964) for the ventromedial and lateral hypothalamic areas of the cat, and are similar to those observed in other parts of the brain (e.g. auditory cortex, Gerstein & Kiang, 1960).

Although the distributions of mean firing rate tend to show an exponential form there cannot be an infinite number of quiescent units, though there are clearly a large number of slow-firing units. Unfortunately, it is not possible to record with equal probability those units which are firing at slow rates ($< 0\cdot5$ spikes/sec.), and the situation becomes more difficult the lower the firing rate. As a consequence, any sample of units from the hypothalamic, preoptic and septal areas will depend in part on the success of monitoring slow-firing units, especially as 40–60 % of units monitored in these areas fired at less than 1 spike/sec. Therefore an experimental treatment which influences the level of 'spontaneous' activity, as occurs with oestrogen feedback, is likely to change the sample of units obtained. Thus, variations in the characteristics of different samples of units may simply reflect that the samples contain different populations of units. The success of monitoring slow-firing units is dependent on the shape and recording properties of the microelectrode and the skill of the operator, both of which are liable to change with time. Unit recording experiments must therefore be carefully designed, and comparisons between experiments should take account of the respective unit samples.

Some encouragement, in view of the difficulties posed by the exponential form of the distribution of mean firing rate (Fig. 2), can be gained from the fact that the large population of slow-firing units is contributing very little to the total spike activity, and thus might be considered of little functional significance under the particular conditions of recording. Alternatively, it could be argued that slow-firing units may be involved in specialized functions, and—in any case—the absence of activity in any unit may be of as much functional significance as the presence of activity.

Certain characteristics of the 'spontaneous' activity described in other papers differ widely from those found in the present study. For example, Nakayama *et al.* (1961) reported firing rates of 3·7–27 spikes/sec. in the anterior hypothalamus of cats under urethane anaesthesia. Such variations could be due to differences in species, recording sites or anaesthesia. However, the dose level of urethane is not critical, at least with rats and rabbits, and supplementary doses of this anaesthetic do not influence the behaviour of hypothalamic neurones (Cross & Silver, 1966).

Attempts to establish the levels of 'spontaneous' activity, fundamental to the investigation of hormonal feedback and homeostatic mechanisms, are thwarted by the exponential form of the unit rate distributions. The levels of 'spontaneous' activity could change considerably without any marked change in the form of these distributions. On the other hand, the mean firing rate per unit is more likely to reflect changes in activity.

The decreases in the total spike activity of the anterior hypothalamic, preoptic and septal areas of the persistent-oestrus and the spayed oestrogen-treated groups, compared with the spayed group, were fairly consistent. Therefore, these changes in activity can be attributed with some certainty to the action of oestrogen.

Everett (1965) postulates that the process of luteinizing hormone (LH) release in the rat involves the transmission of nerve impulses from the septal, preoptic and anterior hypothalamic areas to the basal tuberal region. Furthermore, the threshold of electrical stimulation of the preoptic area for the release of an ovulating quantum of LH was found to be lower in pro-oestrous than late dioestrous rats (Everett, 1964). These differences in threshold may represent changes in the preoptic area, and it is possible that the depression in 'spontaneous' activity that has been observed as the result of oestrogen feedback may be related to the lowered threshold that Everett observed in pro-oestrous rats.

Oestrogen is also known to lower the threshold of electrical stimulation of the anterior hypothalamic-preoptic area necessary for the induction of paradoxical sleep in the rabbit (Kawakami & Sawyer, 1962). However, this threshold is further lowered by a combination of oestrogen and progesterone treatment. In this context, it is interesting to note that the spayed oestrogen-treated rats did not show the same degree of depression in 'spontaneous' activity as the rats with persistent-oestrus, which might indicate that both oestrogen and progesterone are necessary to produce the depression in activity observed in the group with persistent-oestrus.

The reciprocal effects of oestrogen on the levels of activity in the lateral hypothalamic area seem to be in harmony with reports of reciprocal differences between the lateral and ventromedial hypothalamic areas. Stimulation of the lateral hypothalamic area of the rabbit immediately after stimulation of the ventromedial nucleus delays or prevents the ovulation that would be expected from ventromedial stimulation alone (Kurotsu, Kurachi & Ban, 1950; Kurachi & Suchowsky, 1958). Furthermore, Oomura *et al.* (1964) have reported that stimulation of the lateral hypothalamic area of the cat decreased firing rates in the ventromedial hypothalamic nucleus, and vice versa.

I am very grateful to Dr B. A. Cross for providing the experimental facilities, and for helpful advice and criticism. I wish to thank Mr Derek Thurlbourn and Miss Josephine Mallon for technical assistance, and Mrs Valerie Mansfield for care of the animals. The work was supported by the U.S. Public Health Service (Grant no. N.B. 05411) and the Agricultural Research Council.

REFERENCES

Barraclough, C. A. & Cross, B. A. (1963). Unit activity in the hypothalamus of the cyclic female rat: effect of genital stimuli and progesterone. *J. Endocrin.* **26**, 339–359.

Cross, B. A. (1964). The hypothalamus in mammalian homeostasis. In *Symp. Soc. exp. Biol.*, no. 18, pp. 157–193. Ed. G. M. Hughes. Cambridge University Press.

Cross, B. A. & Green, J. D. (1959). Activity of single neurones in the hypothalamus: effect of osmotic and other stimuli. *J. Physiol., Lond.* **148**, 554–569.

Cross, B. A. & Silver, I. A. (1963). Unit activity in the hypothalamus and the sympathetic response to hypoxia and hypercapnia. *Expl Neurol.* **7**, 375–393.

Cross, B. A. & Silver, I. A. (1966). Electrophysiological studies on the hypothalamus. *Br. med. Bull.* **22**, 254–260.

Dafny, N., Bental, E. & Feldman, S. (1965). Effect of sensory stimuli on single unit activity in the posterior hypothalamus. *Electroenceph. clin. Neurophysiol.* **19**, 256–263.

Everett, J. W. (1964). Preoptic stimulative lesions and ovulation in the rat. Thresholds and L.H. release time in late diestrus and proestrus. In *Major problems in neuroendocrinology*, pp. 346–366. Eds. E. Bajusz and G. Jasmin. Basel: S. Karger.

Everett, J. W. (1965). Ovulation in rats from preoptic stimulation through platinum electrodes. Importance of duration and spread of stimulus. *Endocrinology* **76**, 1195–1201.

Gerstein, G. L. & Kiang, N. Y.-S. (1960). An approach to the quantitative analysis of electrophysiological data from single neurons. *Biophys. J.* **1**, 15–28.

Groot, J. de (1959). The rat forebrain in stereotaxic co-ordinates. *Verh. K. ned. Akad. Wet.* (*b*), **52**, no. **4**, 1–40.

Kawakami, M. & Sawyer, C. H. (1959). Induction of behavioral and electroencephalographic changes in the rabbit by hormone administration or brain stimulation. *Endocrinology* **65**, 631–643.

Kawakami, M. & Sawyer, C. H. (1962). Effects of hormones on paradoxical sleep in the rabbit. *Fedn Proc. Fedn Am. Socs exp. Biol.* **21**, 354.

Kurachi, T. & Suchowsky, G. (1958). Zur Frage der Beziehung des Hypothalamus zur Ovulation beim Kaninchen. *Acta endocr., Copenh.* **29**, 27–32.

Kurotsu, T., Kurachi, K. & Ban, T. (1950). Experimental studies on ovulation by electrical stimulation of the hypothalamus of rabbits. *Med. J. Osaka Univ.* **2**, 1–12.

Lisk, R. D. (1960). Estrogen sensitive centres in the hypothalamus of the rat. *J. exp. Zool.* **145**, 197–208.

Lisk, R. D. (1962). Diencephalic placement of estradiol and sexual receptivity in the female rat. *Am. J. Physiol.* **203**, 493–496.

Nakayama, T., Eisenman, J. S. & Hardy, J. D. (1961). Single unit activity of the anterior hypothalamus during local heating. *Science, N.Y.* **134**, 560–561.

Oomura, Y., Kimura, K., Iki, M. & Kuniyoshi, M. (1964). Reciprocal activities of the ventromedial and lateral hypothalamic areas of the cat. *Science, N.Y.* **143**, 484–485.

EFFECTS OF PROGESTERONE ON THE ELECTRICAL ACTIVITY OF THE FOREBRAIN

D. W. LINCOLN

SUMMARY

Unit activity from the hypothalamus and EEG patterns from the cerebral cortex of rats rendered persistently oestrous by exposure to continuous illumination were analysed during the acute infusion of various progesterone preparations.

Infusion of 400 μg. of progesterone in either 0·1 ml. propylene glycol or ethanol caused dramatic changes in the spike activity of many hypothalamic units and precipitated a reproducible change in the EEG pattern. The infusion invariably caused a prolonged synchronization of the EEG, lasting 30–40 min. (i.e. an EEG pattern of large-amplitude slow waves). In addition, a period of high-amplitude high-frequency EEG waves occurred 2–4 min. after the infusion. These EEG changes were usually concurrent with any changes which occurred in the spike activity of hypothalamic units. Similar changes were observed after the infusion of the control materials, i.e. 0·1 ml. of propylene glycol or ethanol. The inclusion of progesterone did not produce changes in brain activity which were substantially different from the control infusions.

Infusion of up to 400 μg. of progesterone in propylene glycol or ethanol did not change the specific response of hypothalamic units to probing the vaginal parts of the cervix. On the other hand, this treatment frequently abolished the non-specific response (i.e. a response which is related to the period of EEG arousal) of these units for a period of 10–30 min. after infusion. The loss of the non-specific response appeared to be associated with an increase in the intensity of stimulus necessary to cause EEG arousal. This change in arousal threshold was caused, at least in part, by the action of the carrier agents.

The infusion of up to 400 μg. of progesterone in a microcrystalline form in saline caused changes in the activity of many units in the anterior hypothalamus and adjacent regions; both excitatory and inhibitory effects were observed. However, every one of these prominent changes in unit activity was associated with a prolonged period of synchronized EEG. There was no evidence to suggest that progesterone was having any selective action on the hypothalamus.

INTRODUCTION

Progesterone has several actions which may involve the central nervous system. These actions may determine, among other things, the process of ovulation and the pattern of reproductive behaviour.

The effects of progesterone on the ovulatory mechanism can be facilitatory as well as inhibitory, the response depending largely on the time of hormone administration. The facilitatory effects were first encountered when Everett (1940, 1943) observed that the daily or periodic treatment of the rat with progesterone restored oestrous cycles and ovulation after a persistent oestrus had developed in old age or under conditions of continuous illumination. Subsequently, Everett (1948) found that ovulation in rats with a 5-day cycle was advanced by 24 hr. when progesterone was given on the third day of dioestrus. Moreover, the response to progesterone was blocked when dibenamine or atropine was given at the same time. Although this fact suggests that a neuroendocrine reflex could be involved in the ovulatory response to progesterone, such a reflex seems fairly complex in neurophysiological terms since the ovulatory release of LH occurs in the mid-afternoon period irrespective of whether progesterone is given at 8.00, 12.00 or 14.00 hr. on the same day (Everett & Sawyer, 1949). These basic observations were recently confirmed by Zeilmaker (1966), though his study indicates that progesterone may advance the critical period by a small amount. The effects of progesterone on rats rendered persistently oestrous by electrolytic lesions of the hypothalamus or by androgen treatment in the neonatal period are not entirely consistent. However, the destruction of the medial preoptic area and the anterior hypothalamus between the anterior commissure and the optic chiasma does appear to abolish the ovulatory response to progesterone (Barraclough, Yrarrazaval & Hatton, 1964). In a similar way, destruction of the ventromedial part of the preoptic area in the domestic fowl prevents progesterone from advancing the time of ovulation (Ralph & Fraps, 1959). The inhibitory or contraceptive action of progesterone on the ovulatory mechanism could also involve the central nervous system, but at present there is no good evidence either for or against this proposition.

The role of progestational steroids in the normal reproductive cycle is a subject of increasing complexity. A pre-ovulatory rise in progesterone and/or 20-hydroxy-pregn-4-en-3-one (20α-OH-progesterone) was detected in the blood of the rat (Eto, Masuda, Shizuki & Hosi, 1962; Feder, Goy & Resko, 1967) and rabbit (Hilliard, Hayward & Sawyer, 1964). These progestational compounds appear to form in the interstitial tissue of the ovary in response to LH (Dorrington & Kilpatrick, 1966). However, there are several situations in which progesterone precipitates ovulation, presumably by causing the release of LH. If this occurred during the normal reproductive cycle, then the feedback of progesterone in the pre-ovulatory period might precipitate further LH release, thereby creating an ovulatory surge in the release of LH. Although such a positive feedback lacks substantial proof, Hilliard, Penardi & Sawyer (1967) established a feedback of a 'supporting' type in which 20α-OH-progesterone maintained the release of LH during the pre-ovulatory period once the ovulatory release of LH had been initiated by coitus. The site at which 20α-OH-progesterone acts to maintain LH levels has not been studied.

There are many other well documented effects of progesterone which involve the central nervous system. In the first place, progesterone and most other steroid hormones have some anaesthetic actions when given in large amounts (Selye, 1941). At more physiological levels, progesterone was shown to modify the thresholds of the reticular activating system (RAS) (Kawakami & Sawyer, 1959*a*, *b*). From this could be predicted a change in the pattern of sleep during any reproductive condition which involved a change in the circulating level of progesterone. Indeed Hartmann (1966) found that the proportion of 'paradoxical' sleep is higher during the luteal phase of the menstrual cycle. The paradoxical phase of sleep is controlled in part at least by the anterior hypothalamus (Kawakami & Sawyer, 1964), the same area which controls ovulation. Studies with progestational compounds labelled with radioactive markers failed, however, to show any selective accumulation of the material in the hypothalamus or any other part of the brain (Seiki, Miyamoto, Yamashita & Kotani, 1969). Although such radiographic studies do not suggest the presence of specific receptors for progesterone in the hypothalamus, the other evidence reviewed indicates that the anterior parts of the hypothalamus are involved at some stage in the mediation of progesterone effects.

In an attempt to throw further light on the means by which progesterone regulates the activity of the brain, the electrical activity of single neurones in the anterior hypothalamus was studied during the acute infusion of progesterone. The experiments were conducted on rats rendered persistently oestrous by continuous illumination.

MATERIALS AND METHODS

Animals and treatments. All experiments were performed on adult female rats of a Wistar strain weighing 210–240 g. These animals were rendered persistently oestrous by exposure to continuous illumination. A persistent oestrus was defined as 10 or more consecutive days of vaginal cornification. No animals were maintained under continuous illumination for more than 35 days at a time.

Recording technique. The equipment for unit recording was essentially the same as that described in earlier communications (Lincoln, 1967, 1969*a*). The electro-encephalogram (EEG) was monitored from bipolar platinum electrodes inserted in an epidural position about 0·5 mm. apart over the frontal cortex. The activity was recorded on a polygraph (Devices M-4) via an EEG preamplifier set to a time constant of 0·1 sec. and filtered to 70 Hz and above.

Surgical procedures. The animals were lightly anaesthetized with a single dose of urethane, injected i.p. as a 25 % aqueous solution at a dose of 1·2 g./kg. The procedure for unit recording was essentially the same as that previously described (Lincoln, 1969*a*). A femoral vein was cannulated to facilitate the administration of the steroid preparations. The catheter was inserted as far as the posterior vena cava.

Steroid preparations. For the initial studies, progesterone was dissolved in either propylene glycol or ethanol (redistilled). The later studies were made with a micro-crystalline suspension of progesterone in normal saline (Luteocyclin M, Ciba). Not more than two infusions of progesterone were given to any animal and at least 2 hr. were allowed between these treatments. The volume of solution administered at each infusion was maintained at 0·1 ml.

Three types of spike waveform were observed in the microelectrode recordings. These waveforms were in complete agreement with those observed and analysed by Bishop, Burke & Davis (1962) and subsequent studies were confined to those recordings which were deemed to represent extracellular spikes from the soma of single cells. These recordings were normally biphasic in waveform and up to 10 mv in amplitude. Sometimes it was possible to continue the recording from one cell for more than 5 hr.

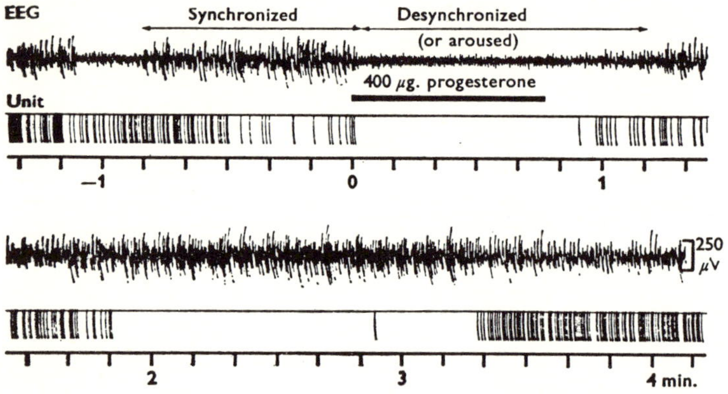

Fig. 1. A continuous polygraph recording showing the effect of an i.v. infusion of 400 μg. progesterone in 0·1 ml. propylene glycol on the activity of a unit in the anterior hypothalamus and the EEG of the frontal cortex. Each deflexion on the unit channel corresponds to one action potential.

The 'spontaneous' rate of spike discharge of units in the anterior hypothalamus ranged from zero to > 50 spikes/sec. The mean firing rates of all the cells examined formed a Poisson distribution with 40% of the recorded cells discharging at less than one spike/sec. One hundred and twenty-four cells were examined for extended periods, i.e. 2 hr. or more, though the total recorded was far greater.

The EEG fluctuated between the three patterns associated with the sleep cycle, and 50% of units in the anterior hypothalamus and adjacent regions displayed gross changes in activity during these fluctuations in EEG pattern, especially during periods in which the EEG showed the correlates of paradoxical sleep. A detailed analysis of the correlations between unit activity in the hypothalamus and the EEG pattern is given elsewhere (Lincoln, 1969*a*). Owing to these spontaneous changes in neural activity, however, it was essential to make prolonged recordings from each unit before giving any infusion.

Effects of progesterone given in propylene glycol or ethanol

A dose of 400 μg. progesterone in 0·1 ml. propylene glycol or ethanol was used initially. The infusion of this material invariably caused a dramatic change in the unitary activity of the hypothalamus and precipitated a reproducible change in the

EEG pattern. A typical effect is shown in Fig. 1. The infusion always caused an immediate desynchronization (arousal) of the EEG, i.e. an EEG pattern of low-amplitude high-frequency waves. This period of desynchronization lasted anywhere from a few sec. to 1–2 min., a duration which was largely determined by the EEG pattern pertaining at the time the infusion was given. The EEG then reverted to the synchronized phase for 30–40 min., i.e. an EEG pattern of large-amplitude slow waves. After this period of changed activity, the EEG returned to the labile state which existed before treatment in which the EEG alternated every few min. between synchronized and desynchronized activity. In addition to the changes already outlined, a period of large-amplitude high-frequency EEG waves usually occurred between 2–4 min. after the infusion. This period of activity is shown in Figs. 1, 3 and 4. The condition is not as obvious as the other EEG changes, but it always occurred at approximately the same time after the infusion and lasted for the same time (1–2 min.).

Changes in the EEG pattern of the frontal cortex are very closely correlated with the patterns of spike discharge of units in the hypothalamus (Lincoln, 1969*a*). Likewise, the changes in EEG pattern after progesterone infusions were usually concurrent with changes in the pattern of cell activity in the hypothalamus. For example, the unit recording shown in Fig. 1 ceased to discharge during the period of the infusion and for a short time after. Activity began to return at about the same time as the EEG reverted to the synchronized form. However, this recording was more interesting than most in that the cell did not cease to discharge completely during periods of EEG arousal which preceded the treatment. The cell also ceased to discharge between 1 min. 50 sec. after infusion; a poriod which coincided with the pattern of large-amplitude high-frequency EEG waves.

Unfortunately, results such as those outlined above were also readily produced by the control infusion of the carrier materials—propylene glycol and ethanol. The inclusion of progesterone did not produce additional changes in brain activity which were of sufficient magnitude or sufficiently reproducible to be ascribed to the action of the hormone. However, the administration of progesterone in propylene glycol or ethanol caused changes in the response of hypothalamic cells to stimulation of the vaginal parts of the cervix. Units in the anterior hypothalamus show two very distinctive forms of response to cervical stimulation: specific and non-specific effects (Lincoln, 1969*b*). Units which show specific responses appear to receive sensory projections from areas localized to the region of the cervix and the response only lasts for the duration of the stimulus. Non-specific effects are related to the period of EEG arousal. These latter effects sometimes last for a prolonged period of time, and apparently identical effects are produced by other forms of stimulation. Fig. 2 shows the complete failure of progesterone to modify the specific response of a unit in the anterior hypothalamic–preoptic area to cervical stimulation. At the same time, the infusion caused all the usual changes in EEG pattern. The period of EEG arousal induced by cervical stimulation was greatly reduced, however, when the test was made 10 min. after the infusion. In some preparations, the stimulus of cervical probing was of insufficient intensity to cause arousal during the period from 10 to 30 min. after infusion. As a result, the non-specific response was abolished during this period, i.e. the response related to the period of EEG arousal. Other

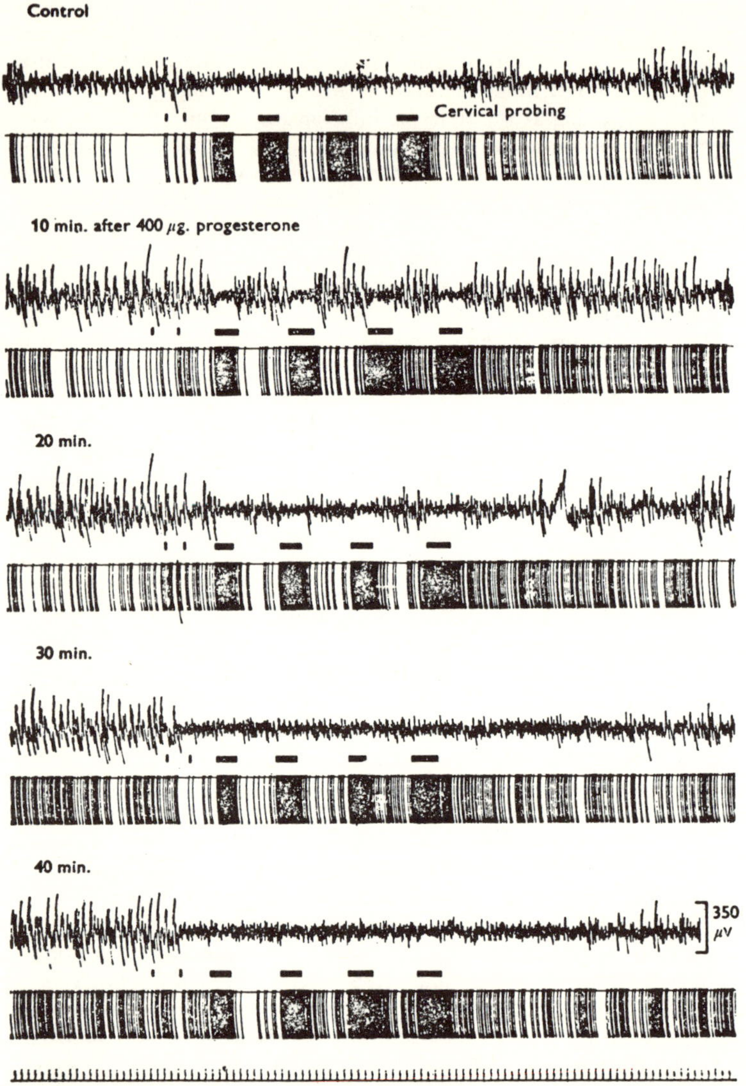

Fig. 2. Polygraph records showing the failure of an i.v. infusion of 400 μg. progesterone in 0·1 ml. propylene glycol to modify the specific response of a unit in the anterior hypothalamic–preoptic area to probing the vaginal regions of the cervix. The stimulus was applied with a tapered glass probe, and the two event marks that precede the periods of cervical probing correspond to lifting the tail and inserting the probe. Note the reduction in the period of EEG arousal when the test was applied 10 min. after the infusion. The time scale is calibrated in 1 sec. intervals.

forms of stimulus such as tail-pinching could still elicit arousal during this period, but tail-pinching is a much stronger stimulus for arousal than cervical probing. Although a tail-pinching usually elicited a response 10–30 min. after infusion, the duration of the response was usually reduced. All this suggests that the infusion raised the threshold of sensory stimulation required to activate the RAS, and it does not mean that the infusion was having any specific effect on the nervous pathway between the reproductive tract and the hypothalamus. Whether specific effects of cervical probing are propagated through to the hypothalamus in the absence of EEG arousal remains to be studied.

Effects of propylene glycol and ethanol

In an attempt to find a carrier for progesterone which did not in itself affect brain activity, various dilutions of propylene glycol and ethanol in 0·9 % NaCl solution were tested. Normal saline had no demonstrable effect when given on its

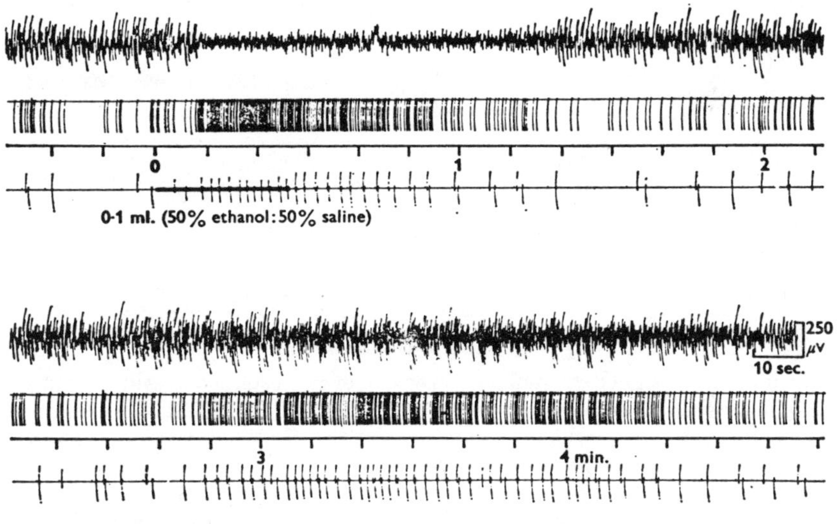

Fig. 3. A continuous polygraph record showing the effect of an i.v. infusion of 0·1 ml. of 50 % ethanol in saline. Both the unit recording and the EEG were taken from the frontal cortex. The third trace in each strip of recording represents a one-in-ten reduction of the activity of the unit. Note the period of large-amplitude high-frequency EEG waves between 1 min. 50 sec. and 4 min. 20 sec. after infusion.

own. The results of two tests with propylene glycol and ethanol are shown in Figs. 3 and 4. In both cases the infusion modified the pattern of brain activity. The effects were quantitated by analysing EEG activity; the proportion of desynchronized EEG pattern was measured at intervals before and after the infusion (Fig. 5). On average, about 40 % of the EEG pattern was in the desynchronized phase before the treatment. All infusions caused an immediate desynchronization of the EEG. However, with propylene glycol and ethanol, this period of desynchronization was followed by 30–40 min. in which the EEG was almost continuously synchronized.

Infusions containing less than 20 % of the solvent had little effect on brain activity, but they would not dissolve an adequate amount of progesterone; the solubility of progesterone falls drastically as the solvent fraction is reduced below 35 %. Such a dilution automatically occurs during an infusion into the bloodstream and it seems very likely that progesterone is precipitated under these circumstances.

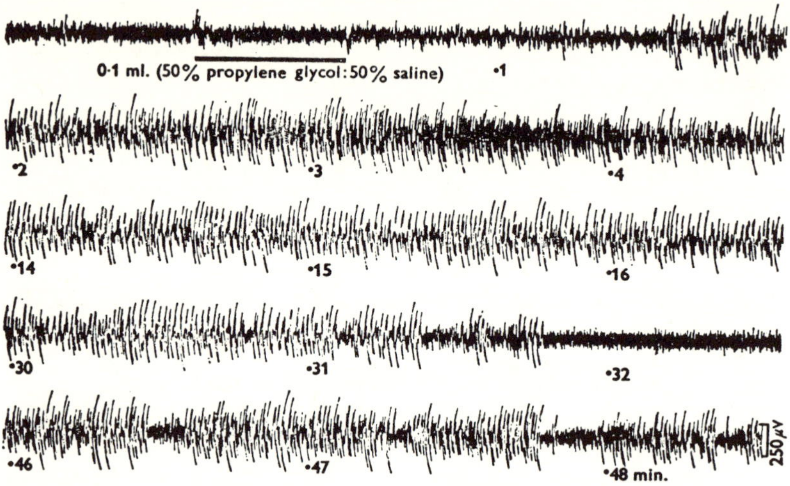

Fig. 4. Polygraph records showing the effect of an i.v. infusion of 0·1 ml. of 50 % propylene glycol in saline on the EEG of the frontal cortex. Note: (i) the EEG reverted to the synchronized form at 1 min. 30 sec., (ii) a period of large-amplitude high-frequency waves occurred between 3 and 4 min., and (iii) the EEG returned to the labile state at 31 min. after infusion.

Effects of progesterone in microcrystalline suspension

The infusion of a microcrystalline suspension of progesterone in saline avoided the effects produced by the organic solvents. At the same time, it is difficult to estimate the amount and rate at which progesterone in this form becomes available to the animal. Doses up to 400 µg. were administered.

From the previous observations, it seemed possible that the EEG pattern might change after the infusion of the microcrystalline preparation of progesterone. The results from ten infusions of 400 µg. were analysed and these showed only a very small increase in the proportion of synchronized EEG. In most cases the infusion caused no measurable change in the EEG pattern. Secondly, the microcrystalline preparation never produced the period of large-amplitude high-frequency waves observed 2–4 min. after the administration of propylene glycol or ethanol.

Many units in the anterior hypothalamus and adjacent regions showed very marked changes in spike activity after the infusion of the microcrystalline preparation of progesterone and both excitatory and inhibitory effects were encountered. The first changes in spike activity were usually seen within 1–2 min. of the infusion and the effects were maximal at 10–20 min. Fig. 6 shows the recording of an anterior hypothalamic unit which increased its rate of spike discharge for 15–20 min. after a progesterone infusion. By contrast, Fig. 7 shows a recording of a unit in the preoptic

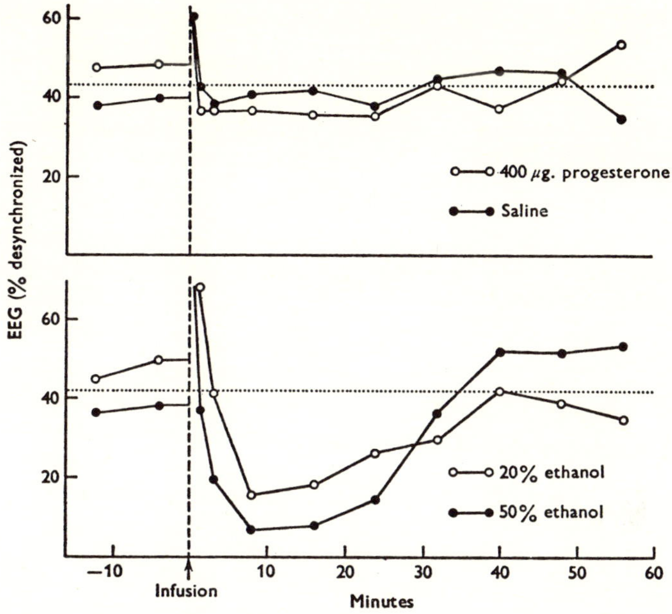

Fig. 5. Effect of progesterone, saline and ethanol on the EEG patterns of the frontal cortex. The data from ten infusions were averaged in the calculation of each graph. Each infusion consisted of 0·1 ml. and the progesterone was given in the microcrystalline form in saline.

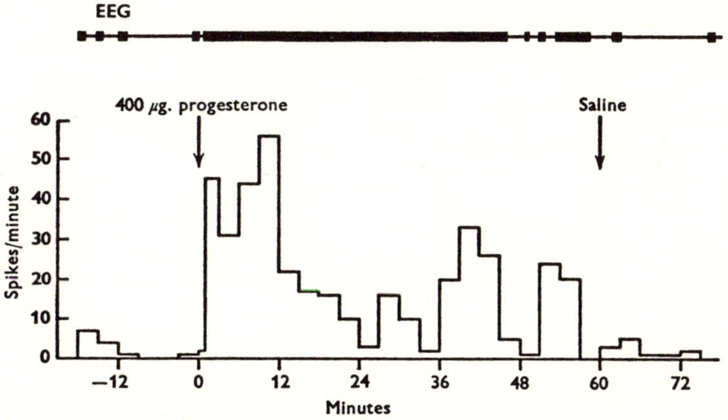

Fig. 6. A diagram illustrating an increase in the spike activity of a unit in the anterior hypothalamus after the i.v. infusion of 400 µg. progesterone (microcrystalline suspension in saline). The periods of synchronized EEG are indicated by the thick lines at the top of the figure.

area in which the rate of spike activity was drastically reduced for about 50 min. after the same treatment. In both cases saline was without effect. However, on all the occasions in which a hypothalamic unit showed a large change in activity after progesterone there was also a prolonged period of synchronized EEG. This indicates that the treatment was causing a widespread change in brain activity. Some recordings were made from single units in the frontal cortex, and, much as expected, some of these units showed changes in spike activity after the infusion of progesterone. It was possible to find examples in which the changes in the spike activity of hypothalamic units and the EEG were not concurrent (Fig. 6). However, such lack of correlation is not outside the range of variation encountered during spontaneous cycles in brain activity.

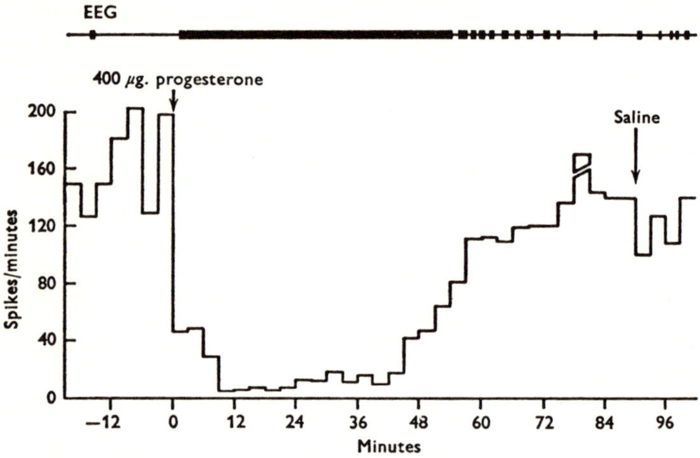

Fig. 7. A diagram illustrating a very marked decrease in the activity of a unit in the preoptic area (or preoptic part of the anterior hypothalamus) after the i.v. infusion of 400 μg. progesterone (microcrystalline suspension in saline).

DISCUSSION

The results stress the need to monitor the EEG during any study of unit activity from the hypothalamus. The conclusions reached in the present series of experiments could have been very different had this not been done. Changes in EEG activity, though closely correlated with the discharge of single hypothalamic units, reflect also on events occurring in many other parts of the central nervous system, particularly in those areas which determine the EEG pattern, e.g. the midbrain.

The effects of propylene glycol and ethanol, whilst interesting in their own right, made the present study very difficult and raised serious doubts about the conclusions which have been reached in other work. Propylene glycol and ethanol appeared to be acting as depressants of central nervous activity. Under urethane, the EEG fluctuates between the synchronized and aroused state, and here the action of the carrier agents was just sufficient to tilt the scales in favour of the synchronized condition. The synchronized state represents a deeper form of anaesthesia and corresponds to Stage I of the sleep cycle. In an unanaesthetized animal these small amounts of propylene glycol and ethanol would probably cause no obvious change in the EEG pattern. The period of large-amplitude high-frequency EEG waves observed between 2 and 4 min. after infusion is difficult to interpret and is almost without any counterpart in the literature. Matsuzaki, Takagi & Tokizane (1964) reported that sodium butyrate and related compounds given i.v. to cats induced a period of paradoxical sleep 3 to 5 min. after the infusion. However, the period of large-amplitude high-frequency waves observed in the present study differed in several ways from the EEG of paradoxical sleep. At present there seems no clear indication as to what this new EEG state represents, but it is very reproducible and does involve changes in the activity of hypothalamic units.

The increase in the EEG arousal threshold 10–30 min. after the administration of propylene glycol or ethanol can cause changes in the response of hypothalamic units to sensory stimulation. This is especially true when the response is of a non-specific type related to the period of EEG arousal, and most hypothalamic responses are of this type. Such a change in arousal threshold could account, at least in part, for the failure of units in the lateral hypothalamus to respond to cervical probing for a period of 30–45 min. after the i.v. infusion of progesterone in propylene glycol (Barraclough & Cross, 1963; Cross & Silver, 1965). Cervical probing is a weak stimulus for EEG arousal and therefore any increase in the EEG arousal threshold means that the stimulus is less likely to create an effect. Ramirez, Komisaruk, Whitmoyer & Sawyer (1967) and Komisaruk, McDonald, Whitmoyer & Sawyer (1967) studied the activity and responsiveness of hypothalamic units after the administration of progesterone in propylene glycol and they also found that this treatment raised the arousal threshold. However, both these studies failed to recognize the possibility that propylene glycol was playing the major part in elevating the arousal threshold.

The use of a microcrystalline suspension of progesterone in saline raises many questions, but at least it avoids the side effects encountered with the usual vehicles. The active concentration of progesterone obtained from an infusion of a microcrystalline suspension is not clear. Presumably, the infusion could create a depot of progesterone which was only slowly rendered available to the animal. In this respect, the infusion could mimic the slow and continuous progesterone production by the ovary. In the present study, however, no changes in hypothalamic activity were observed after these progesterone infusions which did not involve other parts of the brain—as indicated by changes in the cortical EEG. Therefore, the site of action of progesterone could be in the midbrain or brainstem, i.e. in those areas which determine the EEG pattern. These areas send projections into the hypothalamus and information conveyed along these pathways can presumably modulate the pattern of hormone secretion by the pituitary. It was interesting that whenever the infusions of progesterone produced an obvious effect, the response invariably lasted for 30–45 min. However, this time-course probably does not relate directly to the duration of hormone action. The infusion appears to cause an oscillation in brain activity, involving first a long period of EEG synchronization, then desynchronization, then synchronization and so on. The duration of one complete cycle of synchronization and desynchronization lasted 90–120 min. These cycles occurred spontaneously in many preparations, and in other animals they were induced by the infusion of propylene glycol and ethanol and by the i.p. administration of additional urethane. One can only conclude that progesterone can precipitate cyclical changes of the RAS, changes which are propagated rostrally to involve the whole of the hypothalamus.

I wish to express my thanks to Professor B. A. Cross for his help and encouragement and to Mrs A. M. Somerset for her valuable technical assistance. The work was supported by the Lalor Foundation.

REFERENCES

Barraclough, C. A. & Cross, B. A. (1963). Unit activity in the hypothalamus of the cyclic female rat: effect of genital stimuli and progesterone. *J. Endocr.* **26**, 339–359.

Barraclough, C. A., Yrarrazaval, S. & Hatton, R. (1964). A possible hypothalamic site of action of progesterone in the facilitation of ovulation in the rat. *Endocrinology* **75**, 838–845.

Bishop, P. O., Burke, W. & Davis, R. (1962). The identification of single units in central visual pathways. *J. Physiol., Lond.* **162**, 409–431.

Cross, B. A. & Silver, I. A. (1965). Effect of luteal hormone on the behaviour of hypothalamic neurones in pseudopregnant rats. *J. Endocr.* **31**, 251–263.

Dorrington, J. H. & Kilpatrick, R. (1966). Effects of pituitary hormones on progestational hormone production by the rabbit ovary *in vivo* and *in vitro*. *J. Endocr.* **35**, 53–63.

Eto, T., Masuda, H., Shizuki, Y. & Hosi, T. (1962). Progesterone and pregn-4-ene-20-ol-3-one in rat ovarian venous blood at different stages in reproductive cycle. *Jap. J. Anim. Reprod.* **8**, 34–40.

Everett, J. W. (1940). The restoration of cyclic estrus and ovulation in persistent estrous rats by progesterone. *Anat. Rec.* **76**, 21.

Everett, J. W. (1943). Further studies on the relationship of progesterone to ovulation and luteinization in the persistent-estrous rat. *Endocrinology* **32**, 285–292.

Everett, J. W. (1948). Progesterone and estrogen in the experimental control of ovulation time and other features of the estrous cycle in the rat. *Endocrinology* **43**, 389–405.

Everett, J. W. & Sawyer, C. H. (1949). A neural factor in the mechanism by which progesterone advances ovulation in the cyclic rat. *Endocrinology* **45**, 581–595.

Feder, H. H., Goy, R. W. & Resko, J. A. (1967). Progesterone concentrations in the peripheral plasma of cyclic rats. *J. Physiol., Lond.* **191**, 136P.

Hartmann, E. L. (1966). Dreaming sleep (the D-state) and the menstrual cycle. *J. nerv. ment. Dis.* **143**, 406–416.

Hilliard, J., Hayward, J. N. & Sawyer, C. H. (1964). Post-coital patterns of secretion of pituitary gonadotropin and ovarian progestin in the rabbit. *Endocrinology* **75**, 957–963.

Hilliard, J., Penardi, R. & Sawyer, C. H. (1967). A functional role for 20α-hydroxypregn-4-en-3-one in the rabbit. *Endocrinology* **80**, 901–909.

Kawakami, M. & Sawyer, C. H. (1959*a*). Neuroendocrine correlates of change in brain activity thresholds by sex steroids and pituitary hormones. *Endocrinology* **65**, 652–668.

Kawakami, M. & Sawyer, C. H. (1959*b*). Induction of behavioural and electroencephalographic changes in the rabbit by hormonal administration or brain stimulation. *Endocrinology* **65**, 631–643.

Kawakami, M. & Sawyer, C. H. (1964). Conditioned induction of paradoxical sleep in the rabbit. *Expl Neurol.* **9**, 470–482.

Komisaruk, B. R., McDonald, P. G., Whitmoyer, D. I. & Sawyer, C. H. (1967). Effects of progesterone and sensory stimulation on EEG and neuronal activity in the rat. *Expl Neurol.* **19**, 494–507.

Lincoln, D. W. (1967). Unit activity in the hypothalamus, septum and preoptic area of the rat: characteristics of spontaneous activity and the effect of oestrogen. *J. Endocr.* **37**, 177–189.

Lincoln, D. W. (1969*a*). Correlation of unit activity in the hypothalamus with EEG patterns associated with the sleep cycle. *Expl Neurol.* **24**, 1–18.

Lincoln, D. W. (1969*b*). Response of hypothalamic units to stimulation of the vaginal cervix: specific versus non-specific effects. *J. Endocr.* **43**, 683–684.

Matsuzaki, M., Takagi, H. & Tokizane, T. (1964). Paradoxical phase of sleep: its artificial induction in the cat by sodium butyrate. *Science, N.Y.* **146**, 1328–1329.

Ralph, C. H. & Fraps, R. M. (1959). Effect of hypothalamic lesions on progesterone-induced ovulation in the hen. *Endocrinology* **65**, 819–824.

Ramirez, V. D., Komisaruk, B. R., Whitmoyer, D. I. & Sawyer, C. H. (1967). Effects of hormones and vaginal stimulation on the EEG and hypothalamic units in rats. *Am. J. Physiol.* **212**, 1376–1384.

Seiki, K., Miyamoto, M., Yamashita, A. & Kotani, M. (1969). Further studies on the intake of labelled progesterone by the hypothalamus and pituitary of rats. *J. Endocr.* **43**, 129–130.

Selye, H. (1941). Anaesthetic effect of steroid hormones. *Proc. Soc. exp. Biol. Med.* **46**, 116–121.

Zeilmaker, G. H. (1966). The biphasic effect of progesterone on ovulation in the rat. *Acta endocr., Copenh.*

EFFECT OF OESTROGEN ON THE RESPONSIVENESS OF NEURONES IN THE HYPOTHALAMUS, SEPTUM AND PREOPTIC AREA OF RATS WITH LIGHT-INDUCED PERSISTENT OESTRUS

D. W. LINCOLN AND B. A. CROSS

SUMMARY

The responses of septal, preoptic and hypothalamic neurones to pain, cold, changes in ocular illumination and probing of the cervix were recorded in adult female rats under light urethane anaesthesia. Responses in rats with light-induced persistent oestrus were compared with those obtained after ovariectomy, and after ovariectomy with oestrogen treatment.

The majority of units in the lateral hypothalamic area were excited by pain, cold and cervical stimuli, whereas in the lateral septal area most were inhibited. The numbers of units in the anterior hypothalamic and preoptic areas that displayed excitation to these stimuli were approximately equal to those showing inhibition.

The time-course of the responses to pain, cold and cervical stimuli of most hypothalamic and septal units closely corresponded to that of the associated EEG activation (frontal cortex), suggesting that they were non-specific arousal effects. Other responses, usually of brief duration, were not correlated with EEG changes.

Endogenous and exogenous oestrogen increased the percentage of units in the lateral and anterior hypothalamic areas that were inhibited by the pain, cold and cervical stimuli, and decreased the number in the lateral septal area. Oestrogen enhanced the responsiveness of preoptic units to the cervical stimulus, but depressed their responsiveness to pain and cold.

Hypothalamic units inhibited by the pain stimulus had mean 'spontaneous' firing rates of 4–5 spikes/sec. and those which were excited had rates of 1–2/sec.

Light-sensitive units were found mainly in the lateral septal and anterior hypothalamic areas. The usual form of the response was a brief 'on–off' or 'off–on' discharge.

The results are discussed in relation to the central nervous control of ovulation.

INTRODUCTION

Barraclough & Cross (1963), in a study of unit activity in the lateral hypothalamic area in relation to the oestrous cycle in the rat, found that the percentage of units inhibited by pain, cold and cervical stimuli was higher in oestrous than dioestrous animals. Similar differences have since been produced by the administration of oestrogen to dioestrous rats (B. A. Cross and A. L. R. Findlay, see Cross, 1964). These results leave the question as to the site of action of oestrogens in the central nervous system unanswered. Although oestrogen implantation experiments show that the hormone can act directly on the hypothalamus of the cat (Harris, Michael & Scott, 1958) and the rat (Lisk, 1960, 1962), the observations of Kawakami & Sawyer (1959), on the effects of oestrogen on neural thresholds for EEG arousal and the EEG 'after-reaction' response in the rabbit, imply a more diffuse effect of oestrogen in the brain stem.

The implantation studies of Lisk (1960, 1962) and the autoradiographic work of Michael (1965) indicate that the anterior hypothalamic-preoptic area is one of the main sites of oestrogen action. According to Everett (1964) this region is an important component of the neural mechanism controlling the ovulatory release of luteinizing hormone. This paper describes the effects of various stimuli on single neurones in the hypothalamus, septum and preoptic area, and the influence of endogenous and exogenous oestrogen on these responses. The rats, made persistently oestrous by continuous illumination, were the same as those used for the preceding paper (Lincoln, 1967) on the quantitative characteristics of 'spontaneous' unit activity.

MATERIALS AND METHODS

Details of the animals, electrical recording and histological procedures are given in the preceding paper (Lincoln, 1967).

Summary of hormonal treatments. Three groups of 15 rats made persistently oestrous by continuous illumination were treated as follows. (1) *Persistent-oestrus group:* these rats received no further treatment and unit recordings were made forthwith. (2) *Spayed group:* these animals were bilaterally ovariectomized and unit recordings were made 3 days later. (3) *Spayed oestrogen-treated group:* these animals were bilaterally ovariectomized and received 5 μg. oestradiol benzoate (Oestroform, B.D.H.) i.m., twice daily for 3 days. Unit recordings were made 3 days after ovariectomy.

Test stimuli. The three main stimuli of pain, cold and cervical probing were the same as those used by Barraclough & Cross (1963). A manual pinch of the tail was the pain stimulus and ethyl chloride sprayed on the tail provided the cold stimulus. For the cervical stimulus a tapered glass probe was inserted into the vagina and pressed lightly against the cervix. The photic stimulus consisted of an abrupt decrease in intensity of ocular illumination for about 5 sec. The experiments were performed in a semi-darkened room and the eyes of the animal were separately illuminated by two remote sources of light at an intensity similar to that at which they were previously housed. Two glass-fibre light guides (Sunbury Glass Works, Teddington, Middlesex) were used to conduct the light to the eyes.

Each stimulus was applied at least twice and care taken to allow the complete recovery from one stimulus before the application of another stimulus.

Classification of the response. A unit response was classed as excitatory when there was a reproducible increase in the firing rate as the result of a stimulus, inhibitory when the rate was decreased, or as unresponsive if neither change occurred. However, with slow-firing units it was often difficult to distinguish a lack of response from inhibition (see first unit in Fig. 1). The percentages of these equivocal responses were very uniform from one treatment to another, but ranged from 14 % in the septal area to 24 % in the preoptic area. For the purposes of the analyses these units were classed as unresponsive.

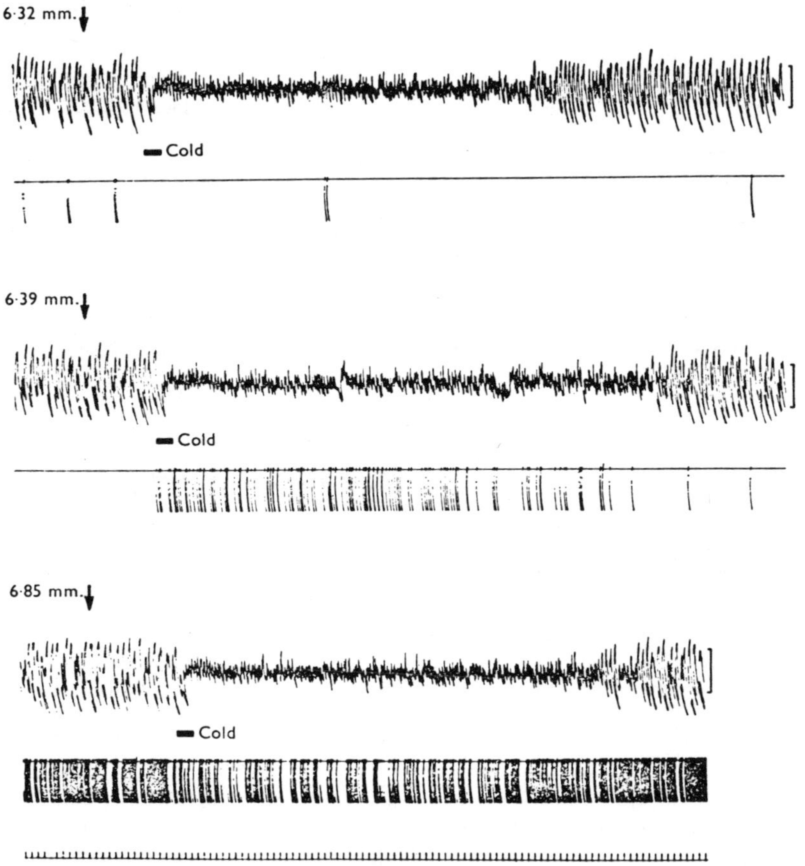

Fig. 1. Polygraph records showing the variations in action potential rate and response of three anterior hypothalamic units recorded on the same electrode track. An EEG of the frontal cortex is shown above each recording. The depth of each unit from the cortical surface is given in millimetres. The lowest trace signals 1 sec. intervals and the EEG calibration is equal to 250 μv.

RESULTS

Behaviour and ovarian status of experimental rats

The light-induced oestrous rats were oestrous behaviourally and displayed no clear diurnal activity pattern. Groups of these animals were test-mated and sperm were found in the vaginal smears of most animals within 24 hr. A few animals became pregnant at the first mating and gave birth to small litters. The majority displayed a pseudopregnancy of variable length and when the animals returned to oestrus they mated and became pregnant.

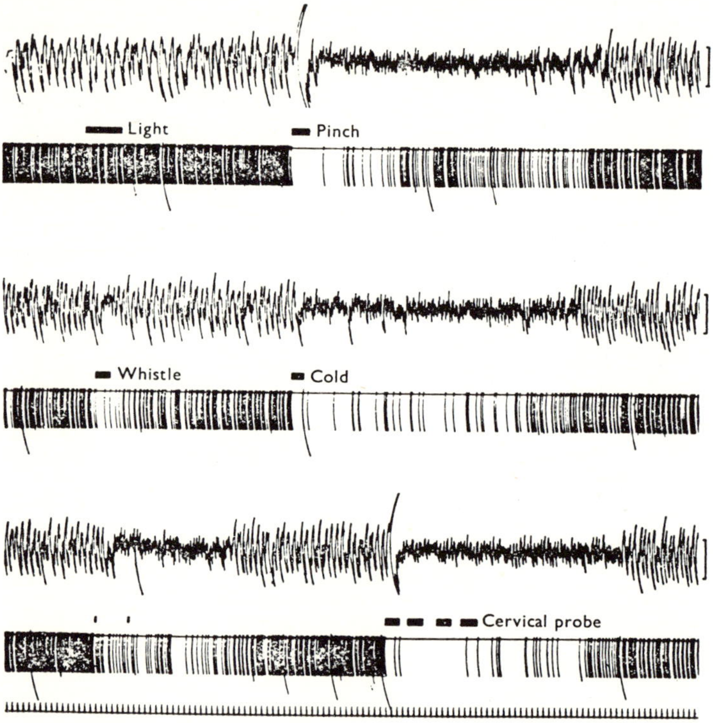

Fig. 2. Polygraph records showing the correlation between the duration of response in an anterior hypothalamic unit and the length of the EEG activation (frontal cortex). The two event marks that precede the cervical probing correspond to lifting the tail and inserting the glass probe into the vagina. The lowest trace signals 1 sec. intervals and the EEG calibration is equal to 250 μv.

The vaginal smears obtained from the rats in the persistent-oestrus and spayed oestrogen-treated groups were of an oestrous type, though some nucleated epithelial cells were often present among the cornified cells in the smears of the persistent-oestrus group. The spayed animals yielded dioestrous smears within 2 days of ovariectomy.

The ovaries of all animals contained many large follicles and no identifiable corpora lutea.

Characteristics of single unit responses

The majority of responsive neurones were affected in the same way by the pain, cold and cervical stimuli (Fig. 2), either by excitation or by inhibition, though the duration of the responses to the different stimuli varied considerably. On the other hand, adjacent units frequently gave contrasting responses to the same stimulus, but of similar duration.

The EEG records from the frontal cortex provided an indication of the state of central nervous excitability. In its most usual form the EEG consisted of high amplitude slow waves (Figs. 1, 2), and upon arousal by the test stimuli this changed to a pattern of low-amplitude high-frequency activity. Therefore the EEG record served as a guide to the threshold intensity of the stimulus necessary for arousal.

For most of the units in the septal and hypothalamic areas the duration of the responses to pain, cold and cervical stimuli, whether excitatory or inhibitory, corresponded fairly closely to that of EEG activation (Figs. 1, 2). This relationship was even more precise in thalamic units (n. anteroventralis thalami and n. ventralis thalami pars anterior), for their responses were invariably coterminous with the period of EEG activation. Most of the EEG-correlated responses were of 5–20 sec. duration, though some lasted much longer. Occasionally during the course of an experiment spontaneous activation of the EEG was recorded, and at such times the firing rates of units usually changed in a manner similar to that elicited by the test stimuli. There appeared to be a relationship between stimulus intensity and the EEG-correlated response of the unit, i.e. a stronger stimulus increased the duration of the unit response without necessarily altering the peak frequency of firing.

In addition to the unit responses that corresponded in duration with that of EEG activation there were some units in the septal, preoptic and hypothalamic areas that gave responses of shorter duration.

Differential responses to pain, cold and cervical stimuli were observed in 8·4 % of all hypothalamic, preoptic and septal units. The commonest type of difference was excitation in response to pain and cold stimuli and inhibition to the cervical stimulus. Most of the units giving this type of response pattern were in the preoptic area and were confined to the persistent-oestrous and spayed oestrogen-treated groups. Other combinations of differential response were rare.

Regional variations in response pattern

Table 1 shows the number of units examined in each area and their responses to pain, cold and cervical stimuli.

The percentages of responsive units in the lateral hypothalamus and septum were similar, though greater than those in the anterior hypothalamic and preoptic areas. A much higher level of responsiveness was observed in the thalamus.

The response patterns of the lateral hypothalamus were characterized by a predominance of excitatory responses whereas those of the septum had an excess of inhibitory responses (Table 1), which were often very pronounced, e.g. there was complete cessation of firing for 5–20 sec. In both the anterior hypothalamic and preoptic areas there were approximately equal numbers of units showing excitatory and inhibitory responses.

In the hypothalamus and septum there were consistent differences in the percentages of units responding to the different stimuli (Table 2). Fewer units responded to the cervical stimulus than to pain or cold, though the percentage showing an inhibitory response to the cervical stimulus was greater than that for the other stimuli.

Table 1. *Distribution of the recorded units and their responses to pain, cold and cervical stimuli*

(The data from the persistent-oestrus, the spayed and the spayed oestrogen-treated groups have been combined.)

	Number of units			Percentage of units		
Stimulus	++	0	−−	++	0	−−
Pain						
LHA	77	57	56	41	30	29
AHA-POA	69	89	66	31	40	29
LS	52	54	78	28	29	43
Cold						
LHA	74	57	43	43	33	24
AHA-POA	60	93	65	27	43	30
LS	56	56	70	31	31	38
Cervical probing						
LHA	64	65	57	34	35	31
AHA-POA	49	103	64	23	48	29
LS	36	70	79	19	38	43

++, Excitatory; 0, unresponsive; −−, inhibitory.
LHA, Lateral hypothalamic area; AHA-POA, anterior hypothalamic area–preoptic area; LS, lateral septum.

Table 2. *Effect of stimulus on response pattern*

(The results from the persistent-oestrus, the spayed and the spayed oestrogen-treated animals for the lateral septal and hypothalamic areas have been combined.)

	Percentage of units responding to stimuli		
	Excitation	Inhibition	Total
Pain	34·8	33·6	68·4
Cold	34·0	32·2	66·2
Cervical probing	26·7	34·6	61·3

Effect of oestrogen on the regional response patterns

The response patterns of the septal, preoptic and hypothalamic areas in the persistent-oestrus and spayed oestrogen-treated groups were very similar, and these 'oestrogen' groups will therefore be dealt with together.

As compared with the spayed group, the lateral and anterior hypothalamic areas of the 'oestrogen' groups showed consistent increases in the percentages of inhibitory responses to pain, cold and cervical stimuli (Fig. 3). There were in addition slight reductions in the percentages of excitatory responses. The presence of oestrogen therefore appeared to be associated with a swing from excitation to inhibition in these areas. In contrast to the hypothalamic units, those in the septum of the 'oestrogen' groups showed a reduction of inhibitory responses as compared with the spayed group.

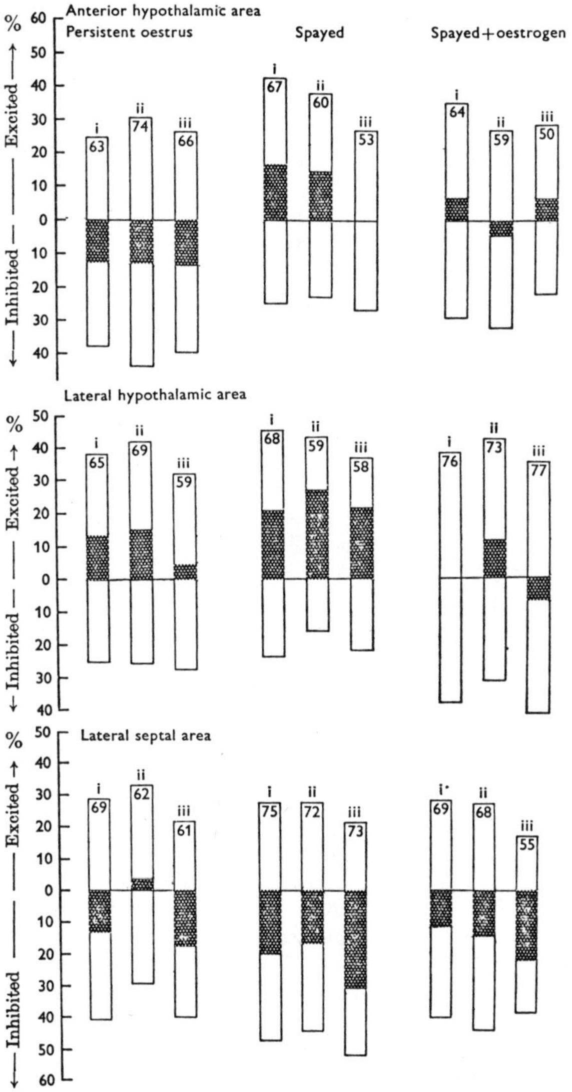

Fig. 3. Histograms showing the effects of the oestrogen treatments on the percentages of units excited and inhibited by the stimuli of (i) pain, (ii) cold, (iii) cervical probing in rats. The total percentages of units that responded to the stimuli are given at the top of each column, and the net response values (excitation–inhibition) are shown by the hatched areas.

The preoptic area was distinguished from the other areas monitored by the fact that oestrogen affected the responses to cervical stimuli in the opposite way to pain and cold responses, i.e. by markedly increasing the percentages of inhibitory responses to cervical stimuli, while reducing the percentages of inhibitory responses to pain and cold (Fig. 4). A further distinctive feature of the preoptic area was that more units responded to cervical stimuli in the 'oestrogen' groups than to pain and cold—the reverse situation to that in the other areas monitored.

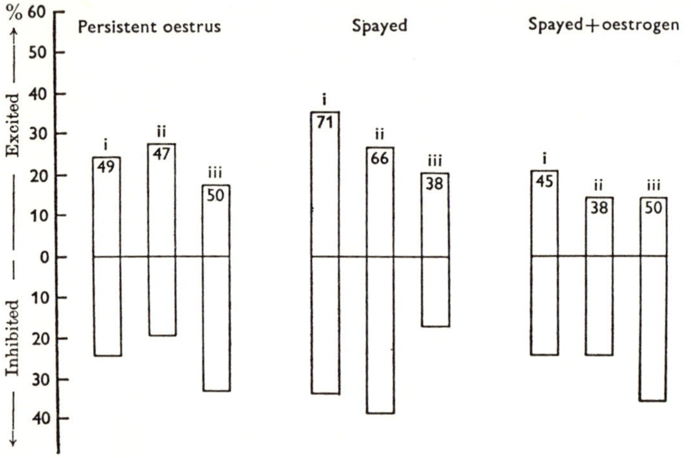

Fig. 4. Histograms showing the effects of oestrogen on the percentages of units in the preoptic area that were excited and inhibited by the stimuli of (i) pain, (ii) cold, (iii) cervical probing.

Responses to photic stimuli

The units that responded to light are considered separately since they were few in number and the responses could not be classified in the same way as those to pain, cold and cervical stimuli.

Photic stimuli rarely altered the EEG, and when activation occurred the effect was not usually repeatable. The responses to light could not therefore be regarded as non-specific arousal effects. The responsive units were widely scattered, but most were found in the lateral septal and anterior hypothalamic areas, namely 3·7 % and 2·7 %, respectively. None were found in the preoptic area.

The responses to the photic stimulus tended to be complex, with both excitatory and inhibitory components. The majority of responses were excitatory and contralateral, though occasionally ipsilateral and bilateral effects were observed (Fig. 5). The responses usually took the form of brief 'on–off' or 'off–on' discharges. Slowly adapting responses were rare, and units which displayed these sustained responses were all slow firing. When the microelectrode penetrated the optic tract the majority of the photic responses from the optic fibres were of the slowly adapting type.

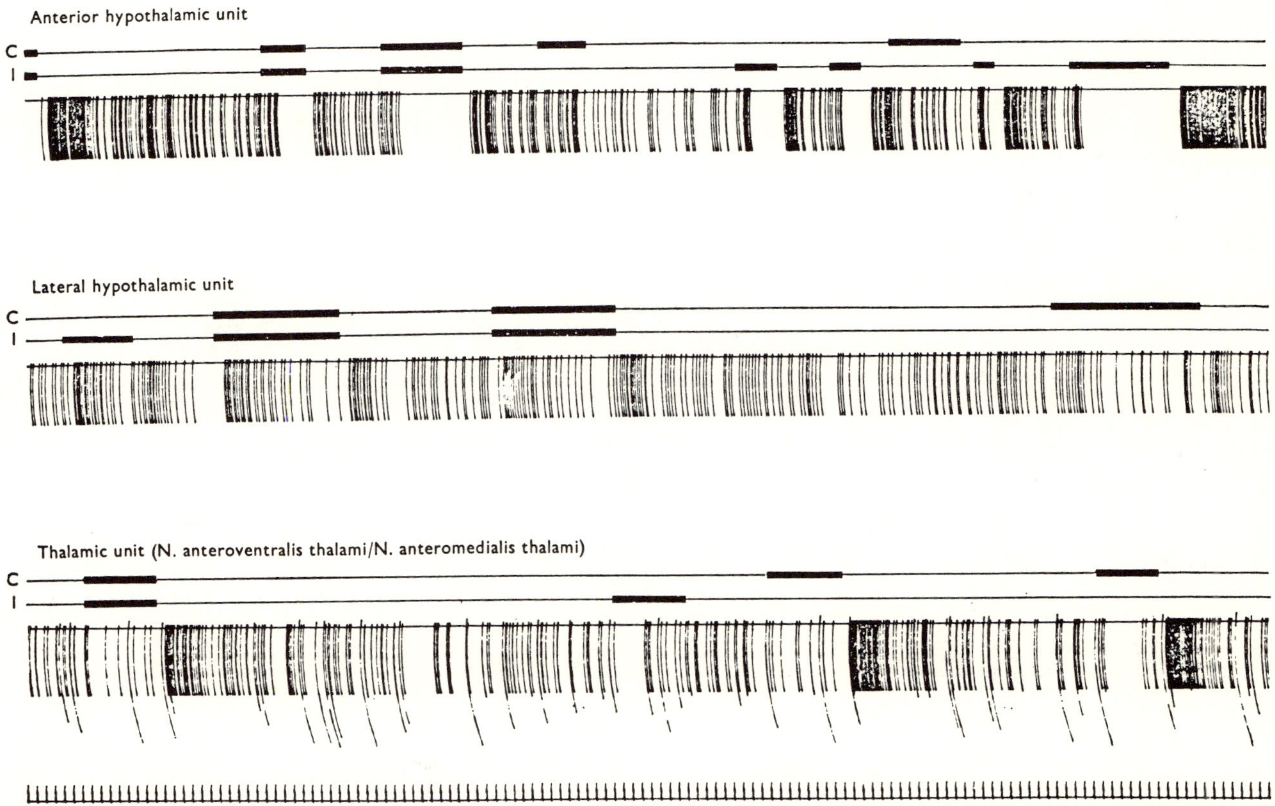

Fig. 5. Polygraph records showing the responses of three units to photic stimuli. The periods of decreased illumination are shown by the thick event marks and the symbols 'C' and 'I' refer to contralateral and ipsilateral stimuli respectively. The anterior hypothalamic unit displays ipsilateral effects, the lateral hypothalamic unit bilateral effects and the thalamic unit contralateral effects. Note the summated deflexions in the recording of the thalamic unit; these are caused by volleys of action potentials and characteristically occur in thalamic units when the EEG of the frontal cortex is showing large-amplitude slow waves.

Relation of 'spontaneous' firing rate to the unit response

In the preceding paper (Lincoln, 1967) a relationship was shown between the rate of 'spontaneous' firing of neurones in the hypothalamus, septum and preoptic area and the frequency of their occurrence. It was of interest therefore to see if any differences could be discerned between the rates of 'spontaneous' firing of those cells that were inhibited by test stimuli compared with those that were excited.

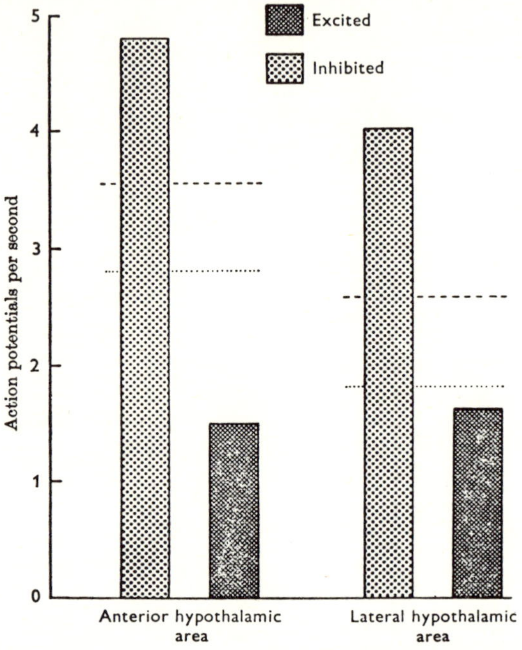

Fig. 6. Histograms showing the relationship between the rate of 'spontaneous' firing and the pain response of anterior and lateral hypothalamic units. The recordings were made when the EEG of the frontal cortex was showing large-amplitude slow waves. The mean firing rates of all units are shown by the dotted lines, and the mean rates excluding units that fired too slowly to determine a clear response are shown by the dashed lines.

Figure 6 summarizes results obtained from 150 units in the anterior and lateral hypothalamic areas that were tested during periods of synchronous EEG recordings and which showed unequivocal responses to pain stimuli. This figure shows that the mean rate of 'spontaneous' firing of the units that were inhibited by the pain stimulus was 4–5 spikes/sec., whereas the mean rate of the units that were excited was 1–2/sec.

DISCUSSION

The observations of Barraclough & Cross (1963) and Cross & Findlay (summarized by Cross, 1964), which indicated that oestrogen increases the percentages of inhibitory responses to pain, cold and cervical stimuli of units in the lateral hypothalamic area of the 'cyclic' rat, are confirmed and extended by this study.

In the present investigations a progressive alteration in the response pattern was observed as the recording electrode monitored units from the lateral hypothalamus, through the anterior hypothalamus and preoptic area to the septum. The lateral hypothalamus contained predominantly units giving excitatory responses, the anterior hypothalamus and preoptic area showed approximately equal numbers of units giving excitatory and inhibitory responses, and in the septum there was a large excess of units giving inhibitory responses. The effects of oestrogen also varied through the same anatomical sequence. In the lateral and anterior hypothalamic areas oestrogen enhanced the inhibitory responsiveness to pain, cold and cervical stimuli, whereas in the septum it decreased the number of inhibitory responses. In the preoptic area oestrogen had an effect intermediate between the anterior hypothalamus and septum, for the responsiveness of units to cervical stimuli was enhanced while that to pain and cold was depressed.

There can be little doubt that the changed responsiveness of units in these forebrain areas is attributable to oestrogen, since the alteration from the pattern in the spayed rats was observed in both animals with persistent oestrus and in the spayed animals treated with oestrogen. The evidence presented in Fig. 6, showing that unit responses may be related to the rate of 'spontaneous' firing, raises the possibility that the oestrogen effects were due to differences in the populations of units in each sample, especially since in the preceding paper (Lincoln, 1967) oestrogen was found to influence the levels of 'spontaneous' activity of units in these forebrain areas. However, this explanation seems unlikely, for though oestrogen changed the resting firing rates of units in the lateral and anterior hypothalamic areas in opposite ways, it nevertheless produced parallel effects on the response patterns of units in these two areas. The sampling problem might be circumvented if it were possible to record acute changes in the same neurone after oestrogen injection, as has been done in the case of progesterone (Barraclough & Cross, 1963; Cross & Silver, 1965). We have so far been unsuccessful in achieving this with oestrogen, and in any case it is possible that the time-course of oestrogen action on nerve cells is too long to make this technically feasible in acute experiments.

Before considering the bearing of our results on the neural mechanisms involved in ovulation it would be helpful to discuss the relationship of the observed patterns of unit activity and response to the brain stem reticular activating system (RAS). The observations reported in the present paper confirm earlier findings of the high degree of sensory convergence on hypothalamic neurones (Cross & Green, 1959; Cross & Silver, 1966)—a known characteristic of reticular units—and further demonstrate the correlation of many unit responses, in terms of duration and intensity, with arousal in the electrocorticogram. These results are fully consistent with the view that the reticular activating system projects rostrally into the hypothalamus (Bernhaut, Gellhorn & Rasmussen, 1953; French, Verzeano & Magoun, 1953). It is questionable how far the unit responses we obtained were directly attributable to such ascending non-specific pathways from the RAS, but the majority of neurones in the lateral hypothalamus were excited by afferent stimuli in a manner consistent with this interpretation. In more rostral regions, however, the proportion of inhibitory responses increased markedly, and such responses would be unlikely to mediate cortical arousal. Nevertheless, even these inhibitory effects were usually of similar duration to the period of EEG activation (Fig. 2) and it is therefore possible that they were caused by inhibitory internuncial pathways from the RAS. If so, we might suppose that during periods of wakefulness unit activity in the hypothalamus would be largely confined to those neurones (in the lateral and, possibly, posterior areas) receiving excitatory connexions from the RAS, whereas in the quiescent period most of the activity would occur in the neurones (in the anterior hypothalamic and preoptic areas) which are inhibited by arousal stimuli.

In the rat, the release of ovulating hormone (LH) occurs between 2 and 4 p.m. (Everett & Sawyer, 1950), which in this nocturnal animal is a period of minimal bodily activity (Richter, 1964). It is possible therefore that spike activity in the neurones firing during this quiescent period, i.e. those inhibited by arousal stimuli, may be a prerequisite for LH release. On this basis the effect of oestrogen in strengthening inhibitory connexions to the anterior hypothalamic and preoptic areas would reduce the probability of ovulation. Such a view is entirely consistent with the fact that rats with light-induced persistent oestrus do not ovulate. The problem would then remain, how to account for ovulation in the normal cyclic animal. Everett (1940, 1943) has established that in rats single injections of progesterone interrupt persistent oestrus induced by continuous illumination. More recently, a preovulatory rise in progesterone secreted from the ovaries has been demonstrated in cyclic rats (Eto, Masuda, Shizuki & Hosi, 1962). It seems likely therefore that progesterone secreted in the preovulatory phase of the oestrous cycle may serve to counteract the inhibitory action of oestrogen. In the earlier experiments of Cross & Silver (1965) on pseudopregnant rats, progesterone was not found to alter the number of inhibitory responses in lateral hypothalamic neurones, but these animals were not under the influence of oestrogen. The action of progesterone on the responses of anterior hypothalamic and preoptic units in oestrogenized rats is now being investigated in this laboratory.

The action of oestrogen in enhancing the response of preoptic units to cervical stimuli while depressing their responsiveness to pain and cold is a feature of some interest. Many of the cervical responses in the preoptic area were of short duration, unlike those elicited by the pain and cold stimuli. These specific effects were mainly observed in the persistent-oestrus and spayed oestrogen-treated groups and may possibly be involved in the pseudopregnancy response.

The comparative scarcity of light sensitive units has been observed in other studies (Cross & Green, 1959; Wendt & Adey, 1960; Barraclough & Cross, 1963) and the responses found in rats with persistent oestrus induced by light did not appear to differ from those of previous reports.

We wish to thank Mr Derek Thurlbourn and Miss Josephine Mallon for technical assistance, and Mrs Valerie Mansfield for care of the animals. The work was supported by the U.S. Public Health Service (Grant no. N.B. 05411) and the Agricultural Research Council.

REFERENCES

Barraclough, C. A. & Cross, B. A. (1963). Unit activity in the hypothalamus of the cyclic female rat: effect of genital stimuli and progesterone. *J. Endocrin.* **26**, 339–359.

Bernhaut, M., Gellhorn, E. & Rasmussen, A. T. (1953). Experimental contributions to problem of conciousness. *J. Neurophysiol.* **16**, 21–35.

Cross, B. A. (1964). The hypothalamus in mammalian homeostasis. In *Symp. Soc. exp. Biol.* no. 18, pp. 157–193. Ed. G. M. Hughes. Cambridge University Press.

Cross, B. A. & Green, J. D. (1959). Activity of single neurones in the hypothalamus: effect of osmotic and other stimuli. *J. Physiol., Lond.* **148**, 554–569.

Cross, B. A. & Silver, I. A. (1965). Effect of luteal hormone on the behaviour of hypothalamic neurones in pseudopregnant rats. *J. Endocrin.* **31**, 251–263.

Cross, B. A. & Silver, I. A. (1966). Electrophysiological studies on the hypothalamus. *Br. med. Bull.* **22**, 254–260.

Eto, T., Masuda, H., Shizuki, Y. & Hosi, T. (1962). Progesterone and pregn-4-ene-20α-OL-3-one in rat ovarian venous blood at different stages in reproductive cycle. *Jap. J. Anim. Reprod.* **8**, 34–40.

Everett, J. W. (1940). The restoration of cyclic estrus and ovulation in persistent-estrous rats by progesterone. *Anat. Rec.* **76**, 21*P*.

Everett, J. W. (1943). Further studies on the relationship of progesterone to ovulation and luteinization in the persistent-estrous rat. *Endocrinology* **32**, 285–292.

Everett, J. W. (1964). Preoptic stimulative lesions and ovulation in the rat. Thresholds and L.H. release time in late diestrus and proestrus. In *Major problems in neuroendocrinology*, pp. 346–366. Eds. E. Bajusz and G. Jasmin. Basel: S. Karger.

Everett, J. W. & Sawyer, C. H. (1950). A 24-hour periodicity in the 'LH-release apparatus' of female rats, disclosed by barbiturate sedation. *Endocrinology* **47**, 198–218.

French, J. D., Verzeano, M. & Magoun, H. W. (1953). An extra-lemniscal sensory system in the brain. *Archs Neurol. Psychiat., Chicago* **69**, 505.

Harris, G. W., Michael, R. P. & Scott, P. P. (1958). Neurological site of action of stilboestrol in eliciting sexual behaviour. In *Ciba foundation symposium on the neurological basis of behaviour*, pp. 236–251. Eds. G. E. W. Wolstenholme and C. M. O'Connor. London: Churchill.

Kawakami, M. & Sawyer, C. H. (1959). Induction of behavioural and electroencephalographic changes in the rabbit by hormone administration or brain stimulation. *Endocrinology* **65**, 631–643.

Lincoln, D. W. (1967). Unit activity in the hypothalamus, septum and preoptic area of the rat: characteristics of spontaneous activity and the effect of oestrogen. *J. Endocrin.* **37**, 177–189.

Lisk, R. D. (1960). Oestrogen sensitive centres in the hypothalamus of the rat. *J. exp. Zool.* **145**, 197–208.

Lisk, R. D. (1962). Diencephalic placement of oestradiol and sexual receptivity in the female rat. *Am. J. Physiol.* **203**, 493–496.

Michael, R. P. (1965). Oestrogens in the central nervous system. *Br. med. Bull.* **21**, 87–90.

Richter, C. P. (1964). Biological clocks and the endocrine glands. *Proc. IInd Int. Congr. Endocrin.*, London. Ed. S. Taylor. *Excerpta Medica Int. Congr. Ser.*, no. 83, pp. 119–123.

Wendt, R. H. & Adey, W. R. (1960). A study of evoked activity in the hypothalamus. *Anat. Rec.* **136**, 301.

Electrocortical Activation by Estrogens

JOHN LOGOTHETIS, M.D., and RICHARD HARNER, M.D.

Introduction

The effect of various steroid hormones upon the electrical activity of the mammalian brain has been the subject of many investigations in the past. Cortisone and corticotropin (adrenocorticotrophic hormone) have been reported to exert convulsive effect in animals [1] and humans,[2,3] although these steroids have recently been used with some success in the treatment of patients with hypsarhythmia.[4,5] Desoxycorticosterone has also been found to exert electrical and clinical anticonvulsant effect in humans [6] and to increase the seizure threshold in animals.[1,7] Other steroids with anticonvulsant properties in animals are progesterone and certain androgenic hormones.[1,7]

We have been unable to find previous reports dealing with the direct effect of estrogens on cerebral electrical activity, although several studies indirectly suggest that ovarian hormones augment convulsive discharge in man and animals. For example, ovariectomy has been reported to give relief of seizures in humans [8-10] and to prevent spread of convulsive discharges in animals.[11]

Materials and Methods

Five normal rabbits and eight rabbits with experimentally produced irritative lesions were studied. In all cases the calvarium was exposed by incising the scalp, using 1% Procaine for local anesthesia. The lesions were made by spraying ethyl chloride through a 4 mm. burr hole on small exposed cortical areas, as described by Morrell and Florenz,[12] or, as modified by Sandler,[13] by applying the ethyl chloride spray to the intact dura. The lesions were termed acute when produced 6 to 8 hours prior to study, subacute when present for 48 hours, or chronic when present for 2 to 3 weeks. All lesions resulted in a persistent spike discharge. An eight-channel EEG recorder (Offner Dynograph) was used to obtain mostly bipolar and few monopolar tracings (reference electrode at the ear) from phonographic needles pinned into the skull in close proximity to the underlying dura. The needle at the site of the lesion was inserted 1-2 mm. from the border of the burr hole. Each animal during the electrical recording was in a dark room placed in a wooden box allowing the head to stick out. The EEG recorder was outside this room; however, close observation of the animal was permitted.

Intravenous effects of Premarin, which is a preparation of water-soluble conjugated estrogens,* were investigated by comparing spontaneous electrical activity, stimulation threshold, and threshold for afterdischarge before and after injection of 10-40 mg. of the hormone. Topical effects were studied by applying Premarin solutions of progressive strength varying from 0.0001% to 1% to cortex with normal and abnormal discharge, using small pieces of filter paper or cotton pledgets soaked in the above solutions. After each observation at the given concentration the exposed cortex was thoroughly rinsed with isotonic saline solution, and enough time was allowed for stabilization of the record to the previous level. Prior to the administration of the hormone electrical recording over a period of at least three hours was taken to establish the basal cerebral activity of each animal.

Thresholds for afterdischarge were determined by stimulating the cortex at five-minute intervals through phonograph needles inserted into the calvarium near the edges of the burr hole. Once the threshold was reached, half-hour intervals were allowed in order to finally establish the threshold afterdischarge. A square wave positive-negative pulse of 1-5 msec. duration recurring at 40-50 cps for 3-4 seconds was used for stimulation at potentials varying from 1.5-100 volts. This large variation in voltage results from a variable resistance at the junction of needle and bone. Thus

This work was aided by a grant from the Teagle Foundation.

* Premarin was kindly supplied by the Ayerst Laboratories.

TABLE 1.—*Study of Afterdischarge in Normal Rabbits Before and After Intravenous Administration of Conjugated Estrogenic Substances (Premarin)*

Rabbit No.	Parameters of Stimulation	Amount Premarin Injected, Mg.	Time Elapsed After Injection, Min.	Threshold Voltage		Freq. of T.A.*		Amplitude of T.A.		Duration of T.A.	
				Before Prem-arin	After Prem-arin	Before Prem-arin	After Prem-arin	Before Prem-arin	After Prem-arin	Before Prem-arin	After Prem-arin
9	40/sec., 5msec.; 3 sec. duration	10	5	5v	5v	2/sec.	5/sec.	$50\mu V$	$50\mu V$	3 sec.	6 sec.
10	40/sec., 5msec.; 3 sec. duration	10	15	5v	5v	2/sec.	5/sec.	$60\mu V$	$40\mu V$	3½ sec.	5½ sec.
11	40/sec., 5msec.; 3 sec. duration	20	4	3v	1½v	1-2/sec.	4-7/sec.	$100\mu V$	$100\mu V$	6 sec.	8 sec.
13	50/sec., 1msec.; 5 sec. duration	10	90	30v	30v	4/sec.	3/sec.	$50\mu V$	$75\mu V$	4 sec.	4 sec.

* T.A. = Threshold afterdischarge.

threshold values may be compared only to others in the same animal and not to values obtained from another animal. Threshold afterdischarges were invariably reproducible once the threshold voltage was reached.

Results

I. Normal Rabbits

Five normal rabbits were used to study the effect of Premarin on the normal electrical activity of the rabbit brain. In all cases the hormone was administered intravenously and in one it was applied topically as well.

A. Intravenous Administration of Premarin.—Five normal rabbits were injected with 10-20 mg. of Premarin. The spontaneous records were studied in all five. Thresholds for afterdischarge were obtained in four of these animals. Of the latter four rabbits, three exhibited an increased cortical response to electrical stimulation occurring 4-90 minutes after the injection (Table 1). This was manifested by increased frequency and duration of afterdischarge (Rabbit Experiments 9, 10, 11), and on one occasion (Rabbit Experiment 11) by decreased afterdischarge threshold. This latter animal received twice as much Premarin as the other; Figure 1, *A* illustrates the record change in one of these animals. Study of the spontaneous electrical activity revealed an activating effect of Premarin in one or possibly two of five animals tested (Table 2). One of these animals studied by monopolar recording Fig. 1, *B*) exhibited bursts of rhythmic spikes at 7 per second and high voltage slow waves occurring diffusely with reversed polarity at the site of the lesion. These changes were first observed 100 minutes after injection of Premarin and lasted until the experiment was arbitrarily terminated 20 minutes later. The left occipital recording was from the site of previous insertion of needles to be used for stimulation at a later time. It may well be that the minimal cortical trauma thus incurred resulted in a local increase in cortical activity which was activated by premarin.

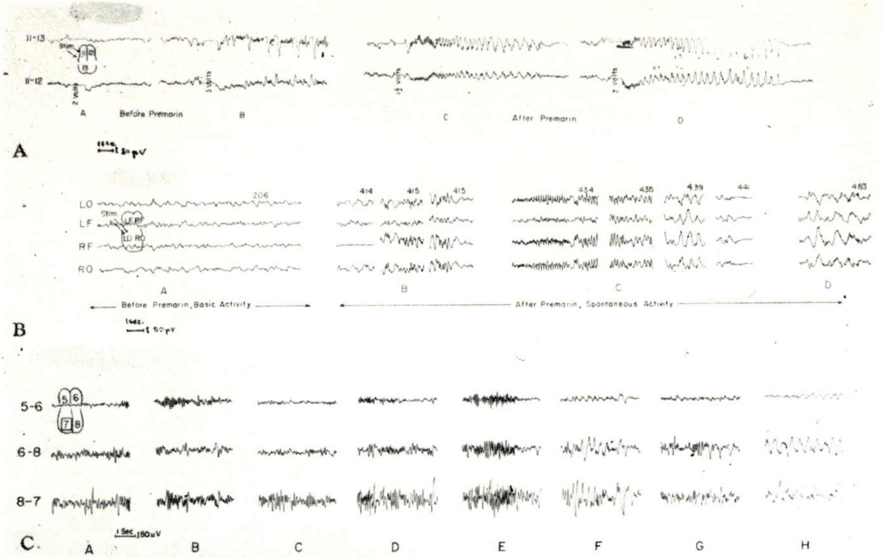

Fig. 1.—*A*. Experiment 11. Electrocortical afterdischarges in normal rabbits before and after intravenous injection of Premarin. Note increase in frequency and duration of afterdischarge and lowering of threshold voltage.

B. Experiment 13. Spontaneous electrocortical activation occurring after intravenous injection of 10 mg. Premarin in normal rabbit. A, Basic activity prior to Premarin. B, 100 minutes after injection of 10 mg. of Premarin, segments of burst of spikes 20 sec. in duration. C, 106 minutes after injection, rhythmic bursts of spikes. Several other similar bursts in next 90 min. D, 120 minutes after injection, record remains abnormal.

C. Experiment 6(*b*), immediate effects of topical application of Premarin to exposed normal left occipital cortex. A, basic record. B,C, no change with 0.0001% and 0.001% solutions. D, 0.01% of Premarin, minimal increase in voltage at site of application. E, 0.1% Premarin, increase in frequency and voltage in posterior leads. F,G,H, 0.2%, 0.1%, and 0.5% of Premarin, high-voltage slow waves over posterior leads.

B. Topical Application of Premarin to the Cortex.—For this experiment the normal animal 6(*a*) was used after a burr hole was placed in the left occipital region under light ether anesthesia and the brain exposed by opening a small window in the

TABLE 2.—*Study of Spontaneous Electrical Brain Activity in Normal Rabbits Before and After Intravenous Administration of Conjugated Estrogenic Substances (Premarin)*

Rabbit No.	Basic Activity Before Premarin	Amt of Premarin Injection, Mg.	Activation After Injection	Time Elapsed After Injection, Min.	Duration of Activation After Premarin, Min.	Duration of Experiment After Injection, Min.
6A	10 μv, 8-10/sec.	20	Bilateral random, short bursts of spikes 50-100 μv	10	110	120
9	10-30 μv, 4-5/sec.	10	None	--	--	50
10	10-20 μv, 4-5/sec.	10	None	--	--	60
11	10 μv, 7-10/sec.	20	None	--	--	25
13	20-50 μv, 3-5/sec.	10	Bursts of spikes and delta waves originating from lt. occip. area	100	20	120

dura. The animal was then called 6(*b*).† Premarin was applied to the exposed pial surface in solutions of increasing concentration (Fig. 1, *C*). Little change in basic activity was observed with concentrations less than 0.01%. With higher concentrations an increase in amplitude and frequency of the resting discharge occurred in a few seconds at the site of application, spreading also to other areas of the cortex. Increase in concentrations up to 0.5% resulted in high-voltage slow waves; little appeared in the way of spike activity.

II. Epileptic Rabbits

Eight rabbits were studied, five with chronic lesions, two with acute lesions, and one with a subacute lesion. The effect of intravenous administration of Premarin was studied in seven of these animals, while topical application at the site of the lesion was carried out in four. In the tables to follow, animals with letters attached to their protocol number were used in more than one experiment.

A. Intravenous Administration of Premarin.—Spontaneous records were studied in all seven animals injected with Premarin; threshold for afterdischarge was determined in one. This latter animal (Fig. 2, *A*) 28 minutes after injection of 10 mg. of Premarin, exhibited a decrease in the threshold for afterdischarge from 2.5 to 1.5 volts, while the afterdischarge itself was greatly increased in voltage, duration, and, to a slighter extent, frequency. An attempt to study a second animal (No. 14)

† We also presented Experiment 6(*b*) elsewhere.[16]

Fig. 2.—*A*. Experiment 8(*a*) Study of stimulation afterdischarge following intravenous injection of 10 mg. Premarin; acute left frontal lesion. Note decrease in threshold, increase in voltage, and frequency of spike discharges (28 min. after injection). Duration of afterdischarge has increased from 70 to 120 seconds.

B, C. Spontaneous electrocortical activation occurring after intravenous injection of Premarin in epileptic rabbits. *B* Experiment 14. Subacute lesion, right occipital. A, prior to injection of 10 mg. of Premarin. B, 85 min. after injection, high voltage spikes and slow waves lasting 12 minutes. *C* Experiment 8. Acute lesion, left frontal. A,B, prior to injection of 10 mg. of Premarin, active focal discharge not exceeding 100μv. C, three minutes after injection of 10 mg. Premarin, bilateral burst of high-voltage spikes leading to clinical seizure. D, 40 minutes after injection, burst of spikes.

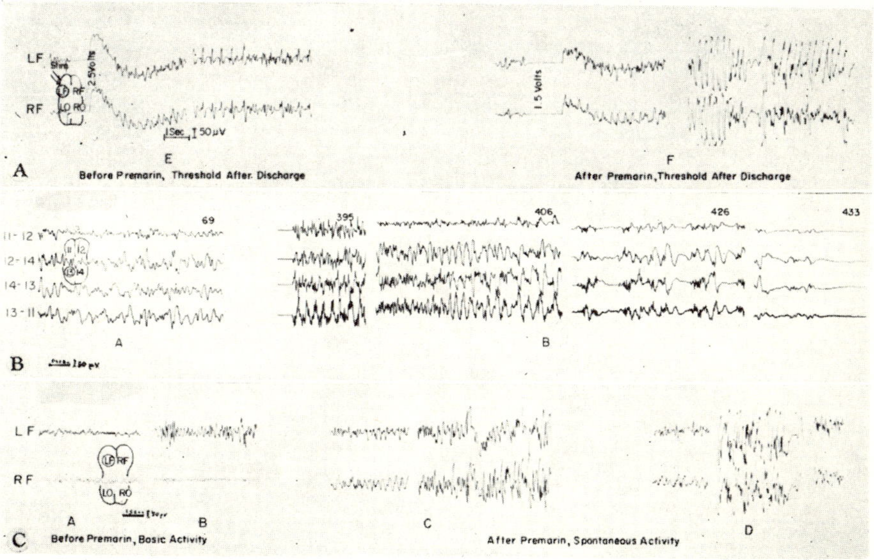

TABLE 3.—*Study of Spontaneous Electrocortical Activity of Rabbits with Epileptic Foci Before*

Animal Protocol	Type & Location of Lesion	Amount of Premarin Injected, Mg.	Time Elapsed After Injection, Min.	Duration of Electrical Change, Min.	Duration of Experiment After Injection, Min.
1A	Chronic right occipital	20	60	180	240
2A	Chronic right occipital	20	70	110	180
3A	Chronic right occipital	20			300
4A	Chronic right occipital	20			90
5	Chronic right occipital	20×2 within 3 hr.	3 after 2d injection	4 (death)	7 after 2d injection
8	Acute left frontal	10	3	60	63
14	Subacute left occipital	10	85	12 (death)	91

Chronic lesion: 2-3 weeks old; Acute lesion: 6-8 hours old; Subacute lesion: 48 hours old.

in similar fashion was terminated because the rabbit began convulsing continuously shortly after receiving the Premarin and continued to do so until the experiment was terminated. Examination of the spontaneous recordings in the seven animals (Table 3) revealed activation of the epileptic discharge after injection of Premarin in five. The activation appeared 3-85 minutes after the injection of 10-40 mg. of Premarin and lasted until the end of the experiment. This electrical activation appeared in the form of paroxysmal bursts of high-voltage spikes and superimposed delta activity lasting for several seconds, recurring at varying intervals up to three hours. The activation was simultaneous in the primary and mirror area, i.e., homologous opposite cortex, in three of the five animals (Nos. 5, 8, 14); the mirror focus alone was activated in one rabbit (2[*a*]) and activation at the site of the lesion with subsequent spread to the mirror focus was observed in one animal (1[*a*]). Three of these animals (5, 8, 14) convulsed a few minutes after activation of the record; two of them (5, 14) subsequently died in status epilepticus. Figure 2, *B-C,* illustrates two examples of this group.

B. Topical Application of Premarin.—Premarin applied to the cortex of four epileptic rabbits in concentrations varying from 0.1% to 1% produced bursts of high-voltage spike activity in all animals. Three of four animals (Nos. 1, 3, 6[*c*]) initially exhibited spike activity in the mirror area with subsequent spread to the site of application. Only in the record (No. 4) did abnormal discharge appear first at the site of application of Premarin. Three of the animals convulsed; two of them died in status epilepticus. Figure 3 illustrates examples of this experiment.‡

During the topical applications it was noted that, as the highest concentrations were applied, rinsing and longer time were required for recovery of the preapplication electrical activity. With concentrations of 0.5% or more a persistent residual activation usually remained, presumably due to some diffusion from the earlier applications. It is possible that the convulsions observed in the three animals with lesions was the result of more than a local effect.

The following is a brief review of the above experimental results: The intravenous administration of estrogens in the form of Premarin brought about activation of electrocortical afterdischarges in three of four normal animals studied and activated spontaneous electrocortical potentials in one of five animals tested. Topical application of the hormone to normal cortex of one animal resulted, as well, in electrical activation. In the epileptic group intravenous

‡ We also presented Experiment 3 elsewhere.[16]

and After Intravenous Administration of Conjugated Estrogenic Substances (Premarin)

Activity at Lesion		Activity Mirror Focus		Clinical Seizure		Death After Premarin
Before Premarin	After Premarin	Before Premarin	After Premarin	Before Premarin	After Premarin	
Few spikes	Bursts rhythm. spikes	Few spikes	Sharp waves, 100µv	No	No	No
Few spikes	Voltage depres.; no spikes	No spikes	Spikes; delta waves	No	No	No
Spikes	No change	No spikes	No spikes	No	No	No
Spikes	No change	No spikes	No spikes	No	No	No
Random spikes 100µv	Bursts spikes 300µv	Few spikes, 100µv	Bursts spikes, 300µv	No	Yes	Yes
Bursts spikes 100µv	Bursts spikes 200µv	No spikes	Bursts spikes, 200µv	No	Yes	No
Spikes; slow waves, 100µv	Cont. spikes 200µv	Spikes; slow waves, 100µv	Cont. spikes 200µv	No	Yes	Yes

administration of estrogens produced activation of electrocortical afterdischarges in one animal studied, and activated spontaneous discharges in five of seven animals tested. Three of the animals with irritative lesions convulsed, and two died, presumably as a result of the excessive activation. Topical application of the hormone to the

Fig. 3.—Immediate effect of topical application of Premarin over exposed epileptic cortex.

A. Experiment 3. Chronic lesion, right occipital. A, prior to Premarin, few spikes. B, effect of diluent alone. C, 0.1% Premarin, no definite effect. D, 0.2% Premarin, burst of spikes in mirror area. E,F, 1% Premarin, high-voltage spikes right hemisphere spreading all areas.

B. Experiment 4. Chronic lesion, right occipital. A, prior to Premarin, occasional spikes and slow waves at site of lesion. B, 0.1% Premarin, low spikes at site of lesion. *C*. Experiment 6(*c*) Acute lesion, left occipital. A, prior to Premarin, spikes at site of lesion. B, 0.2% Premarin, no effect. C-F, 1% Premarin, high voltage spikes starting at mirror area accompanied by clinical seizure.

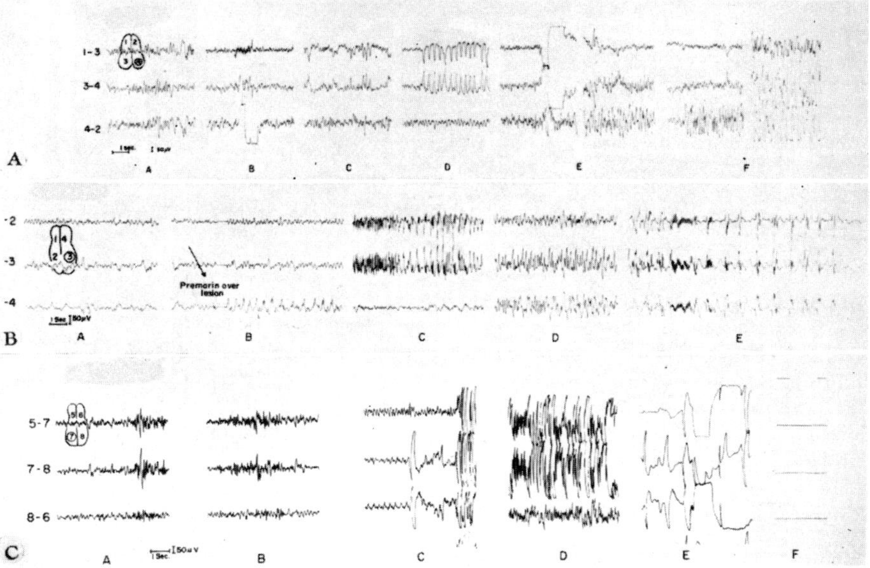

site of epileptic lesion in four animals produced uniform electrocortical activation; three convulsed and two died in status epilepticus shortly after application of Premarin.

Comment

In would appear from the above studies that estrogens in the form of Premarin stimulate abnormal electrocortical activity in the rabbit when administered intravenously or applied directly to the cortex. High-voltage spike discharges, clinical seizures, and even death in status epilepticus resulted in some animals. Topical application was more effective than intravenous injection in producing these abnormalities. Although activation was seen in both normal rabbits and those with experimentally produced irritative lesions, it is quite clear that the latter animals were much more sensitive to Premarin. Futhermore, while only minimal change in spontaneous recording occurred in five normal animals given the hormone, definite increase in amount of afterdischarge was seen in three of these animals following electric stimulation. Activation of the mirror focus in animals with focal lesions was a prominent finding following both intravenous injection and application of Premarin at the site of the lesion.

It is clear that at this stage of the investigation there are several questions remaining unanswered. However, one might speculate as to the circumstances under which estrogens can get into the central nervous system and the mechanism by which they produce activation. The fact that the activating effect of Premarin is more easily demonstrable in the presence of either a cortical lesion or electrocortical stimulation suggests that some change in the cerebral cortex, either anatomic or physiologic, is necessary for estrogens to act upon electrocortical discharge. The possibility that such alteration may be in fact an increase in the permeability of the blood-brain barrier is tempting and will bear further study. The observation that the mirror area is so greatly activated by the estrogenic hormones, even when applied locally to the primary focus, suggests that the effect of Premarin may be mainly to facilitate spread of the abnormal cortical activity, while discharges occurring at the primary focus are influenced to a much less degree. Neurochemical investigations regarding estrogens are few, but two studies indirectly suggest that estrogens have an inhibitory effect on cholinesterase activity with subsequent build-up of acetylcholine.[14,15]

The amounts of estrogens used in this experiment, both for injection and for topical cortical application, are obviously unphysiological for the animals and reflect a pharmacologic rather than physiologic action. In a previous communication[16] dealing with the effects of estrogens on human epileptics it was reported that 11 of 16 patients studied showed activation of their electroencephalographic abnormality and 4 had convulsions when given 20-40 mg. of Premarin intravenously. These results coupled with those of the present study should warn against excessive use of estrogens in patients with convulsive disorders.

Summary and Conclusions

Estrogenic hormones in the form of Premarin were shown to have an activating effect on the electrocortical discharges of the rabbit brain. This activation was in the form of paroxysmal spike discharges and occurred after topical or intravenous administration.

The above effect was more marked in rabbits with experimentally produced irritative cortical lesions.

Activation of the mirror focus in the opposite hemisphere prior to activation of the primary epileptic focus was a prominent finding in the epileptic group.

These findings coupled with previous studies in humans should warn against excessive use of estrogens in patients with convulsive disorders. •

University of Minnesota Medical School.

REFERENCES

1. Costa, P. J., and Bonnycastle, D. D.: The Effect of DCA, Compound E, Testosterone, Progesterone and ACTH in Modifying "Agene-Induced" Convulsions in Dogs, Arch. Internat. Pharmacodyn. 91:330, 1952.

2. Geppert, L. J.; Dietrick, A. C.; Johnston, E. H., and Lind, C. J.: Fatal Convulsive Seizures Associated with Cortisone Therapy: Report of a Case, A.M.A. Am. J. Dis. Child. 84:416, 1952.

3. Dorfman, A.; Apter, N. S.; Smull, K.; Bergenstal, D. M., and Richter, R. B.: Status Epilepticus Coincident with Use of Pituitary Adrenocorticotrophic Hormone: Report of 3 Cases, J.A.M.A. 146:25, 1951.

4. Sorel, L., and Dusaucy-Bauloye, A.: A Propos de 21 cas de hypsarhythmia de Gibbs: Son traitement spectaculaire par l'ACTH, Acta neurol. et psychiat. belg. 58:130, 1958.

5. Stamps, F. W.; Gibbs, E. L.; Rosenthal, I. M., and Gibbs, F. A.: Treatment of Hypsarrhythmia with ACTH, J.A.M.A. 171:408, 1959.

6. Aird, R. B., and Gordon, G. S.: Anticonvulsive Properties of Desoxycorticosterone, J.A.M.A. 145:715, 1951.

7. Spiegel, E., and Wycis, H.: Anticonvulsant Effects of Steroids, J. Lab. & Clin. Med. 30:947, 1945.

8. Everke, C.: Uber ovarielle Epilepsie, Monatsschr. Geburtsh. u. Gynäk. 61:256, 1923.

9. Russel, A. W.: Epileptische Anfälle der doppelseitigen ovarial Tumor, Zentralbl. Gynäk. 33:1044, 1905.

10. Rebattu, Mollon, and Sêdaillean: Epilepsie et fonctions ovariennes, Lyon méd. 131:1028, 1922.

11. Longo, V.: Epilessia sperimentale e glandole endocrine: influenza dell' attività delle glandole sessuali sulla predisposizione del cane all'epilessia riflessa da eccitamenti afferenti, Riv. pat. nerv. 57:432, 1941.

12. Morrell, F., and Florenz, A.: Modifications of Freezing Technique for Producing Experimental Epileptogenic Lesions, Electroencephalog. & Clin. Neurophysiol. 10:187, 1958.

13. Sandler, B.: Personal communications to the authors, 1959.

14. Christiansen, E. G.: Correlation Between Variation in Amount of Estrogen and Cholinesterase Activity in Human Serum, Thesis, Copenhagen, 1956.

15. Reynolds, S. R. M.: Cholinergic Action of Oestrin, Science 87:537, 1938.

16. Logothetis, J.; Harner, R.; Morrell, F., and Torres, F.: The Role of Estrogens in Catamenial Exacerbation of Epilepsy, Neurology 9:352, 1959.

THE TIME COURSE OF EFFECTS OF SEX HORMONES ON ELECTRICALLY-EVOKED POTENTIALS IN THE FROG FOREBRAIN

By

Kiyoshi Oshima and Aubrey Gorbman

ABSTRACT

In the frog, over a period of up to 12 days, the effects of a single injection of steroid hormone were measured on potentials evoked in the olfactory lobe and telencephalon after electrical stimulation of the olfactory nerve. Response amplitudes in the olfactory lobe and telencephalon were depressed by 10 μg doses of progesterone whether given alone, or in combination with 10 μg of oestradiol. In the olfactory lobe the change in response induced by progesterone was significant by 2 days and reached a peak by 6 to 8 days after injection. In the telencephalon the peak effect of progesterone was also at about 6 days, but no significant change from the control could be found before 4 days.

In contrast, oestradiol, when given alone, augmented the response to olfactory stimulation detected in the olfactory lobe and telencephalon. The time relations were about the same as for progesterone.

Effects of the two hormones on stimulus threshold were relatively modest and in general were correlated with the effects on response amplitude.

Similarity in time course of effects of progesterone and oestradiol, and the dominance of the progesterone effect over that of oestradiol suggests that despite their opposite actions, at least part of their influence is on the same elements in the olfactory response system.

Relatively little is yet known of olfactory-evoked central nervous activity in amphibians, or of the influences that regulate it. Histological and anatomical

---

This study was aided by a grant, NB 04887, from the National Institutes of Health, U. S. Public Health Service.

data have been provided by *Allison* (1953*a,b*) concerning centripetal olfactory tracts. *Takagi & Shibuya* (1960) and *Takagi* (1962) have traced such tracts in the frog brain by following olfactory evoked potentials. In our own earlier work we have been concerned with the modification of evoked olfactory bulbar responses by prior sex hormone injections (*Oshima & Gorbman* 1966*a,b,* 1968) in goldfish.

Against this background of research indicating a responsiveness of olfactory function to certain hormones, we have undertaken experiments to investigate hormonal sensitivity of similar central nervous functions in anuran amphibians. In these experiments responses in the olfactory bulb and in the telencephalon (hippocampal region, *Herrick* 1933) of frogs were evoked by electrically stimulating the ipsilateral olfactory nerve. The peak to peak amplitudes of these evoked potentials and threshold intensities (voltage) of stimuli were measured every two days for twelve days after single injections of progesterone and/or oestradiol at a dosage of 10 μg for the purpose of observing the time course of effects of these hormones.

MATERIAL AND METHODS

One hundred and thirty seven frogs (*Rana pipiens*) of both sexes were used in experiments; they were kept at a relatively well controlled temperature (22°C ± 1°C) throughout the period March–May, 1967. The frogs were obtained from a commercial breeder (J. R. Schettle Frog Farm, Inc., Stillwater, Minnesota). Animals weighing between 25–40 g were treated in one of four ways: one group was given 10 μg progesterone; a second group was given 10 μg progesterone and 10 μg oestradiol; a third group was given 10 μg oestradiol; a fourth group was given an equivalent volume (0.05 ml) of the hormone vehicle, sesame oil. Animals from each of these groups were tested at 2 day intervals, up to 12 days after a single intramuscular injection of hormone. Pentobarbital sodium (Nembutal®, 100 μg/10 g body weight) was used in some experiments to compare its known depressive effects with the observed actions of the several tested hormones. The frogs were fed mealworms daily.

After moderate ether anaesthesia and immobilization (gallamine-triethiodide, 40 μg per 10 g body weight, subcutaneously) the brain was exposed and the dura and arachnoid dissected from the dorsal side. The preparation was protected under a layer of mineral oil. Bipolar stainless steel electrodes (*Oshima & Gorbman* 1966*a,b*) were used for surface EEG recording of several parts of brain (shown in Fig. 1) and for electrical stimulation of the left olfactory nerve.

Electroencephalograph recording and electrically evoked responses in the several parts of brain following olfactory nerve stimulation were amplified by a Grass 5P5 amplifier and displayed on a Grass Model 5 Polygraph and Tektronix No. 502 oscilloscope. The electrical stimuli for the left olfactory nerve, separated from the olfactory epithelium, were 0.1 ms sweep-synchronized square pulses provided by a Grass S4 stimulator. The oscilloscope was triggered by the stimulator and in some instances approximately 3 to 5 superimposed traces of the response were photographed by a Grass kymograph camera.

The experiments were conducted in a quiet room in which the temperature was regulated near 23°C. Measurements were made of the peak-to-peak amplitudes of the maximum recorded components of the responses evoked in the olfactory bulb and in the hippocampal region of the telencephalon. Measurements were made also of the threshold voltage to induce the evoked response in the olfactory bulb and in the telencephalon in some animals.

RESULTS

Representative evoked responses in several parts of the forebrain in control animals are shown in Fig. 1. The evoked potentials appeared largest in the homolateral olfactory bulb (137.9 ± 8.2 μV) with a delay of 40–50 ms following a stimulus of 7 V (Fig. 1, Ad). The evoked responses in the homolateral hippocampal region following stimuli of 7 V were 91.1 ± 12.4 μV in amplitude and 60–80 ms in latency (Fig. 1, Cd). Pentobarbital sodium given in a dose of 100 μg per 10 g body weight depressed amplitudes of these evoked potentials extremely (Fig. 1, Ae and Ce). Treshold voltages to evoke typical potentials in the olfactory bulb and the hippocampal region in control animals were 2.8 ± 0.5 V and 3.5 ± 0.6 V, respectively (Fig. 1, Ac and Cc). The evoked responses in the homolateral mid-posterior portion of the telencephalon and contralateral hippocampal region (see Fig. 1 for loci) appeared smallest (40–50 μV in amplitude and complex in pattern.

The time course of effects of progesterone and oestradiol on amplitudes of evoked potentials in the olfactory bulb and the hippocampal region to 7 V nerve stimuli at the olfactory nerve are shown in Fig. 2. Progesterone appeared to depress the amplitudes of evoked potentials 2 days (92.4 ± 6.6 μV, $P < 0.005$), 4 days (94.6 ± 4.4 μV, $P < 0.025$), 6 days (56.1 ± 7.3, $P < 0.001$), 8 days (80.9 ± 15.7 μV, $P < 0.025$) and 12 days (94.1 ± 12.4, NS) after injection. A significant depressant effect of progesterone on evoked potentials in the hippocampal region, however, was not obtained until 6 days after treatment (42.9 ± 0.5 μV, $P < 0.005$). In contrast with progesterone, oestradiol increased the amplitude of evoked potentials in both the olfactory bulb and hippocampal region, but its actions on these two parts of the forebrain had different time courses. Mean amplitudes of potentials evoked in the olfactory bulb 2, 4, 6, 8 and 12 days by 7 V stimuli after oestradiol application were 182.6 ± 13.4 μV ($P < 0.025$), 207.9 ± 9.9 μV (NS), 201.3 ± 25.0 μV ($P < 0.05$), 245.5 ± 25.7 μV ($P < 0.005$) and 183.1 ± 10.2 μV ($P < 0.01$), respectively. Responses with largest amplitudes were obtained 8 days after oestradiol treatment.

The most marked facilitatory effect of oestradiol on response amplitudes of the hippocampal region were seen 6 days (174.9 ± 16.5 μV, $P < 0.005$) and 8 days (151.8 ± 9.9 μV, $P < 0.001$) after oestrogen treatment. Combined injection of progesterone and oestradiol yielded effects similar to those of progesterone alone. However, a significant difference in the olfactory bulbar

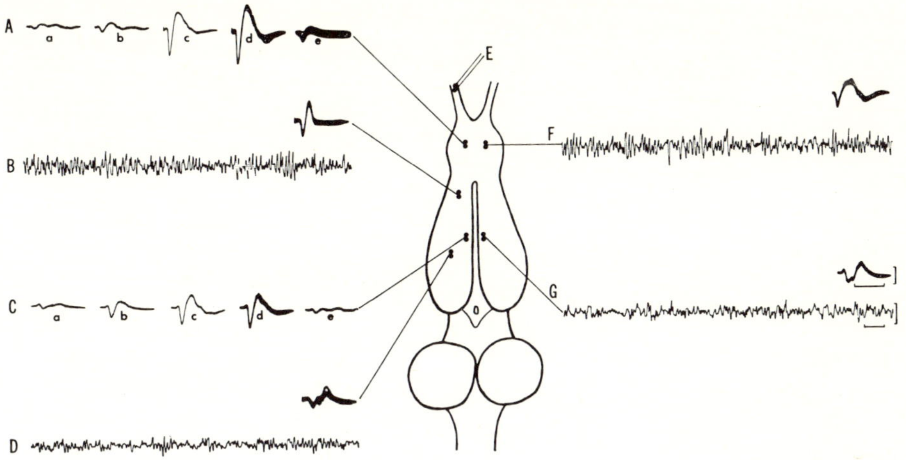

Fig. 1.

Spontaneous EEG and evoked responses in different parts of the frog forebrain following electrical stimulation of the olfactory nerve. Recording electrode positions shown in diagram.

A. Evoked responses in ipsilateral olfactory bulb to electrical stimulation of the olfactory nerve at a voltage of 1 V (a), 2 V (b), 3 V (c), 7 V (d). Stimulus onset is coincident with the beginning of each trace. At 7 V, 3 responses were superimposed. (e) Superimposed responses evoked by stimulating the olfactory nerve at 7 V, 20 min after intraperitoneal injection of pentobarbital sodium at a dosage of 100 μg/10 g body weight.

B. Spontaneous EEG and several superimposed evoked responses in the anterior part of the telencephalon following 7 V electrical stimulation of the ipsilateral olfactory nerve.

C. Responses in the hippocampal region of the telencephalon evoked by olfactory nerve stimulation at 3 V (a), 4 V (b), 6 V (c) and 7 V (d, e).
(e) same as in A.

D. Spontaneous EEG and superimposed single responses evoked in the posterior part of the telencephalon following 7 V electrical stimulation of the ipsilateral olfactory nerve.

E. Locus of electrical stimulation of the olfactory nerve.

F. Spontaneous EEG and several superimposed single responses in the olfactory bulb evoked by 7 V electrical stimuli to the contralateral olfactory nerve.

G. Spontaneous EEG and superimposed single evoked responses in the hippocampal region following 7 V electrical stimulation of the contralateral olfactory nerve.

Calibration: Oscillographic tracings: 50 μV and 200 ms; polygraphic (EEG) recordings. 50 μV and 1 s.

response was obtained only 6 days after injection (66.1 $\pm$ 11.1 μV, $P < 0.005$). A significant decrease in response amplitude in the hippocampal region was found also 6 days after progesterone-oestradiol treatment as well as after progesterone injection alone (35.0 $\pm$ 8.5 μV, $P < 0.001$).

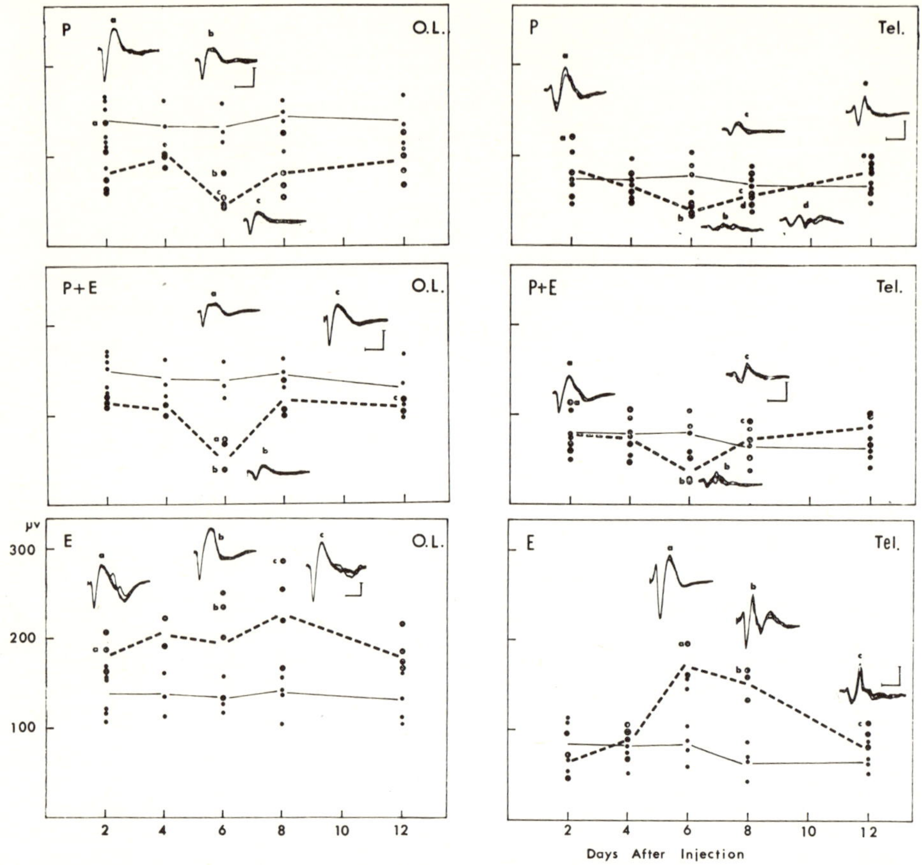

Fig. 2.

Time course of effects of a single injection of sex hormones on amplitudes of olfactory bulbar and telencephalic responses evoked by 7 V electrical stimuli applied to the ipsilateral olfactory nerve. Key to symbols on individual charts: P: progesterone, 10 μg injected animals; P + E: Progesterone 10 μg and oestradiol 10 μg combined injection; E: oestradiol 10 μg injection; O. L.: ipsilateral olfactory bulb recorded evoked potentials. Tel.: hippocampal region of ipsilateral telencephalon.

Oscillographic recordings of superimposed single evoked responses are shown over the curves approximately over the abscissa time interval at which they were evoked. Small letters next to a dot on the curves correspond to the illustrated responses above them in each instance. Larger dots and broken lines indicate hormone-injected animals; smaller dots and solid lines indicate sesame oil-injected controls. Calibration: 50 μV and 200 ms.

Fig. 3 illustrates the time course of effects of progesterone and oestradiol on the threshold intensity for evocation of electrical potentials in the olfactory bulb and in the hippocampal region to olfactory nerve stimuli. There was never

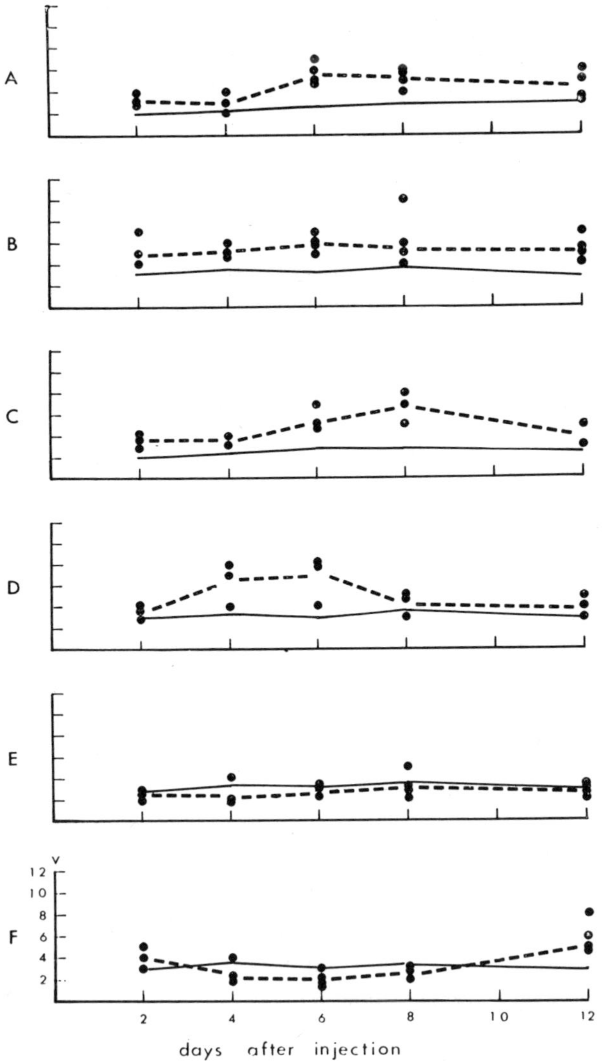

Fig. 3.
Time course of effects of sex hormones on threshold voltage for evocation of ipsilateral olfactory and hippocampal responses to nerve stimulation. Broken lines and dots represent data from experimental animals, and solid lines indicate controls. A: progesterone-treated animals; recording from the olfactory bulb; B: progesterone, hippocampal region; C: progesterone and oestradiol, olfactory bulb; D: progesterone and oestradiol, hippocampal region; E: oestradiol, olfactory bulb; F: oestradiol, hippocampal region.

a significant decrease of threshold voltages in any of the hormone treated frogs (Fig. 3, E, F). However, significantly increased threshold voltages were seen in animals treated with either progesterone or the progesterone-oestradiol combination. Data from some of the points which in Fig. 3 appeared to indicate significant changes are further analyzed in Table 1. The largest increase in

Table 1.
Mean threshold voltages. Time relationships after sex hormone treatment.

Part of brain	Treatment	Days after injection	Number of animals	Mean threshold voltage ± SE	*P*
Olfactory bulb	Control		10	2.8 ± 0.5	
	Progesterone	6	4	5.8 ± 0.2	< 0.001
	Progesterone	8	4	5.3 ± 0.2	< 0.001
	Progesterone + oestradiol	6	3	6.3 ± 0.7	< 0.005
	Progesterone + oestradiol	8	3	6.7 ± 0.8	< 0.005
Telencephalon	Control		10	3.5 ± 0.6	
	Progesterone	6	4	6.0 ± 0.2	< 0.005
	Progesterone	8	4	6.8 ± 1.2	<0.025
	Progesterone + oestradiol	4	3	6.3 ± 1.2	N. S.
	Progesterone + oestradiol	6	3	6.6 ± 1.3	N. S.

threshold voltage in the olfactory bulb appeared 6 to 8 days after progesterone or progesterone-oestradiol treatment. In the hippocampal regions, only progesterone produced a remarkable increase of threshold voltage (6 to 8 days after injection).

DISCUSSION

In a study we have made of oestrogenic hormone dose-response relationships in fish (*Oshima & Gorbman,* in press) and in unpublished research with progesterone (*Oshima & Gorbman,* unpubl.), we have found that higher dosages frequently reverse the effects found at lower dosages. The possible biphasic actions of hormones on the central nervous system, dependent on dosage, must be born in mind in interpreting any experiments, such as the present ones, in which only one level of hormonal dosage has been employed. Although the 10 μg dosages of hormone per 25 to 40 g of body weight would seem to be in the upper range of »physiological« level dosage no assumptions about this can be made without further study. Nevertheless, under these testing conditions it is clear that progesterone decreased the amplitudes of electrically evoked potentials in the forebrain of frogs and it increased threshold intensity; oestradiol increased response amplitudes, but had a similar effect on thresholds.

The depressant action found for pentobarbital sodium on evoked potentials (Fig. 1, Ae and Ce) coincided well with results of *Ottoson* (1959). *Ottoson* (1959) has reported progressively depressant action of Nembutal® given intraperitoneally at a dosage of 125 mg per frog upon olfactory bulbar potentials induced by electrical stimulation of the nasal mucosa. Depression of the evoked response patterns by progesterone was in our tests similar to the action of Nembutal®.

The inhibitory effect of progesterone and the facilitatory effect of oestradiol on amplitudes of evoked potentials in the olfactory bulb appeared by 2 days after hormone treatment and persisted up to 12 days after injection. On the other hand, hormonally influenced effects in the telencephalon were limited to a period about 6 to 8 days after treatment as shown in Fig. 2. This time-dependent difference of effects of sex hormones would seem to be explicable on the basis of specific regional properties in frog brains. However, the most significant changes in amplitude of the olfactory bulbar response generally occurred also 6 to 8 days after hormone treatment. The time course of changes in the threshold voltages, as shown in Fig. 3 and Table 1, concur roughly with these generalizations, but there are some apparent exceptions: relatively later changes in the bulb than in the hippocampal region.

With respect to response amplitude of steroid hormone-treated frogs, it seems possible to generalize that response properties of the olfactory bulb change more quickly than in telencephalon, but that the maximal changes in responsiveness of both of these parts of the brain peak at the same time, around 6 to 8 after hormone treatment.

Kawakami & Sawyer (1967) reported that the inhibitory effect of progesterone (2 mg) and certain other progestational compounds (1–25 mg) on the EEG after-reaction occurred 1–5 days after injection into female rabbits weighing 3 to 5 kg. *Kobayashi et al.* (1962) have reported that a few minutes after intravenous injection, progesterone (10–20 mg) had a marked depressant effect on the arousal reaction of the hippocampal EEG to posterior hypothalamic stimulation in rats weighing 150 to 250 g.

Clearly, the time course of effects of sex hormones on central nervous function depends upon species of the animal studied, on the parts of the brain tested, on the nature of the hormones, and the manner of their administration as well as on other experimental conditions.

When progesterone and oestradiol were given together, only 6 days after injection a significant decrease in response amplitude was seen in the olfactory bulb. This result indicates that the inhibitory effect of progesterone is dominant (at these dosage levels) over the stimulatory action of oestrogen alone and that the sensitivity to the time-dependent effects of sex hormones is reduced when the two hormones are given simultaneously.

In oestradiol-treated animals, threshold voltages were equal to, or below the control values; no significant difference could be obtained between experimentals and controls in spite of an increase in amplitudes of evoked potentials. These results are not like those in progesterone-treated animals. It is possible that oestradiol doses larger or smaller than 10 μg have affected threshold voltage as well as response amplitude.

Takagi (1962) has found that prior electrical stimulation of the anterior diencephalon inhibits the wave in the olfactory bulb evoked by stimulation of the olfactory nerve in frogs. He also found that facilitation occurred in a few cases. Considering these findings with respect to the present experiments, the inhibitory effects of progesterone on evoked potentials in the olfactory bulb may be due to its action on the centrifugal inhibitory mechanism, including the anterior parts of the diencephalon. Facilitatory effects of oestradiol can be explained in the same way. Furthermore, it is suggested that the dominant effect of progesterone over oestrogen can be due to differential sensitivities of the facilitatory and inhibitory centrifugal olfactory bulb regulating nervous mechanisms. As the centrifugal nervous system generally inhibits the afferent olfactory signals in the telencephalon (*Takagi* 1962; *Hara & Gorbman* 1967), inhibitory effects of progesterone on the evoked potentials in the telencephalon could presumably be due to an inhibitory mechanism in the olfactory bulb as well.

REFERENCES

Allison A. C.: J. comp. Neurol. *98* (1953*a*) 309.

Allison A. C.: Biol. Rev. *28* (1953*b*) 195.

Hara T. J. & Gorbman A.: Comp. Biochem. Physiol. *21* (1967) 185.

Herrick C. J.: Proc. Nat. Acad. Sci. *19* (1933) 7.

Kawakami M. & Sawyer C. H.: Endocrinology *80* (1967) 857.

Kobayashi T., Takezawa S., Oshima K. & Kawamura H.: Endocr. jap. *9* (1962) 302.

Oshima K. & Gorbman A.: Gen. comp. Endocr. *7* (1966*a*) 398.

Oshima K. & Gorbman A.: Gen. comp. Endocr. *7* (1966*b*) 482.

Oshima K. & Gorbman A.: J. Endocr. *40* (1968) 655.

Ottoson D.: Acta physiol. scand. *47* (1959) 160.

Takagi S. A.: Jap. J. Physiol.*12* (1962) 365.

Takagi S. A. & Shibuya T.: Jap. J. Physiol. *10* (1960) 99.

Effects of Sex Hormones on Photically Evoked Potentials in Frog Brain[1]

KIYOSHI OSHIMA AND AUBREY GORBMAN

Sites in the frog's optic tectum, diencephalon, and telencephalon were found to yield evoked patterns of electrical response to light flashes. In frogs treated with estradiol, testosterone, or progesterone in different doses, the amplitudes and latencies of these electrical responses were altered, each hormone having a particular and different action in different parts of the brain. It was concluded that the loci of hormonal responsiveness for each hormone are, at least in part, different and characteristic for the type of hormone. Furthermore, the optically evoked forebrain potentials varied greatly during the year, arguing for a natural cycle of humoral control over this phenomenon.

In earlier work dealing principally with fishes we have sought for and found phases of central nervous function that appear to be subject to endocrine regulation (Hara *et al.*, 1965; 1966; Oshima and Gorbman, 1966a,b; 1968). The nervous phenomena which lend themselves most readily to such analysis are evoked electrical responses of particular parts of the brain, since they are generally limited in time and subject to measurement. One of the difficulties in such exploratory work with lower vertebrates derives from the fact that descriptions of the properties of sensory evoked central phenomena often are few and sometimes controversial. An example of this situation may be seen in the descriptions of light-evoked responses of the forebrain.

Responses to photic stimulation have been recorded in the telencephalon outside the primary visual cortex in various lower vertebrates, in reptiles (Smirnov, 1961; Karamian *et al.*, 1966; Zagorulko, 1957; Mazurskaya *et al.*, 1967), amphibians

[1] This study was aided by a grant from the National Institutes of Health, No. NB 04887.

(Karamian *et al.*, 1966; Zagorulko, 1957; Boldyreva and Grindel, 1959; Voronin and Gusselnikov, 1959), and fishes (Enger, 1957). However, no cortical visual responses were observed in the forebrain of frogs by Buser (1955) or by Smirnov and Manteifel (1962), or Smirnov (1961). As for the regulation of the telencephalic responses to photic stimulation by hormones or similar agents in lower vertebrates, there is no published information.

This report will record the results of exploration in the frog's forebrain hippocampal region, in the diencephalon, and in the optic tectum for potentials evoked by photic stimulation in experiments conducted during several seasons of 1 year. Further, a comparison is made of the form, size, and latency of these responses between "normal" frogs, and specimens treated with exogenous progesterone, estrogen, or testosterone.

METHODS

Throughout the period August 1965 to April 1966 observations were made on a total of 109 frogs (*Rana pipiens*) of both sexes obtained from a commercial breeder (J. F. Schettle Frog Farm, Inc., Stillwater, Minnesota). Animals weighing between 25–40 g were treated in one of four ways: One group was given a total of either 5 or 50 μg of estradiol benzoate divided over 5 days; a second group similarly was given a total of either 5 or 50 μg of progesterone; a third group was given 50 μg testosterone propionate; a fourth group was given an equivalent volume of the hormone vehicle, sesame oil. These animals received an intramuscular injection of each hormone in a 0.05-ml volume or vehicle every day for 5 days and they were studied 7 days after the final injection. The number of animals in each group was 17–21. Pentobarbital sodium (Nembutal) (100 μg per 10 g body wt) was used in some experiments to compare its known depressive effects with the observed actions of the several tested hormones.

Animals were kept in an environment saturated with moisture at a relatively well controlled temperature (22 $\pm$ 1°) and with automatically limited periods of artificial lighting (10 hr daily). They were fed mealworms once a day. After moderate ether anesthesia and immobilization (gallamine-triethiodide, 0.04 mg per 10 g body wt, subcutaneously) the brain was exposed and the covering dura and arachnoid dissected from the dorsal side. The preparation was protected under a layer of mineral oil. Bipolar recording electrodes were made of two stainless-steel insect pins (No. 00) insulated by enamel except at sharpened tips (0.3-mm tip separation) (Oshima and Gorbman, 1966a). Bipolar surface recording of the EEG and photically evoked responses in the telencephalon, diencephalon, and optic tectum were amplified through Grass 5P5 amplifiers and displayed on a Grass Model 5 Polygraph or Tektronix #502 Oscilloscope.

Single photic stimuli of four different intensities (instrument setting 1, 2, 4, and 8) and of 10 μ sec duration were given by use of a Grass Photic Stimulater (Model PS-2) placed 100 cm from one of the eyes with the pupils dilated by topically applied atropine (horizontal candle power estimated approximately 1.5×10^6 with the instrument intensity setting at 16). The experiments were conducted in a darkened room in which the temperature was regulated near 22°.

Measurements were made of the peak to peak amplitudes of the maximum recorded component of the evoked response. Measurements were made also of the latency of the primary component after onset of the flash. The mean response amplitudes and latencies were computed for each of the test conditions. Usually 8–12 responses were recorded at each electrode position.

Throughout the Spring-Summer period May to July 1966, a separate group of 49 animals was tested at six intervals, about 8 animals at each time (the numbers of animals in each group are shown in Table 1). At each test frogs were given single intramuscular injections of one of the following: 10 μg progesterone, 10 μg testosterone propionate, 10 μg estradiol benzoate, 10 μg thyroxine, 10 μg progesterone combined with 10 μg estradiol, or sesame oil. Seven days after the hormone or hormone vehicle injection the frogs were tested for production of photically evoked potentials in the telencephalon. As additional indicators of seasonal variability in the telencephalic photically evoked response, 36 control animals given single injections of sesame oil were used throughout the autumn–winter period August 1965 to April 1966.

RESULTS

As illustrated in Fig. 1, photically evoked potentials recorded from the fore-

TABLE 1

SEASONAL CHANGES IN THE APPEARANCE OF PHOTICALLY EVOKED RESPONSES OF THE FROG TELENCEPHALON AND THEIR MODIFICATION BY SEX HORMONE TREATMENT

Period of experiments	Treatment[a]	% of Animals responsive to single light flashes[b]	Number of animals tested[c]
August 1965 to April 1966	Controls given Sesame oil	100%	36
May–July 1966	Controls given Sesame oil	30%	10
	Progesterone 10 μg	100%	8
	Progesterone 10 μg and estradiol 10 μg in Sesame oil	50%	8
	Testosterone 10 μg in Sesame oil	43%	7
	Estradiol 10 μg in Sesame oil	25%	8
	Thyroxine 10 μg in saline solution	25%	8

[a] Hormone was given by intramuscular single injection. Animal was tested 7 days after hormone administration.

[b] Photostimulator setting at intensity 8.

[c] 2–4 animals of each group were tested each month.

brain and the diencephalon differ from the evoked potentials in the midbrain optic tectum in form as well as latent period. Maximum amplitude of the responses increased in parallel with increasing intensity of the light flashes in all cases. In the optic tectum (except in testosterone-treated animals) usually a relatively more complex evoked wave form was found, as compared with the telencephalon or diencephalon. The evoked diencephalic

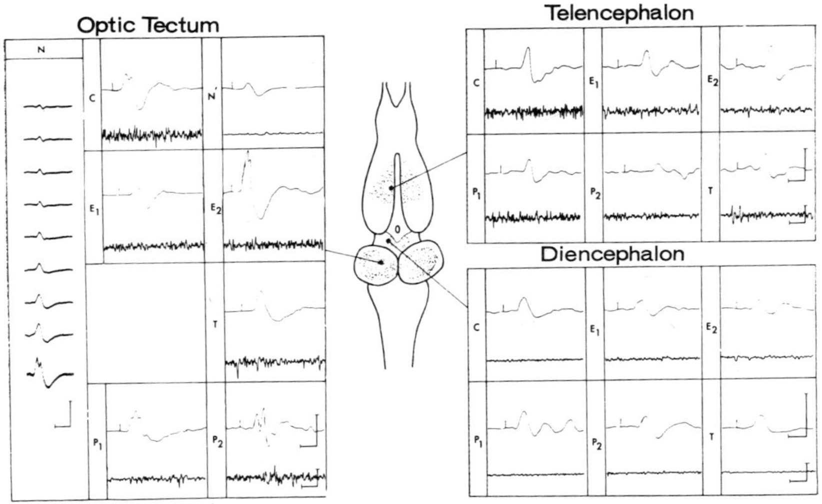

FIG. 1. EEG changes and electrical responses evoked by single light flashes in the forebrain, diencephalon, and optic tectum, and their alteration by steroid hormone treatment or by Nembutal. In the column at the left are oscillographic records. Calibration: 50 μV (vertical), 50 msec (horizontal). The remaining are pairs of polygraph recordings, the upper ones in each pair are single flash responses (calibration: 50 μV, 100 msec) and the lower ones are spontaneous EEG records (calibration: 50 μV, 1.0 sec) from the same animals. Previous treatment of the animals whose recordings are shown is represented by the following letters: C, sesame oil-injected control; N, Nembutal (0.2 mg per 10 g body wt); E_1, 5.0 μg estradiol benzoate; E_2, 50 μg estradiol benzoate; T, 50 μg testosterone propionate; P_1, 5.0 μg progesterone; P_2, 50 μg progesterone. Further details concerning dosage are in the text.

The time of the light flashes is at the indicated beginning of the oscilloscope records, and it is shown by a vertical mark on the polygraph tracings. The series of oscilloscope records at the left represent the single flash evoked responses in the optic tectum at successive 1-min intervals (reading upward) in one frog. The additional Nembutalized response shown (N′) is a polygraph record 4 min after injection of the anesthetic.

Stippling of the diagram showing a dorsal view of the frog brain indicates the areas from which photically evoked responses could be recorded readily.

responses were more stable but lower in amplitude. Typical examples are illustrated in Fig. 1. No striking or consistent changes of spontaneous EEG of the different brain regions followed the administration of sex steroids. Only in the optic tectum was there an obvious depression of spontaneous EEG after either Nembutal or progesterone treatment.

The focal zones within which photically evoked potentials can be obtained readily in responsive areas of the frog brain are shown in Fig. 1. Anatomically, these areas in the frog telencephalon appear to involve mainly the primordium hippocampi (15, 16). The electrically active area in the diencephalon may correspond to the habenula or the region of the dorsal nucleus of the thalamus, but more precise anatomical localization is not possible at this time.

Intraperitoneal injection of Nembutal in doses of 0.1–0.2 mg/10 g body wt led to decrease in amplitude and a prolonging of the latency of response (Fig. 1). For example, optic tectal responses initially occurring with latencies of 40–50 msec and with maximum amplitudes of 38–70 μV, have 60- to 90-msec latency periods and 15- to 36-μV amplitudes within 4–7 min after the administration of 0.2 mg/10 g body weight of Nembutal. Over a subsequent period of 50 min there is a gradual increase in intensity and variability in height of amplitude of the evoked response. Decrease in the maximum amplitude (compared with control) of photically evoked responses was characteristic of the optic tectum of animals treated with estrogen in doses of 5 μg and also in the telencephalon of animals given progesterone in doses of 50 μg in comparison with the control group as shown in Fig. 2. Estrogen in doses of 50 μg, on the other hand, increased the maximum amplitude of the responses in the optic tectum ($p < .01$, 50 μg estrogen vs. control). The photically evoked potential of the diencephalon did not change in amplitude following the administration of any of the test hormones.

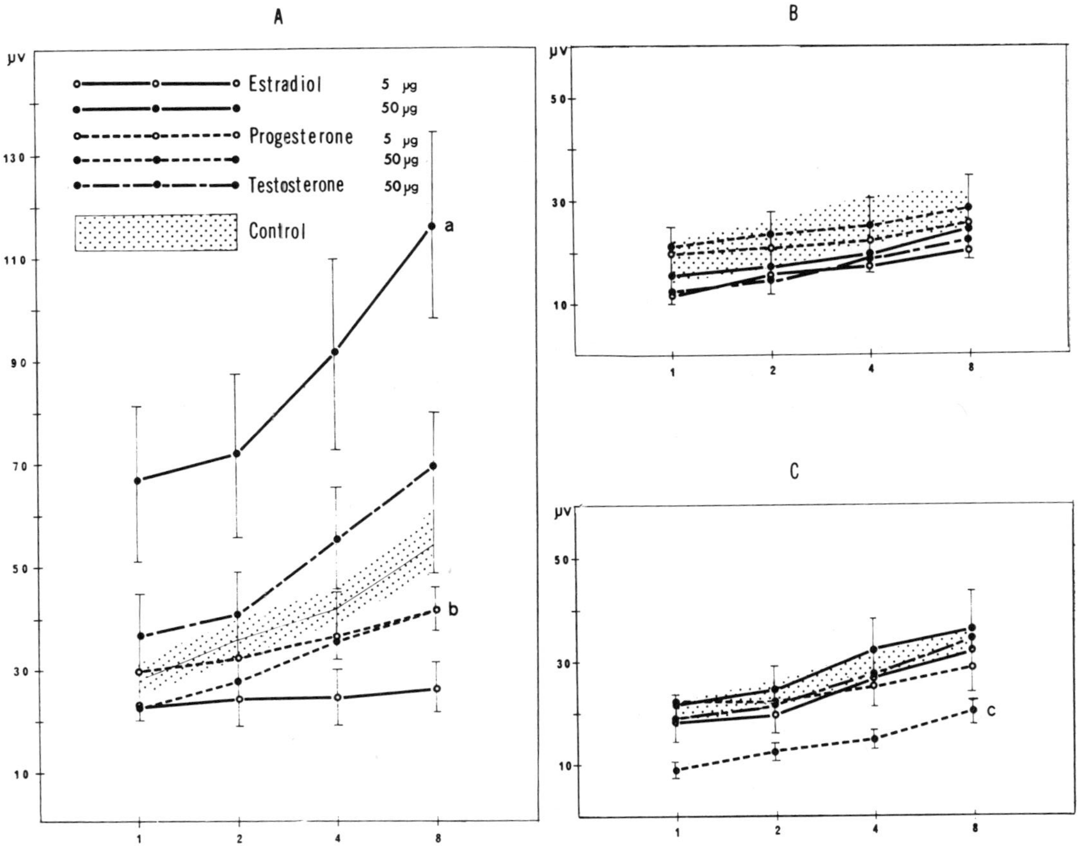

FIG. 2. Effects of sex hormones upon mean maximum amplitudes of the optic tectal (A), diencephalic (B), and telencephalic (C) photically evoked potentials at four different stimulus intensities (stimulator settings 1, 2, 4, and 8). Vertical limits of each point indicate standard error. a, $p < .01$; b, $p < .005$; c, $p < .05$ (t test).

In control frogs the mean latency of the telencephalic response to a single light flash at setting 8 was 144.0 ± 4.2 msec. The latency of the diencephalic response to the same stimulus was 83.8 ± 4.7 msec. The latency of the tectal response to such a stimulus was 47.6 ± 1.9 msec. The latency of the optic tectal evoked response was approximately 33% of that of the telencephalic response. Accordingly, it seems that the tectal process may play a primary role in the changes of latency of elements in the visual process. Also these findings provide evidence that a multisynaptic pathway is probably involved.

As illustrated in Fig. 3, a significant increase in latency of the photically evoked response in the optic tectum occurred in frogs previously treated with 50 μg progesterone (compared with control, $p < .001$). In the diencephalon, latency of the photically evoked potential increased in animals treated with 50 μg progesterone (98.9 ± 3.3 msec, $p < .025$) compared to control); an opposite effect on latency was obtained in animals given only 5 μg progesterone (68.6 ± 4.1 msec, $p < .05$ vs. control). A marked increase in latency of the photically evoked potential in the telencephalon occurred only in progesteronized frogs given doses of 50 μg. The prolonged telencephalic response latency was 163.1 ± 4.7 msec ($p < .01$ vs. control). On the other hand, a relatively remarkable decrease in telencephalic latency of photically evoked responses was obtained in animals treated with 50 μg testosterone (128.7 ± 3.6 msec, $p < .01$).

Throughout the period from August 1965 to April 1966 electrical responses could be photically evoked in the telencephalon in 100% of the experimental frogs tested. However, from May 1966 to July 1966 light flashes did not consistently evoke such responses in the telencephalon, while electrical responsiveness of the optic tectum remained unchanged. During this relatively unresponsive period, in only 30% of tested frogs did photic stimulation evoke

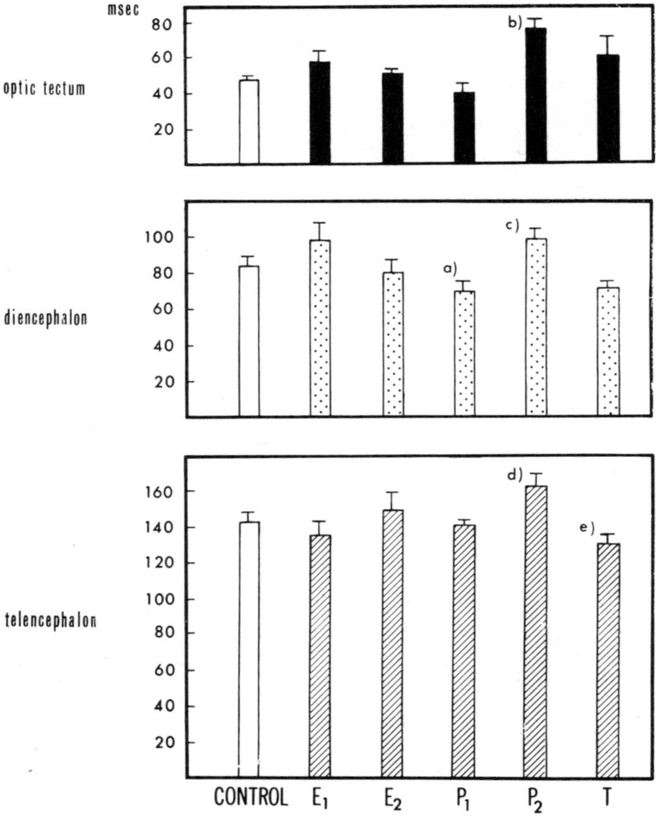

FIG. 3. Mean latencies in milliseconds ± standard error of photically evoked potentials from optic tectum, diencephalon, and telencephalon, following sex hormone treatment. Control, sesame oil-treated; E_1, 5 μg estrogen-treated; E_2, 50 μg estrogen-treated; P_1, 5 μg progesterone-treated; P_2, 50 μg progesterone-treated; T, 50 μg testosterone-treated. a, $p < .05$; b, $p < .001$; c, $p < .025$; d and e, $p < .01$ (t test).

a telencephalic electrical response. In the May–June 1966 period, injection of 10 μg of progesterone stimulated uniform telencephalic responsiveness to single light stimuli, but thyroxine, testosterone, or estrogen were not similarly effective (Table 1).

DISCUSSION

Our data show that there is a distinct annual cycle of responsiveness of the frog telencephalon to photic stimuli. This fact implies that there is some kind of seasonal humoral regulation of telencephalic activity. It also may serve to reconcile some of the apparent disagreement between different authors (cited in the introduction) who argue whether or not optic stimulation can evoke electrical forebrain responses in amphibians. As to which hormones are responsible for increased telencephalic responsiveness in non-summer seasons, or for decreased responsiveness in summer, the data presented here offer some possible enlightenment but perhaps no complete explanation. Progesterone in relatively small single doses, 10 μg, overcame the apparent inhibition for photic responses in the frog telencephalon in summer, while thyroxine, estradiol and testosterone were ineffective. In goldfish, Hara *et al.* (1965, 1966) have found that thyroxine facilitates responsiveness of the midbrain optic tectum to light flashes, and in lungfish Godet and Dupé (1965) have reported that thyroxine activates the telencephalic phase of an evoked olfactory response. Thus, if it is true, as our data suggest, that progesterone, but not thyroxine, facilitates the summer telencephalic photic response, then an apparent paradox exists: Thyroxine, which in many other kinds of situations acts as a nervous stimulant (Hara *et al.*, 1965, 1966; Godet and Dupé, 1965; Wilson *et al.*, 1964; Short *et al.*, 1964) is without effect, while progesterone, a nervous depressant or anesthetic (Sawyer and Kawakami, 1961; Woolley and Timiras, 1962; Kobayashi *et al.*, 1962) has a facilitatory effect. Even in other phases of the present series of experiments (Figs. 2 and 3), progesterone has a slightly inhibitory action on photic response amplitude in the telencephalon and tends to prolong response latency. It is of interest that Segura and DeJuan (1966) found in toads that electrical responses to photic stimulation are enhanced in spring and summer but diminished in winter. We have no explanation for the opposite character of the seasonal responsiveness of these two anuran species, but it deserves further study.

Endocrine modulation of optically evoked central nervous electrical events has been studied only to a limited extent. Most of the initial interest has centered on the influence of thyroid state in man upon responses to light flicker, recorded by EEG techniques. Lansing and Trunnel (1963), Wilson *et al.* (1964), and Oomura *et al.* (1963) found in such clinical trials that thyroid hormone has a sensitizing effect. In experimental animals, Bradley *et al.* (1960) found a potentiating influence of thyroxine (rats), and Hara *et al.* (1965, 1966) found in goldfish that thyroxine was stimulatory to various phases of the optic tectal response. It is of interest here that Hara *et al.* were unable to alter the character of optic tectal responses in goldfish by pretreatment with sex steroids.

In our experiments with three sex steroids given to frogs at two dose levels, estradiol produced the most remarkable changes in central photic responsiveness. These changes were greatest in the optic tectum and were related to hormonal dosage level (Figs. 2 and 3). The higher dose (50 μg of estradiol benzoate) facilitated the amplitude of response to the optic tectum but did not affect response latency. The lower dose, 5 μg depressed the response amplitude (with respect to the normal control frog) and slightly prolonged the latency. Estradiol did not appreciably alter the telencephalic response. Its only effect upon the diencephalic phase of the photic response was to prolong latency (lower dose only, Fig. 3).

Progesterone had relatively little effect

on photic response amplitude at the three recording sites, except for a depression of the response in the diencephalon by the higher (50 μg) dose. Progesterone affected response latency at all three points in the brain studied. Lower doses (5 μg) slightly shortened the latency, but 50-μg doses consistently prolonged the response latency (Figs. 2 and 3).

The biphasic dose-related responses of different nervous functional parameters to hormones appears to be quite general (Oshima and Gorbman, 1966a,b, 1968). We have found for both thyroxine and estradiol that several nervous effects characteristic of low doses of hormone increase up to a particular hormone dosage and then are more and more strongly reversed with further increases in hormone dosage. Reversal in phase of response by increasing hormone dosage must in itself indicate some basic general feature of the action of hormones on nerve cells and it should be studied in greater detail.

Testosterone given in a 50-μg dose, like the same dose of estradiol, facilitated the amplitude of the photic response in the frog optic tectum. Its action was limited to the optic tectum, however, unlike estradiol and progesterone which did produce some changes in the diencephalon and telencephalon (Figs. 2 and 3).

The long latency of the telencephalic photic responses recorded by us (130–160 msec) argues that they are propagated through polysynaptic pathways. Furthermore, the relatively shorter latencies of the diencephalic and optic tectal photic responses argues that these are primary events from which nervous pathways project to the telencephalon. In our own experiments, in considering the possible sites of hormonal sensitivity and hormonal responsiveness in the brain, more than this presumably direct pathway must be accounted for. For example, Brown and Marco (1967) have shown that thalamic stimulation in the cat increases the amplitude of evoked photic potentials in the visual cortex. Redding (1967) has observed a decrease in amplitude of cortical visual potentials after hippocampal stimulation. He interpreted this as a result of an inhibitory influence by the hippocampus on the brain stem reticular activating system.

Because of the complexity of the regulatory interrelationships between the diencephalon and forebrain, and other centers like the reticular formation, it is difficult on the basis of our observations to decide where the hormones are exerting their influence. Thus, because we found changes in photic response amplitude and/or latency in certain areas of the diencephalon or forebrain we could not justifiably claim that these areas are themselves the hormone-receptive sites. Further work will be needed in order to identify precisely the loci of steroid hormone sensitivity.

Meanwhile, it is clear that steroid hormone sensitivity exists in the brain, and that it can be expressed in terms of altered properties of the evoked photic response. The fact that such hormone sensitive loci are specific can be deduced from the fact that each hormone produces a different pattern of changes in amplitudes and latencies at particular points along the retino-telencephalic pathway of the photic response.

The importance of these results in specific terms of behavior and reproductive function remains to be evaluated. Photo-neuroendocrine mechanisms are basic in regulating and scheduling reproductive cycles (1964). Modulation of light-evoked potentials by sex hormones could be interpreted to mean that the primary sensitivity for triggering neuroendocrine reflexes to light changes is itself controlled by endocrine state. Our clear evidence of an annual cycle of photic responsiveness of the frog's telencephalon is a good example of this. These observations indicate that endocrine factors, probably different from those we actually tested (estradiol, testosterone, progesterone) are responsible for natural cycles of light responsiveness in the forebrain. Furthermore, since different tested sex steroids appear to have qualitatively different patterns of influence on features of the photic response in the brain, it is likely that these responses and their derivative phenomena are subject to a complex of alternative and interacting controls.

REFERENCES

Boldyreva, G. N., and Grindel, O. M. (1959). Investigation of the electrical activity of different areas of the brain in the frog. *Fiziol. Zh. Sechenov SSSR* **45,** 1037–1044.

Bradley, P. B., Eayrs, J. T., and Schmalbach, L. S. (1960). The electroencephalogram of normal and hypothyroid rats. *Electroencephalog. Clin. Neurophysiol.* **12,** 467–477.

Brown, T. S., and Marco, L. A. (1967). Effects of stimulation of the superior colliculus and lateral thalamus on visual evoked potentials. *Electroencephalog. Clin. Neurophysiol.* **22,** 150–158.

Buser, P. (1955). Analyse des réponses éléctriques du lobe optique a la stimulation de la voie visuelle chez quelques vertébrés inférieurs. Doct. Thèse, University Press, Masson, Paris.

Enger, P. S. (1957). The electroencephalogram of the codfish (*Gadus callarias*). *Acta Physiol. Scand.* **39,** 35–72.

Godet, R., and Dupé, M. (1965). Quelques aspects des relations neuroendocriniennes chez Protopterus annectens (poisson dipneuste). *Arch. Anat. Microscop. Morphol. Exptl.* **54,** 319–330.

Hara, T. J., Ueda, K., and Gorbman, A. (1965). Influences of thyroxine and sex hormones upon optically evoked potentials in the optic tectum of goldfish. *Gen. Comp. Endocrinol.* **5,** 313–319.

Hara, T. J., Gorbman, A., and Ueda, K. (1966). Influence of thyroid state upon optically evoked potentials in the midbrain of goldfish. *Proc. Soc. Exptl. Biol. Med.* **122,** 471–475.

Kappers, C. U. A., Huber, G. C., and Crosby, E. C. (1960). "The Comparative Anatomy of the Nervous System of Vertebrates, Including Man," Vol. III. Hafner, New York.

Karamian, A. I., Vesslkin, N. P., Belekhova, M. G., and Zagorulko, T. M. (1966). Electrophysiological characteristics of tectal and thalamocortical divisions of the visual system in lower vertabrates. *J. Comp. Neurol.* **127,** 559–576.

Kobayashi, K., Kobayashi, T., Takezawa, S., Oshima, K., and Kawamura, H. (1962). Electrophysiological studies on the feed-back mechanism of progesterone. *Endocrinol. Japon.* **9,** 302–320.

Lansing, R. W., and Trunnell, J. B. (1963). Electroencephalographic changes accompanying thyroid deficiency in man. *J. Clin. Endocrinol. Metabol.* **23,** 470–480.

Mazurskaya, P. Z., Davydova, T. V., and Smirnov, G. D. (1967). Functional organization of exteroceptive projections in the forebrain of the turtle. *Neuroscience Translations No. 1,* 109–117.

Noble, G. K. (1931). "The Biology of the Amphibia." McGraw-Hill, N. Y.

Oomura, Y., Ogata, S., and Ozaki, S. (1963). The effect of sodium on the slow muscle fiber. *Japan. J. Physiol.* **13,** 319–331.

Oshima, K., and Gorbman, A. (1966a). Influence of thyroxine and steroid hormones on spontaneous and evoked unitary activity in the olfactory bulb of goldfish. *Gen. Comp. Endocrinol.* **7,** 482–491.

Oshima, K., and Gorbman, A. (1966b). Olfactory responses in the forebrain of goldfish and their modification by thyroxine treatment. *Gen. Comp. Endocrinol.* **7,** 398–409.

Oshima, K., and Gorbman, A. (1968). Modification by sex hormones of the spontaneous and evoked bulbar electrical activity in goldfish. *J. Endocrinol.* **40,** 556–566.

Redding, F. K. (1967). Modification of sensory cortical evoked potentials by hippocampal stimulation. *Electroencephalog. Clin. Neurophysiol.* **22,** 74–83.

Sawyer, C. H., and Kawakami, M. (1961). Interactions between the central nervous system and hormones influencing ovulation. *In* "Control of Ovulation" (C. A. Villee, ed.), Pergamon Press, New York.

Scharrer, E. (1964). Photo-neuroendocrine Systems: General Concepts. *Ann. N. Y. Acad. Sci.* **117,** 13–22.

Segura, E. T., and DeJuan, A. (1966). Electroencephalographic studies in toad. *Electroencephalog. Clin. Neurophysiol.* **21,** 373–380.

Short, M. J., Hein, P., and Wilson, W. P. (1964). Thyroid hormone and brain function. III. Influence of triiodothyronine on evoked potentials of the cortex and reticular formation and upon the interrelationship of caudate and reticular activity of the cat. *Electroencephalog. Clin. Neurophysiol.* **17,** 414–419.

Smirnov, G. D. (1961). *In* "Brain and Behavior." Am. Inst. Biol. Sci., Washington, D. C.

Smirnov, G. D., and Manteifel, Y. B. (1962).

Comparative electrophysiological investigation of the brain over the evolutionary scale of vertebrates. *USP. Sov. Biol.* **54,** 309–332.

VORONIN, L. G., AND GUSSELNIKOV, V. I. (1959). Some comparative physiological data on bioelectrical brain reactions. *Zh. Vysshei Nervnoi Deatel'nosti Pavlova* **9,** 398–408.

WILSON, W. O., JOHNSON, J. E., AND FEIST, F. W. (1964). Thyroid hormone and brain function. II. Changes in photically elicited EEG responses following the administration of triiodothyronine to normal subjects. *Electroencephalog. Clin. Neurophysiol.* **16,** 329–331.

WOOLLEY, D. E., AND TIMIRAS, P. S. (1962). The gonad-brain relationship; effect of female sex hormones on electroshock convulsion in the rats. *Endocrinology* **70,** 196–209.

ZAGORULKO, T. M. (1957). On the localization of cerebral centers of the visual analyses in the frog. *Fiziol. Zh. Sechenov. SSSR* **43,** 1156–1165.

Olfactory Coding in Olfactory Bulb and Medial Forebrain Bundle of Normal and Castrated Male Rats

D. W. PFAFF AND E. GREGORY

PREVIOUS STUDIES of olfactory coding in vertebrates (4, 5, 8, 16–19) have indicated that few neurons in the olfactory system respond exclusively to a single odor or a small well-defined group of odors. This finding could mean that appropriate "elementary" odors have not been identified. In searching for such odors as would yield specific responses by olfactory neurons in rats, we have used natural odors which play an important role in guiding the rat's behavior. If the rat's olfactory system is organized to favor discrimination of behaviorally relevant odors important for survival, then perhaps such odors would yield the most specific responses. The odor of urine from behaviorally receptive female rats ("estrous females") evokes intense behavioral exploratory responses from male rats, while urine odors from behaviorally unreceptive females (ovariectomized females) evoke less intense behavioral responses (24). Also, rats can detect and discriminate odors of excretions from other rats which have been frightened by painful electric shock (9, 32, 34). In this study, urine samples from estrous and ovariectomized females, and from castrated and intact males (untreated or frightened by electric shock) were used as odor sources. Since the relevant volatile chemicals in rat urine have not been separated and identified, the use of these odors introduces problems of intensity control. In the present experiment the parameter controlled was dilution of the odor relative to odor-staturated air, because the absolute concentrations of the odorants in moles per liter could not be determined. This approach was chosen because previous work emphasizing the use of chromatographically purified nonbiological odorants has not by itself proved sufficient to yield specific responses by olfactory receptors (19). Also, beginning work with well-chosen but initially crude stimuli in other chemosensitive systems—namely, olfaction in the silkmoth *Bombyx* (27) and taste in the carp (11)—led to further understanding of those sensory systems.

Recording in this study included single-unit analysis in the preoptic region as well as in the olfactory bulb. The preoptic region is an anterior extension of the hypothalamus which has been linked to the hormonal control of reproductive functions by ablation and stimulation results (12, 26, 31) and by significant uptake of radioactive sex hormones (13, 14, 20, 21, 35). Neurons in the preoptic area—including many units in and around the medial forebrain bundle—respond to olfactory bulb shocks, and give truly olfactory responses to odors (as opposed to trigeminal or arousal responses) (23). This electrophysiological evidence of strong olfactory input to the preoptic area agrees with anatomical studies which show olfactory input to the medial forebrain bundle at the preoptic level (25, 28, 33) and with previous electrophysiological work on the medial forebrain bundle (1, 30).

Finally, since the preoptic region has been implicated in the control of pituitary function and mating behavior by sex hormones, recording was carried out both in normal and castrated male rats to look for effects of testicular androgens on olfactory coding. Earlier experiments suggested that acute testosterone injections in castrated male rats affect absolute levels of responses to odors, but do not consistently affect olfactory coding (23).

Thus, the three purposes of this study were *a*) to search for specific responses to odors, *b*) to compare recording in the olfactory bulb and preoptic area, and *c*) to search for androgenic hormone effects on olfactory coding.

METHODS

A total of 40 intact male rats and 67 males which had been castrated at least 2 weeks before were used for recording experiments. All were Sprague-Dawley rats weighing between 225 and 375 g and were sexually inexperienced. The rats were anesthetized with urethan (1.5 g/kg, ip). Before surgery and at 3-hr intervals during experimentation atropine was administered (0.3 mg/kg, sc).

After tracheotomy, a PE-205 polyethylene tube was pushed up the trachea from the site of tracheotomy into the back of the nose. Then and during the experiment air was drawn through the nose by applying a vacuum to this polyethylene tube. A rotating valve interposed in the vacuum line caused an intermittent application of the vacuum (an "artificial sniffer"), with a peak flow rate for each "sniff" of 3 liters/min.

Recording procedures and odor presentation

The head of the rat was stabilized in a stereotaxic instrument. After incision and retraction of the skin, the frontal bone dorsal to the olfactory bulb or the appropriate cortical region was thinned by drilling. The deepest layer of bone and the dura were then removed carefully with forceps.

Single units were recorded extracellularly with micropipettes filled with 3 M sodium chloride. Tip diameters were between 1 and 5 μ, with d-c resistances between 0.5 and 5 megohms. The reference electrode was clipped to the retracted skin. The micropipette was positioned using a micromanipulator according to a stereotaxic atlas (10).

Conventional recording procedures were used. Input from the micropipette was led, via a cathode follower, to a high-gain push-pull preamplifier, and then was displayed on an oscilloscope. Frequencies below 400 and above 10,000 Hz were filtered out. Permanent records of spike discharges were made on magnetic tape or on film (Grass kymograph camera). The frequency of spike discharges was quantitatively evaluated using a spike-frequency histogram generator equipped with a Schmitt trigger and a counting circuit. Adequacy of the counting procedure was monitored routinely on the oscilloscope. The output of the histogram generator was displayed on a Grass model 7 polygraph. The electroencephalogram and rectal temperature were monitored routinely.

For olfactory stimulation, air from a high-pressure line was cleaned by passing it through silica gel and activated charcoal, humidified by bubbling through distilled water, and passed by the nose of the rat at a rate measured with a flowmeter. A Harvard infusion pump was used to add measured amounts of odor-saturated air from a syringe to the stream of cleaned air. The odor-saturated air came from liter odorant-storage bottles with Teflon tops and stainless steel fittings that matched the 50-ml syringes used for odor delivery. Each odorant was contained in its own liter storage bottle and had its own 50-ml syringe to avoid cross contamination. Successive samplings from a given odorant's bottle were separated by more than 10 min, which was considered sufficient to resaturate the air in the closed bottle after a sample was withdrawn. In addition, to ensure saturation, the closed bottle was shaken after each use. Successive stimulus presentations to the rat were separated by more than 2 min, to avoid problems of adaptation.

Since the volatile chemicals in the rat urine stimuli used have not been separated and identified, it was not possible to specify physical concentration of odorants in moles per liter. Instead, the parameter controlled was dilution relative to saturated air. The relative dilution of a stimulus was specified as (ml/min odor-saturated air from syringe)/(cleaned air, ml/min + odor-saturated air, ml/min). In these experiments odors were diluted to between 1/100 and 1/10 of saturation. Stimuli were usually 12 or 24 sec long. Different stimuli were always compared at the same duration and relative dilution. Each stimulus was presented between 3 and 5 times during recording from each cell.

The 10 odorants used in this study are listed in Table 2. Nonurine odorants were the best grades available from a variety of chemical companies. Urine for use as odorant was collected from female (200–350 g) or male (300–450 g) Sprague-Dawley rats. Estrous females were brought into a state of receptivity (verified through behavioral testing with stud males) by subcutaneous injections of 0.2 mg estradiol benzoate in 0.2 ml sesame oil 48 hr before the beginning of urine collection, and 0.5 mg progesterone in 0.5 ml sesame oil at the beginning of urine collection. Other females had been ovariectomized at least 3 weeks before urine collection and received only injections of sesame oil. The male rat urine sources were either intact ("normal males"), or had been castrated at least 3 weeks before urine collection. Another group of intact males ("frightened males") were subjected to 5 min of painful intermittent electric foot shock (1–1.5 ma, 60 cycles) to frighten them immediately before the beginning of urine collection. The five groups of urine-source rats (estrous females, ovariectomized females, normal males, castrated males, frightened males) each consisted of four rats, a number considered large enough to minimize effects of individual differences unrelated to experimental treatment. Urine was collected over a 24 hr period in standard metabolism cages equipped with feces screens. It was used fresh or after storage in a frozen state for 24 hr.

Histological procedures and data analysis

During experiments, the coordinates of each track and depth of each cell were recorded. The bottoms of most electrode tracks were marked by lesions at the tip of the pipette (50 μa dc, for 50 sec). After the experiment, the brain was fixed by cardiac perfusion with 10% formalin. Serial sections 50 μ thick were cut, serially mounted, and stained with Weil or cresyl violet. Projected images of sections with electrode tracks were drawn and the position of each cell in a given track of known depth was calculated.

Spike frequencies were quantitatively determined from the writeout of the spike-frequency histogram generator or by counting spikes on film. The existence of a response to an odor was determined by magnitude of deviation away from resting activity compared to the variability of resting activity. When it was difficult to tell whether a deviation from average resting activity constituted a response or merely reflected random variation, standard parametric statistics were used to determine the statistical significance of the deviation. Units which did not respond to any odors were not included in tabulating the results unless other units in the same preparation did respond; i.e., negative results from completely unresponsive preparations are not included. Analyses were performed on the average peak-response magnitude determined from the several presentations of each stimulus for each cell. The average response magnitude was categorized in one of the following size classes: 25–49% change from resting activity, 50–74%, 75–99%, or 100+%.

Responses to odors could not always be categorized as simple excitation or inhibition. Occasionally a unit showed a biphasic response, usually with the excitation phase first, in response to a high odor concentration. Also, a few units showed weak excitatory responses when the resting activity was low, and weak inhibitory responses when resting activity was high. These various complex responses are designated as "mixed" responses in Table 2.

Recordings from normal male rats were from 38 units in the olfactory bulb and 38 units in the preoptic area, all of which were tested for responses to all 10 odorants used in this study. Recordings from castrated male rats were from 51 olfactory bulb units and 79 preoptic area units, each of which was tested for responses to five odors or less.

Recordings from the units tested with all 10 odorants were analyzed to determine whether the probability of response to 1 odorant was independent of the probabilities of responses to the other 9 odorants. The method of analysis depends on the fact that if the probabilities of responses to stimuli A and B are P_A and P_B, and if responses to A and B are independent of each other, then the probability of a neuron responding both to A and to B is $P_A \cdot P_B$ (ref 7, p. 133). For each possible pair of odors used, the probability of units responding to both odors of the pair was predicted by multiplying the proportions of units responding to each odor in the pair. The predictions from this method—which assumes independence of responses to the two odors—are plotted for each possible odor pair (10 odors, 45 possible odor pairs) on the abcissa of Fig. 1. On the ordinate is plotted, for each odor pair, the observed proportion of units which responded to both odors in the pair.

Recordings from both normal and castrated male rats were analyzed to determine the proportion of units which responded differently to the two odors in each possible pair. For each odor pair, a checklist of the type shown in Table 1 was constructed, and each unit which was tested for responses to both odors was tabulated in one of the four mutually exclusive categories shown. Differential response on the basis of response direction was scored if the response to one odor was excitatory, and to the other odor, inhibitory or mixed. Differential response on the basis of response magnitude was scored only if the two responses were in different response-size classes (see above) and if, in successive paired presentations of the two odors, responses to the same odor were always larger. When all the units were thus analyzed for that odor pair, the proportion of units responding differentially to the members of that pair was calculated by the method shown in Table 1. Then the entire procedure was repeated for a second odor pair, etc., until all possible odor pairs were analyzed. Some pairs compared two urine odors (e.g., estrous vs. ovariectomized female); other pairs compared two nonurine odors (e.g., amyl acetate vs. cineole, amyl acetate vs. benzaldehyde, cineole vs. benzaldehyde); finally, other pairs compared

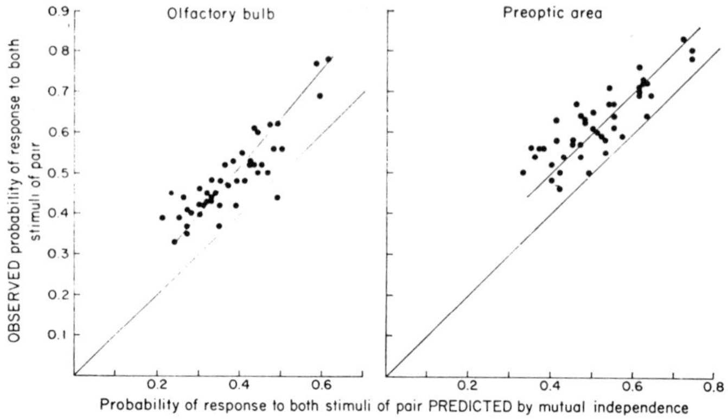

FIG. 1. Observed probabilities that units responded to both odors of a pair, compared to the probabilities expected from mutual independence of responsiveness to different odors (see METHODS). Each point represents results from 38 units for 1 odor pair. The 45 points in each graph represent the 45 possible pairs of 10 odorants. Analysis does not take into account whether response is excitatory or inhibitory. The line through the origin is that on which all points would fall if perfect independence was found. Best-fit (least-squares) lines are drawn through sets of data points.

urine with nonurine odors (e.g., estrous female urine vs. amyl acetate).

Differences between proportions of units in cell samples were tested for statistical significance with a standard parametric test (ref 7, p. 208). Best-fit lines were calculated by the least-squares method (ref 15, p. 119–123).

RESULTS

Occurrence of responses to odors

High percentages of both preoptic area units and olfactory bulb units responded to the various rat urine and nonurine odors (Table 2). The preoptic area sample included many units in and around the edges of the medial forebrain bundle. Table 2 includes combined results from normal and castrated male rats because there were no reliable differences between them in percentages of responding units.

Significantly more preoptic area units than olfactory bulb units responded to the female rat urine odors, primarily because of an increase in the number of inhibitory responses (Table 2). In general, preoptic units tended to give more responses to urine odors and to give more inhibitory responses to all odors than olfactory bulb units.

No units were found which responded with absolute specificity to one odor. Among 79 olfactory bulb units and 91 preoptic area units which were tested with three or more odors, all responded to at least two. However, five preoptic units and one olfactory bulb unit gave larger responses to estrous female urine odor than to any other odor; and five preoptic units and two olfactory bulb units responded in the opposite direction to the female urine odors, compared to responses to the other odors.

Units tested with all 10 odorants were analyzed to determine whether the probability that a unit responds to one odorant was independent of the probabilities of responses to the other nine odorants (see METHODS;

TABLE 1. *Method of tabulating differential responses by single units to two odors*

	Differential Response: Yes	Differential Response: No
Response to one and not the other	√	
Excited by one and inhibited the other?	√	
Responses in same direction but of consistently different magnitude?	√	
None of the above		√
Totals	A	B units

Percent units responding

$$\text{differentially} = \frac{A}{A + B} \times 100$$

TABLE 2. *Percent of units in male rat olfactory bulb and preoptic area responding to various odors*

	Olfactory Bulb					Preoptic Area				
	No. units tested	% Units respond	Direction of Response, % units			No. units tested	% Units respond	Direction of Response, % units		
			Exc	Inhib	Mix			Exc	Inhib	Mix
Urine odors										
Estrous ♀	89	65	47	12	6	116	88*	55	30*	3
Ovariectomized ♀	79	64	44	15	5	88	79†	49	29†	1
Normal ♂	38	53	28	17	8	38	65	39	23	3
Castrated ♂	38	44	18	18	8	38	63	37	18	8
Frightened ♂	38	57	42	12	3	38	58	42	13	3
Nonurine odors										
Amyl acetate	84	88	70	11	7	102	90	61	27†	2
Cineole	72	80	54	19	7	95	80	51	25	4
Benzaldehyde	53	72	56	8	8	44	81	39	40*	2
Heptane	38	76	47	11	18	38	73	47	23	3
Phenethyl alcohol	38	58	42	11	5	38	56	32	21	3

Data in this table are from normal and castrated male samples combined because there were no significant differences between them. Respond = responding. Exc = excited, Inhib = inhibited, Mix = mixed. Different from olfactory bulb. *$P < .005$. †$P < .05$.

N = 38 olfactory bulb units and 38 preoptic area units). In Fig. 1 the observed probability of response to both odors in a pair is plotted against the probability expected if responses to the two odors were mutually independent. The 45 points in each graph represent the 45 possible odor pairs. No single point by itself in either graph is significantly different from the probability expected from mutual independence. However, in both the olfactory bulb and the preoptic area, the points for virtually all odor pairs are regularly arranged above the predicted line, thus indicating a degree of mutual dependence among all the odors used in this experiment.

Differential response analyses

Recordings from normal and castrated male rats were analyzed for differential responding by each unit for each possible odor pair. Responses of a unit to two odors could be counted as different on the basis of any one of three criteria: a) presence versus absence of response, b) excitation versus inhibition, or c) consistent difference of response magnitude (see METHODS, Table 1). For example, Fig. 2 shows a preoptic area unit in the medial forebrain bundle which responded differentially to three odors on the basis of response magnitude.

A high proportion of preoptic area units responded differently to estrous female urine odor than to ovariectomized female urine, whereas only a low proportion of olfactory bulb units did so (Fig. 3). The opposite was true for discrimination among nonurine odors: a higher proportion of olfactory bulb units than preoptic area units responded differentially to the members of each pair of nonurine odors (Fig. 3). A high proportion (70–80%) of all units, both in the olfactory bulb and in the preoptic area, responded differently to urine odors than to nonurine odors. The results of these differential response analyses were essentially the same in castrated as in normal male rats.

Additional results from the larger set of urine odors used for recording from normal males (Table 3) indicated that the sharpened urine odor discrimination by preoptic area units was specific for the female urine odors. No other combination of urine odors showed the significant increase of discrimination from olfactory bulb to preoptic area units shown by estrous versus ovariectomized female urine odors. Use of these additional urine odors also revealed interesting differences among the urine discriminations by olfactory bulb units. Whereas only a low percentage of olfactory bulb units

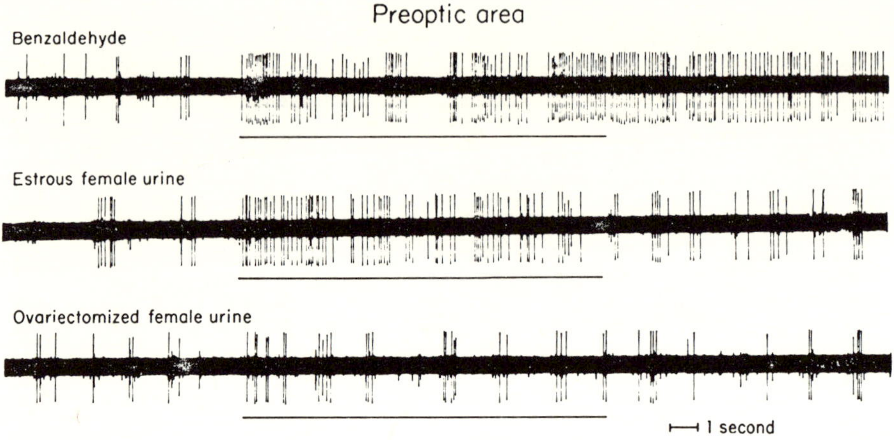

FIG. 2. Responses by a unit in the medial forebrain bundle to three odors (dilution: $\frac{1}{10}$ of saturation). Benzaldehyde regularly gave the largest responses, and ovariectomized female urine odor the smallest reponses from this unit.

responded differentially to two urine odors from the same-sex rat (estrous vs. ovariectomized female; normal vs. castrated male), a significantly higher percentage responded differentially if the two urine odors were from rats of different sex (Table 3).

The extent of the preoptic region and medial forebrain bundle recorded from is shown in Fig. 4. Recordings were distributed throughout the area shown. Neither units which responded to female urine odors nor those which gave differential responses to the two female odors were distinguished by locations clearly different from locations of other units. Olfactory bulb recordings were almost always in or near the mitral cell layer. They were distributed along the length of the bulb from the anterior tip, back to the frontal sinus, but no major aspect of the results seemed to depend on how far anterior the cell was located.

DISCUSSION

Many responses to odors of estrous and ovariectomized female urine were recorded from units in the olfactory bulb and preoptic area. However, no units were found which responded exclusively to either urine stimulus. Such specific-responding cells may not exist in the rat brain. However, failure to find such units could also be due to difficulty in isolating them with the recording techniques used, to an unfortunate selection of recording sites or stimuli, poor preservation of the natural products used, or to complicating effects of anesthesia. Another qualification is that, since odor concentration was not measured in terms of moles per liter (in fact, the relevant volatile chemicals in urine have not been identified), units may actually have been responding to very low absolute concentrations of urine odors. Responses by single units in the female mouse to male mouse urine odors (29) are similar to rats in that no absolutely specific responses were found in the olfactory bulb or medial forebrain bundle.

The probabilities of mutual responsiveness to different odors by individual cells were higher than what would be expected if the distribution of responsiveness for each odor were independent of the distributions for other odors. Probabilities close to the expected distribution have been reported for recording from peripheral taste nerves (6). Two limitations on the inferences from this kind of statistical analysis should be noted. First, the deviation of the entire set of points from the mutual independence line may be a statistical artifact of pooling results from large numbers of preparations which vary among

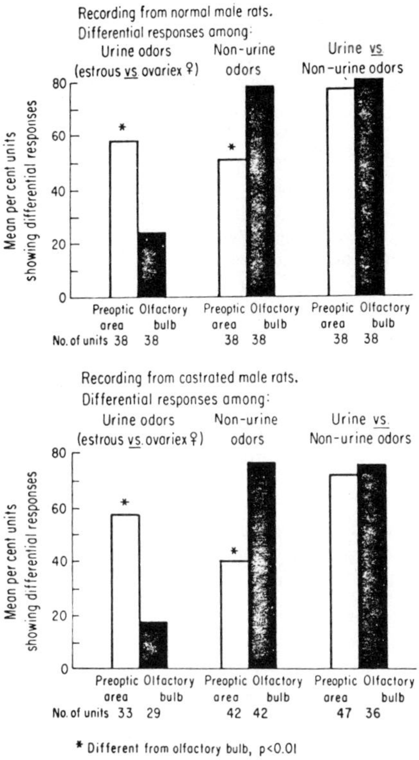

FIG. 3. Differential responses between female urine odors were more prevalent in the preoptic area than olfactory bulb. The opposite was true of differential responses among nonurine odors. The pair of bars on the left shows differential responses to estrous, compared to ovariectomized female urine odor. The pair of bars in the middle shows differential responses between nonurine odors (e.g., amyl acetate vs. cineole). The pair of bars on the right shows differential responses between odors in a pair, where each pair compared one urine and one nonurine odor (e.g., estrous female urine vs. amyl acetate).

themselves in overall sensitivity to olfactory stimulation (22). Second, the pair-by-pair analysis is not an exhaustive analysis for mutual independence, which would require considering all possible response combinations for the 10 odorants taken 10 at a time. The latter was not performed because thousands of cells would have been required in order to assess the relative numbers in each of the 2^{10} response categories.

Differential response analyses, taking into

TABLE 3. *Percent units showing differential responses among urine odors*

Odor Discrimination	Percent Differential Responses: Olfactory bulb	Preoptic area
Within a sex:		
Estrous vs. ovariex ♀	24	58*
Normal vs. castrate ♂	28	38
Between sexes:		
Castrate ♂ vs. ovariex ♀	48	54
Castrate ♂ vs. estrous ♀	60†	65
Normal ♂ vs. ovariex ♀	61†	59
Normal ♂ vs. estrous ♀	59†	75
Fear (electric shock)		
Frightened vs. normal ♂	50	64
Frightened vs. castrate ♂	52	56
Fear + sex difference		
Frightened ♂ vs. estrous ♀	66†	58
Frightened ♂ vs. ovariex ♀	69†	62

Data are recordings from normal male rats. * Preoptic area different from olfactory bulb, $P < .01$. † Differential responses significantly greater than "within a sex" discriminations, $P < .01$.

account the direction and magnitude of response, showed that cells in the preoptic area gave more differential responses to female urine odors than cells in the olfactory bulb, even though the opposite was true for nonurine odors (Fig. 3). This is particularly interesting since the preoptic

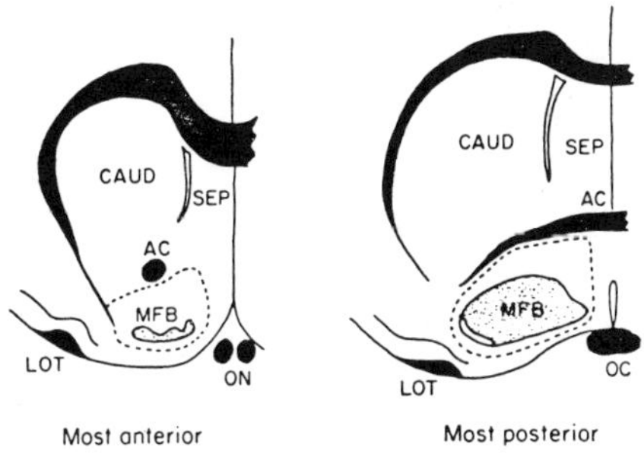

FIG. 4. Dotted lines show extent of recording sites in preoptic area around medial forebrain bundle. The coronal sections drawn represent the most anterior (*left*) and most posterior (*right*) sites of recording in preoptic area. CAUD, caudate nucleus; SEP, septum; AC, anterior commissure; MFB, medial forebrain bundle; LOT, lateral olfactory tract; ON, optic nerves; OC, optic chiasm.

area has been implicated in the control of mating behavior and pituitary function (see introduction).

The enhanced discrimination for female urine odors by preoptic area units was not androgen dependent, for similar results were seen in normal and castrated male rats. This is consistent with previous results of injecting testosterone acutely while recording from castrated males (23). In the previous experiments, even though spontaneous activity or absolute magnitudes of olfactory responses by preoptic area units were often affected by testosterone injection, there was no regular tendency for responses to the two female odors to be affected differently from each other; i.e., responses to the two odors were not regularly made more or less discriminable from each other. These electrophysiological results are paralleled by behavioral results. Although the behavioral preference of male rats for female urine odors, measured by the amount of time they spontaneously investigate such odors, is androgen dependent (24); the detection and discrimination of female urine odors by male rats is not androgen dependent (2, 3). Thus, it is possible that the differential responses by single units, reported above, are related to behavioral functions of detection and discrimination, and that neither the differential responses nor the behavioral discrimination depend on androgen levels.

SUMMARY

1) A high proportion of units in the olfactory bulb and preoptic area (including medial forebrain bundle) of male rats responded to odors from female rat urine as well as to other odors. *2*) No units were observed which responded only to one odor. *3*) The proportions of units in the olfactory bulb and preoptic area responding to either member of odor pairs were higher than those predicted from mutual independence of responses to different odors. *4*) More units in the preoptic area than in the olfactory bulb responded differentially to estrous compared to ovariectomized female urine odors. The opposite was true of differential responses to nonurine odors. *5*) A high proportion of all units, in the olfactory bulb and preoptic area, responded differently to any given urine odor compared to any given nonurine odor. *6*) Proportions of responding units and differential responses were essentially the same in castrated as in normal male rats.

ACKNOWLDEGMENTS

This study was supported by the Biomedical Division of the Population Council, by National Science Foundation Grant GB-4198X to C. Pfaffmann and by National Institutes of Health Grant NS-08902-01.

We thank Miss Minna Spencer and Mr. Charles Marboe for excellent assistance, and Dr. Carl Pfaffmann, Dr. Marion Frank, and Dr. Robert O'Connell for helpful suggestions concerning the experiments and manuscript.

REFERENCES

1. Barraclough, C. and Cross, B. Unit activity in the hypothalamus of the cyclic female rat: effect of genital stimuli and progesterone. *J. Endocrinol.* 26: 339–359, 1963.
2. Carr, W. J. and Caul, W. F. The effect of castration in rat upon the discrimination of sex odours. *Animal Behavior* 10: 20–27, 1962.
3. Carr, W. J., Solberg, B., and Pfaffmann, C. The olfactory threshold for estrous female urine in normal and castrated male rats. *J. Comp. Physiol. Psychol.* 55: 415–417, 1962.
4. Döving, K. B. An electrophysiological study of similarities of homologous substances. *J. Physiol., London* 186: 97–109, 1966.
5. Döving, K. B. Analysis of odour similarities from electrophysiological data. *Acta Physiol. Scand.* 68: 404–418, 1966.
6. Frank, M. and Pfaffmann, C. Taste nerve fibers: a random distribution of sensitivities to four tastes. *Science* 164: 1183–1185, 1969.
7. Freund, J. E. *Modern Elementary Statistics.* Englewood Cliffs, N.J.: Prentice-Hall, 1952.
8. Gesteland, R. C., Lettvin, J. Y., and Pitts, W. H. Chemical transmission in the nose of the frog. *J. Physiol., London* 181: 525–559, 1965.
9. King, M. G. Stimulus generalization of conditioned fear in rats over time: olfactory cues and adrenal activity. *J. Comp. Physiol. Psychol.* 69: 590–600, 1969.
10. König, J. F. and Klippel, R. A. *The Rat Brain.* Baltimore: Williams & Wilkins, 1963.
11. Konishi, J. and Zotterman, Y. Taste functions in fish. In: *Olfaction and Taste, I,* edited by Y. Zotterman, New York: Pergamon, 1963, p. 215–233.
12. Lisk, R. D. Sexual behavior; hormonal control. In: *Neuroendocrinology,* edited by L. Martini and W. Ganong. New York: Academic, 1967, vol. 2, p. 197–239.
13. McEwen, B. S. and Pfaff, D. W. Factors in-

fluencing sex hormone uptake by rat brain regions. I. Effects of neonatal treatment, hypophysectomy and competing steroid on estradiol uptake. *Brain Res.* 21: 1–16, 1970.
14. McEwen, B. S., Pfaff, D. W., and Zigmond, R. E. Factors influencing sex hormone uptake by rat brain regions. II. Effects of neonatal treatment and hypophysectomy on testosterone uptake. *Brain Res.* 21: 17–28, 1970.
15. McNemar, Q. *Psychological Statistics.* New York: Wiley, 1962.
16. Moulton, D. G. Electrical activity in the olfactory system of rabbits with indwelling electrodes. In: *Olfaction and Taste, I,* edited by Y. Zotterman. New York: Pergamon, 1963, p. 71–84.
17. Moulton, D. G. Spatio-temporal patterning of response in the olfactory system. In: *Olfaction and Taste, II,* edited by T. Hayashi. New York: Pergamon, 1967, p. 109–117.
18. Mozell, M. M. Olfactory discrimination: electrophysiological spatiotemporal basis. *Science* 143: 1336–1337, 1964.
19. O'Connell, R. J. and Mozell, M. M. Quantitative stimulation of frog olfactory receptors. *J. Neurophysiol.* 32: 51–63, 1969.
20. Pfaff, D. W. Uptake of estradiol-17B-H^3 in the female rat brain. An autoradiographic study. *Endocrinology* 82: 1149–1155, 1968.
21. Pfaff, D. W. Autoradiographic localization of radioactivity in rat brain after injection of tritiated sex hormones. *Science* 161: 1355–1356, 1968.
22. Pfaff, D. W. Statistical effects of sensitivity differences among neurophysiological preparations. *J. Theoret. Biol.* In press.
23. Pfaff, D. W. and Pfaffmann, C. Olfactory and hormonal influences on the basal forebrain of the maie rat. *Brain Res.* 15: 137–156, 1969.
24. Pfaff, D. W. and Pfaffmann, C. Behavioral and electrophysiological responses of male rats to female rat urine odors. In: *Olfaction and Taste, III,* edited by C. Pfaffmann. New York: Rockefeller Univ. Press, 1969, p. 258–267.
25. Powell, T. P. S., Cowan, W. M., and Raisman, G. The central olfactory connexions. *J. Anat.* 99: 791–813, 1965.
26. Sawyer, C. H. Reproductive behavior. In: *Handbook of Physiology. Neurophysiology.* Washington, D.C.: Am. Physiol. Soc., 1960, sect. 1, vol. II, chapt. 49, p. 1225–1240.
27. Schneider, D. Electrophysiological investigation of insect olfaction. In: *Olfaction and Taste, I,* edited by Y. Zotterman. New York: Pergamon 1963, p. 85–103.
28. Scott, J. W. and Leonard, C. M. The olfactory connections of the lateral hypothalamus in the rat, mouse and hamster. *J. Comp. Neurol.* In press.
29. Scott, J. and Pfaff, D. W. Behavioral and electrophysiological responses of female mice to male mouse urine odors. *Physiol. Behav.* 5: 407–411, 1970.
30. Scott, J. and Pfaffmann, C. Olfactory input to the hypothalamus: electrophysiological evidence. *Science* 158: 1592–1594, 1967.
31. Szentagothai, J., Flerko, B., Mess, B., and Halasz, B. *Hypothalamic Control of the Anterior Pituitary.* Budapest: Akademiai Kiado, 1968.
32. Valenta, J. G. and Rigby, M. K. Discrimination of the odor of stressed rats. *Science* 161: 599–601, 1968.
33. Valverde, F. *Studies on the Piriform Lobe.* Cambridge: Harvard Univ. Press, 1965.
34. Weiss, J. M., McEwen, B. S., Silva, M. T. A., and Kalkut, M. F. Pituitary-adrenal influences on fear responding. *Science* 163: 197–199, 1969.
35. Zigmond, R. E. and McEwen, B. S. Selective retention of estradiol by cell nuclei in specific brain regions of the ovariectomized rat. *J. Neurochem.* 17: 889–899, 1970.

CORRELATION BETWEEN PRE-OPTIC AREA UNIT ACTIVITY AND THE CORTICAL ELECTROENCEPHALOGRAM: DIFFERENCE BETWEEN NORMAL AND CASTRATED MALE RATS[1]

DONALD W. PFAFF AND ESTELLE GREGORY

Some neurons in the mesencephalic reticular formation (Schlag and Balvin 1963; Pfaff and Pfaffmann 1969), hypothalamus (Komisaruk *et al.* 1967; Ramirez *et al.* 1967; Lincoln 1969a) and pre-optic area (Pfaff and Pfaffmann 1969) exhibit significant changes in resting discharge rates when the cortical EEG shows the sudden transitions between synchrony and desynchrony (activation) typical of the urethane-anesthetized rat preparation. The correlation of neuron discharge rates with cortical EEG state affects the interpretation of hormone-induced changes in neuronal activity, especially limiting claims for specificity of hormone effect on the brain (Komisaruk *et al.* 1967; Lincoln 1969b). We report here evidence that the correlation, itself, between pre-optic unit activity and the cortical EEG is affected by circulating androgens in male rats. Further observations were made to describe functional characteristics of EEG-correlated pre-optic neurons.

METHODS

Experiments were performed on eighty-three Sprague-Dawley rats obtained from Charles River Breeding Laboratories, weighing between 200 and 350 g. None was sexually experienced. Rats were either intact ($N = 42$), or were castrated ($N = 41$) at least 2 weeks before being used, in order to reduce endogenous levels of testicular androgens. The rats were anesthetized with urethane (1.5 g/kg, i.p.). Before surgery and at 3 h intervals during experimentation, atropine (0.3 mg/kg, s.c.) was administered to reduce mucus secretion.

A routine tracheotomy was performed. Then, one PE205 polyethylene tube was inserted for respiration, and a second was inserted from the site of tracheotomy into the back of the nose to draw air through the nose for olfactory stimulation. To this second tube was attached a vacuum line running through a rotating valve, thus applying an intermittent, controlled vacuum to the back of the nose, creating an "artificial sniffer". The air drawn through the nose was either from a cleaned air stream or a mixture of cleaned and odor-saturated air. Other details of the olfactory stimulation procedures have been described (Pfaff and Pfaffmann 1969; Pfaff and Gregory 1971).

Recording procedures

The head of the rat was stabilized in a stereotaxic instrument. After incision and retraction of the skin, the bone dorsal to the olfactory bulb or the appropriate cortical region was thinned by drilling. The deepest layer of bone and the dura were then removed carefully with forceps.

Single units were recorded extracellularly with micropipettes filled with 3 *M* sodium chloride. Tip diameters were between 1 and 5 μ, and DC resistances were between 0.5 and 5 MΩ. The reference electrode was clipped to the retracted skin. The micropipette was positioned with the

[1] Supported by National Institutes of Health (NIH) Grant NS-08902-01, and by NSF grant 4198X to C. Pfaffmann. The second author is a post-doctoral trainee with a stipend from the NIH Training Grant GM-01789-03 BHS.

use of a micromanipulator (La Précision Cinématographique), according to the stereotaxic atlas of Konig and Klippel (1963), except for the olfactory bulb, for which an atlas was not required. Input from the micropipette was led to a Grass P6 pre-amplifier and then to a Tektronix 502 oscilloscope and an audio monitor. Frequencies below 400 and above 10,000 c/sec were filtered out. Permanent records of spike discharges were made on magnetic tape (Magnecord model 1048) or on film (Grass Kymograph Camera). The frequency of spike discharges was evaluated quantitatively with the use of a spike frequency histogram generator equipped with a Schmitt trigger and a counting circuit. The output of the counting circuit was displayed above the EEG on a Grass Model 7 polygraph. The cortical EEG was recorded from two screws set in the bone over the cortex, one in the parietal bone and the other in the frontal bone on the same side. Frequencies below 1 and above 75 c/sec were filtered out, and the EEG was amplified with the Grass 7P3A pre-amplifiers on the polygraph.

During experiments the coordinates of each track and depth of each cell were recorded. The bottoms of most electrode tracks were marked by lesions at the tip of the pipette (50 μA DC, for 50 sec). After the experiment the brain was fixed by cardiac perfusion with 10% neutral formalin. Serial sections 50 μ thick were cut, serially mounted and stained with Weil or cresyl violet. Projected images of sections with electrode tracks were drawn, and the position of each cell in a given track of known depth was calculated.

Data analysis

Relations between unit activity and the EEG were evaluated with spike frequencies determined quantitatively by the histogram generator and displayed above the cortical EEG record. Only records 20 min or longer (ranging to a maximum of 3 h 10 min) were selected for analysis. Unit activity and EEG both during "resting" and "stimulated" (usually olfactory) states were included, but almost all of the samples analyzed, in practice, came from the resting activity. The median spike frequency was determined for each record. The distinction between EEG synchrony (predominant large amplitude, low frequency activity) and desynchrony ("activation"; predominant small amplitude, high frequency activity) is almost always obvious in the urethanized rat preparation, since the transitions are abrupt and large. The few intermediate EEG samples were discarded. Ten sec samples were selected at regular intervals in the record, spaced such that the entire record would yield 40–80 samples for χ^2 analysis. Each sample showed unit activity either above or below the median rate, and the EEG either in synchrony or desynchrony. The data for each cell were thus subjected to a 2×2 χ^2 analysis (Siegel 1956). For instance, a unit that reliably increased firing rate during EEG activation would have high numbers of samples in the "activity above median—EEG desynchrony" and "activity below median—EEG synchrony" boxes and low numbers of samples in the "activity below median—EEG desynchrony" and "activity above median—EEG synchrony" boxes, yielding a significant χ^2 value. The proportion of units showing significant relation to the EEG from normal males was compared to the proportion from castrates using a standard parametric method for differences between proportions (Freund 1952).

Records from the 37 cells in the normal male's pre-optic area which showed significant correlations with EEG state—the largest group of EEG correlated cells—were analyzed to see which changed first at each EEG transition, the activity of the unit or of the EEG. For this analysis, EEG transitions from desynchrony to synchrony were treated separately from transitions from synchrony to desynchrony, since precedence relations for one type of transition could be different from those for the other. At each EEG transition the point of sudden EEG change (if any) was identified and marked. Then if unit activity changed significantly from its pre-transition average before this point, "cell changed first" was recorded. If unit activity remained at its pre-transition level until after the EEG change and then was altered, "EEG changed first" was recorded. An "indeterminate" category had to be established in order to record those cases in which: (a) unit firing before EEG transition was so variable that the exact second of unit change could not be determined; (b) the transitions (EEG and unit) were gradual and overlapping;

(c) there may have been a small time difference between EEG and unit transition, but this could not be proven clearly with the slow paper speed used; or (d) the unit did not change at all, with that particular EEG transition. Differences between proportions of transitions in which EEG changed first were tested with a standard parametric method (Freund 1952). The difference in the pattern of precedence relations between "desynchrony to synchrony" and "synchrony to desynchrony" transitions was tested with the 2×2 χ^2 test (Siegel 1956).

responses and excitation during EEG activation —was tested using the 3×3 χ^2 test (Siegel 1956). It should be noted that the physiological alterations giving rise to the EEG correlations were not predominantly the olfactory responses themselves but were spontaneous changes.

RESULTS

Comparison of normal and castrated males

Some units in the pre-optic area showed resting activity changes correlated with cortical

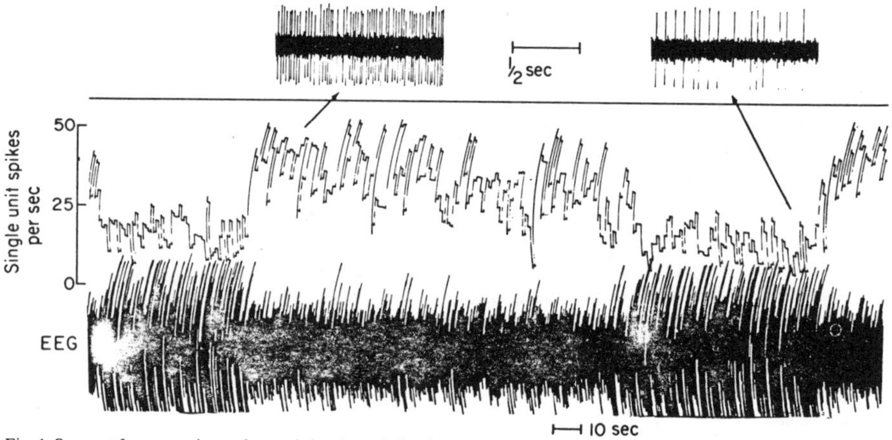

Fig. 1. Segment from experimental record showing relation between resting discharge of a pre-optic area single unit and the cortical EEG. Unit tended to increase firing rate during EEG desynchrony (activation). Recording from urethane-anesthetized normal male rat. Above: photographic samples of single unit activity during EEG activation (left) and EEG synchrony (right). Center: spike frequency histogram. Below: cortical EEG.

Results from normal male pre-optic area cells ($N=53$) were tabulated according to whether the cell gave excitatory or inhibitory responses to odors (the stimulus modality most frequently tested) and whether the cell showed significantly increased or decreased activity during EEG activation. The results of this tabulation were the same regardless of the odor for which responses were tabulated. Therefore, an average response direction for all odors was used. The deviation from chance expectation of the grouping of these two properties—excitatory olfactory

EEG changes (Fig. 1). The proportion of pre-optic units showing significant correlation to the EEG was significantly larger in normal male than in castrated male rats (Fig. 2). A similar comparison for recording from olfactory bulb units showed no difference between normal and castrated males. In the pre-optic area, the higher proportion of EEG-correlated cells in normal males resulted from the larger number of cells (than in the castrate) showing the relation typical of reticular formation cells (Schlag and Balvin 1963; Pfaff and Pfaffmann 1969); *i.e.*, there were

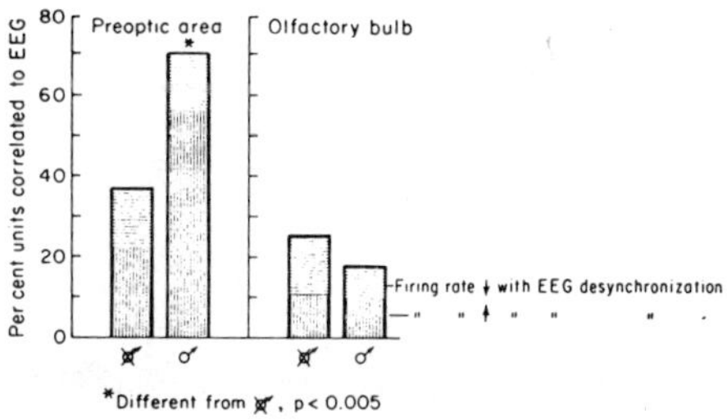

Fig. 2. Percent of units in pre-optic area and olfactory bulb whose resting discharge rate showed significant relation to cortical EEG state. In pre-optic area, significantly more units were related to EEG in normal male (♂) than in castrated male (☿) rats. Number of units sampled: Pre-optic area ♂ 53; ☿ 34; olfactory bulb ♂ 40, ☿ 32 units.

more cells that increased activity significantly during EEG activation ($P < 0.005$).

Characteristics of EEG-correlated cells

Records from cells in the normal male pre-optic area which showed significant correlations to the EEG state were analyzed to see which changed first at each EEG transition, the unit's activity or the EEG. During transitions from EEG desynchrony to EEG synchrony, pre-optic unit activity changed first significantly more often than the EEG (Table I). However, during transitions from EEG synchrony to EEG desynchrony there was a slight tendency in the opposite direction. The EEG tended to change

TABLE I

Analysis of order of change between unit and EEG in EEG transitions during recording from EEG-correlated cells in normal male pre-optic area

No. of transitions in which:	Desynchrony to synchrony	Synchrony to desynchrony
Unit activity changed first	230*	79
EEG changed first	47	128
Indeterminate**	217	299

* For transitions from EEG desynchrony to synchrony, unit-first greater than EEG-first, $P < 0.001$ (test for difference between proportions, Freund 1952). Desynchrony to synchrony transitions different from synchrony to desynchrony, $P < 0.001$ (χ^2 test).

** Due to unit firing rate variability, gradual transitions, or small time differences with slow paper speed.

first slightly more often than the pre-optic cell. These results showing whether unit activity or the EEG changed first for each type of EEG transition tended to be the same whether the unit's EEG correlation came from increased or from decreased activity during EEG activation. Pre-optic cells appeared to change activity significantly as few as 2 sec and as much as 7–8 sec before the EEG changed. Cells in the olfactory bulb probably followed the same pattern of results in this analysis, but the smaller number of correlated cells prevented us from reaching a definite conclusion.

In the normal male pre-optic area, the presence and type of correlation between the spontaneous activity of a unit and the EEG state was related to the unit's responses to odors. Those units which showed a typical reticular cell type of EEG correlation (increased activity during EEG desynchrony) tended to be those which gave excitatory responses to odors (Table II).

TABLE II

Comparison between responses to odors and EEG correlation during recording from cells in normal male pre-optic area

Response of single unit to odors	Change in single unit firing rate during EEG desynchronization		
	Increase	Decrease	None
Excitatory	22 units	2	4
Inhibitory	4	1	7
None	4	1	6

$P < 0.05$ (χ^2 test).

Some pre-optic and olfactory bulb units whose activity was significantly correlated to the EEG responded to odors, especially urine odors, in a characteristic way (Fig. 3). After the initial, direct response to the odor, the activity of such a cell then usually dropped below baseline gradually, whereas the EEG changed from a desynchronized to a synchronized state. The secondary response of the cell—the inhibition correlated with EEG synchronization—began as early as the second half of the odor presentation or as late as 20–40 sec after the odor presentation.

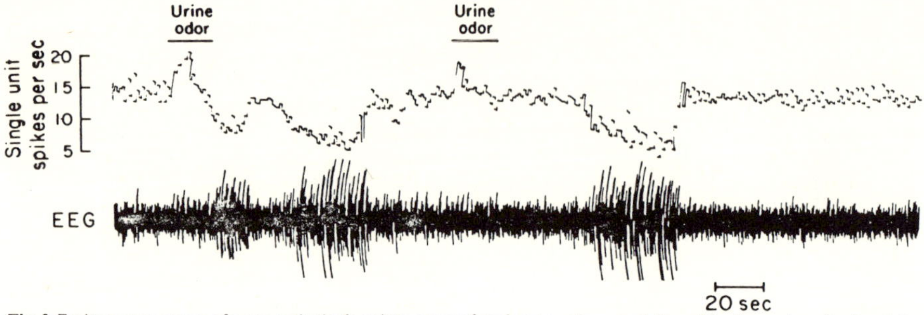

Fig. 3. Excitatory responses of a pre-optic single unit to estrous female urine odor were followed by depression of unit activity and correlated cortical EEG synchrony. Recording from urethane-anesthetized normal male rat.

Cells whose activity was significantly correlated to the EEG were not located in a clearly different pre-optic subregion from cells which were not. Nor were cells whose activity increased during EEG activation clearly separated from cells whose activity decreased. Rather, the histological results were like those reported for hypothalamic recording (Komisaruk *et al.* 1967; Lincoln 1969a); cells that showed different relations to EEG could be found very close to one another. A possible exception to this conclusion was the slight (non-significant) tendency for cells that increased activity during EEG activation to be located above the medial forebrain bundle at posterior pre-optic levels (under the anterior commisure). The extent of the basal forebrain sampled is shown in Fig. 4.

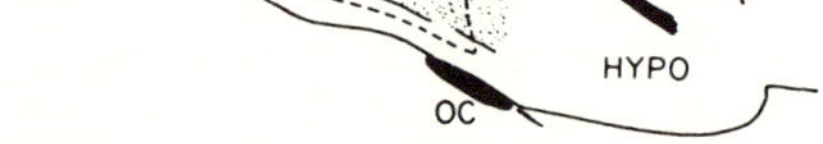

Fig. 4. Broken lines show extent of recording sites in pre-optic area medial forebrain bundle (MFB) in schematic sagittal section. AC, anterior commissure; FX, fornix; OC, optic chiasm; CC, corpus callosum; MT, mamillothalamic tract; FR, fasciculus retroflexus; HYPO, hypothalamus; OLF, olfactory bulb; SEP, septum.

DISCUSSION

Correlations observed between pre-optic area neuronal activity and the cortical EEG in these experiments extend previous reports (Komisaruk *et al.* 1967; Lincoln 1969a) of similar correlations observed during hypothalamic recording. Our own previous recording results from castrated male rats (Pfaff and Pfaffmann 1969) contrasted midbrain reticular formation neurons with both pre-optic area and olfactory bulb neurons. A high percentage of midbrain reticular formation cells (82%) were correlated to EEG, primarily increasing activity during EEG activation. A lower percentage of pre-optic and olfactory bulb units were EEG-correlated, and the correlated cells were split more evenly between those that increased and those that decreased during EEG activation. Our present recording from castrated males confirms the earlier results with castrates; approximately 37% of pre-optic units and an even lower percentage of olfactory bulb units were EEG-correlated. However, in the present recording from normal males, a high percentage of pre-optic cells were EEG-correlated, primarily increasing activity during EEG activation. Since olfactory bulb units in normal males were approximately the same as in castrates, completely non-specific factors may not be the explanation for the difference in the pre-optic area between normal and castrated animals. Thus, in normal males, pre-optic area but not olfactory bulb neurons had EEG correlations much like the mesencephalic reticular formation neurons recorded in earlier experiments.

What factors change as a result of higher androgen levels in the normal male to bring pre-optic units into a more reticular-like relation with the cortical EEG? Three possible causal relations are: (1) In the normal male, reticular formation neurons could exert a more powerful control over pre-optic neurons than in the castrate, thus enforcing a greater similarity between reticular and pre-optic relations to the EEG. (2) In the normal male, pre-optic neurons could exert a more powerful control over reticular neurons than in the castrate, and in doing so play a greater role in controlling the EEG. (3) Finally, in the normal male, a third brain region could exert more control over both reticular and pre-optic neurons, causing greater similarity between their functional characteristics. These possibilities are not mutually exclusive. Their interest lies in the possibility that they constitute mechanisms by which non-specific reticular arousal systems are related to neurons in the pre-optic area controlling mating behavior (Lisk 1967). The first possibility, a greater control of reticular activating circuits over a possible pre-optic mating behavior mechanism, suggests a mechanism for the demonstrations of Larsson (1963), Barfield and Sachs (1968) and Caggiula and Eibergen (1969) that non-specific activation can enhance mating performance in male rats. In fact, receptive females sometimes bite inactive males around the head and ears, which often stimulates the males to resume mating. Possibility (1) could also underlie the theoretical suggestion (Beach 1956, 1958) of an arousal mechanism necessary for normal male rat mating behavior. The second possibility, greater control by a pre-optic mating behavior mechanism over the EEG, is consistent with the idea that olfactory (Pfaff and Gregory 1971) and other stimuli affecting pre-optic neurons so as to promote mating behavior, can play a greater role (through pre-optic control over the reticular formation) in determining the arousal of the entire brain of the normal male. Thus, the secondary responses by pre-optic neurons to odors, correlated with EEG responses (Fig. 3), could play an important role in the arousal qualities of odors.

The analysis of which measure changed first, pre-optic unit activity or the EEG (Table I), has some limited power to distinguish among the different possible causal relationships. During EEG transitions from desynchrony to synchrony, many pre-optic units whose activity was related to EEG state tended to change (usually to decrease) firing rate before the EEG became synchronized, whereas the EEG rarely synchronized before the unit activity change occurred. Thus, it is possible that pre-optic activity changes helped to cause EEG synchronization, whereas the reverse possibility is unlikely. This suggestion is comparable with evidence from other laboratories showing that low frequency stimulation (Sterman and Clemente 1962; Clemente and Sterman 1963; Hernandez-Peon and Chavez-Ibarra 1963), or chemical stimulation (Hernandez-Peon *et al.* 1963; Hernandez-Peon and Chavez-Ibarra 1963) of the pre-optic area induces cortical EEG synchrony and sleep, whereas large pre-optic lesions (Nauta 1946; McGinty and Sterman 1968) abolish sleep. Moreover, local hormonal stimulation of the hypothalamus can induce EEG synchrony (Morelli 1968), and sex hormones are, in fact, concentrated by cells in the pre-optic area and hypothalamus (Pfaff 1968). In the present "which-changed-first" analysis, EEG transitions from synchrony to desynchrony gave quite different results from those of transitions from desynchrony to synchrony (Table I). Although no uniform pattern was evident, EEG desynchrony tended to precede pre-optic changes, making it quite unlikely that pre-optic changes cause EEG desynchrony.

Two specific limitations on the strength of these implications about causality are: first, the evidence in the present experiment is strictly correlational. Deliberate experimental manipulations of one variable to cause changes in the other are required to establish causal relations between pre-optic activity and EEG. The second limitation derives from factors other than causal relations which could yield the present results in the "which-changed-first" analysis (Table I). For instance, in a case where decreases in pre-optic unit discharge regularly preceded EEG synchronization, and EEG desynchronization regularly preceded increase in pre-optic firing, one possible interpretation would be that inhibition of pre-optic acitivity causes EEG synchronization, and EEG desynchronization excites pre-optic neurons. However, the same results could be explained by a third controlling both pre-optic activity and EEG synchrony, if it were assumed that the threshold for pre-optic inhibition by this third system is lower than that for initiating EEG synchrony, so that pre-optic inhibition would start sooner and end later than EEG synchrony.

Part of the tendency for pre-optic cell activity to show or not show correlations with EEG state can be ascribed to the state of the preparation. If one pre-optic cell in a normal male rat preparation showed good EEG correlation, there was a greater chance that most of the other cells in the preparation would also show it. Whether androgen-dependent factors in the state of the preparation played a role in producing the difference between normal male and castrated male pre-optic recording remains a question for further study. However, obvious conditions such as anesthetic dose were kept constant between normal male and castrated male preparations. Secondly, it was not the case that an extremely small number of preparations contributed all of the EEG-correlated cells; among the normal male pre-optic area experiments, no preparation contributed more than 4 EEG-correlated cells. Finally, the failure of the olfactory bulb to show a difference between normal and castrated animals suggests (although not conclusively) that non-specific factors in the state of the preparation were not the determining influences in producing the androgen effect.

SUMMARY

1. Some neurons in the pre-optic area of urethane-anesthetized male rats showed activity changes correlated with cortical EEG changes.

2. A larger proportion of pre-optic neurons in normal males than in castrates showed these significant correlations to EEG state. The larger proportion in normal males resulted from the greater number of pre-optic cells showing the EEG correlation typical of mesencephalic reticular formation units: higher firing rate during EEG desynchrony ("activation"). During recording from olfactory bulb units, no difference between normals and castrates in EEG correlation was observed.

3. Pre-optic units whose activity was related to the EEG tended to change firing rate slightly before the EEG changed from desynchrony to synchrony but not before the EEG changed back from synchrony to desynchrony.

4. Pre-optic units that increased firing rate during EEG activation tended to be the same units that showed excitatory responses to odors.

5. Pre-optic units showing correlation to the EEG tended to be located among units showing no correlation rather than being restricted to a clearly defined pre-optic subregion.

The authors thank Miss Minna Spencer for excellent technical assistance and Drs. Henry Edinger and Ralph Norgren for their critical suggestions about the manuscript.

REFERENCES

BARFIELD, R. D. and SACHS, B. D. Sexual behavior: stimulation by painful electrical shock to skin in male rats. *Science*, **1968,** *161*: 392–395.

BEACH, F. A. Characteristics of masculine "sex drive". In M. R. JONES (Ed.), *Nebraska symposium on motivation.* Univ. Nebraska Press, Lincoln, Neb., **1956:** 1–32.

BEACH, F. A. Neural and chemical regulation of behavior. In H. F. HARLOW and C. N. WOOLSEY (Eds.), *Biological and biochemical bases of behavior.* Univ. Wisconsin Press, Madison, Wisc., **1958:** 263–284.

CAGGIULA, A. R. and EIBERGEN, R. Copulation of virgin male rats evoked by painful peripheral stimulation. *J. comp. physiol. Psychol.*, **1969,** *69*: 414–419.

CLEMENTE, C. D. and STERMAN, M. B. Cortical synchronization and sleep patterns in acute restrained and chronic behaving cats induced by basal forebrain stimulation. *Electroenceph. clin. Neurophysiol.*, **1963,** *Suppl. 24*: 172–187.

FREUND, J. E. *Modern elementary statistics.* Prentice Hall, Englewood Cliffs, N.J., **1952.**

HERNANDEZ-PEON, R. and CHAVEZ-IBARRA, G. Sleep induced by electrical or chemical stimulation of the forebrain. *Electroenceph. clin. Neurophysiol.*, **1963,** *Suppl. 24*: 188–198.

HERNANDEZ-PEON, R., CHAVEZ-IBARRA, G., MORGANE, P. J. and TIMO-IARIA, C. Limbic cholinergic pathways involved in sleep and emotional behavior. *Exp. Neurol.*, **1963,** *8*: 93–111.

KOMISARUK, B. R., MCDONALD, P. G., WHITMOYER, D. I. and SAWYER, C. H. Effects of progesterone and sensory stimulation on EEG and neuronal activity in the rat. *Exp. Neurol.*, **1967,** *19*: 494–507.

KÖNIG, J. F. R. and KLIPPEL, R. A. *The rat brain.* Williams and Wilkins, Baltimore, **1963.**

LARSSON, K. Non-specific stimulation and sexual behaviour in the male rat. *Behaviour*, **1963,** *20*: 110–114.

LINCOLN, D. W. Correlation of unit activity in the hypothalamus with the sleep cycle. *Exp. Neurol.*, **1969**a, *24*: 1–18.

LINCOLN, D. W. Effects of progesterone on the electrical activity of the forebrain. *J. Endocr.*, **1969**b, *45*: 585–596.

LISK, R. D. Sexual behavior: hormonal control. In L. MARTINI and W. GANONG (Eds.), *Neuroendocrinology, Vol. 2.* Academic Press, New York, **1967:** 197–239.

MCGINTY, D. J. and STERMAN, M. B. Sleep suppression after basal forebrain lesions in the cat. *Science*, **1968,** *160*: 1253–1255.

MORELLI, L. Effeti electrocorticografici di microiniezioni di benzoato di estradiolo nell'ipotalamo. *Arch. Sci. biol. (Bologna)*, **1968,** *52*: 325–335.

NAUTA, W. J. H. Hypothalamic regulation of sleep in rats. An experimental study. *J. Neurophysiol.*, **1946,** *9*: 285–316.

PFAFF, D. W. Autoradiographic localization of radioactivity in rat brain after injection of tritiated sex hormones. *Science*, **1968,** *161*: 1355–1356.

PFAFF, D. W. and GREGORY, E. Olfactory coding in the olfactory bulb and medial forebrain bundle of normal and castrated male rats. *J. Neurophysiol.*, **1971,** *34*: 208–216.

PFAFF, D. W. and PFAFFMANN, C. Olfactory and hormonal influences on the basal forebrain of the male rat. *Brain Res.*, **1969,** *15*: 137–156.

RAMIREZ, V. D., KOMISARUK, B. R., WHITMOYER, D. I. and SAWYER, C. H. Effects of hormones and vaginal stimulation on the EEG and hypothalamic units in rats. *Amer. J. Physiol.*, **1967,** *212*: 1376–1384.

SCHLAG, J. and BALVIN, R. Background activity in the cerebral cortex and reticular formation in relation with the electroencephalogram. *Exp. Neurol.*, **1963,** *8*: 203–219.

SIEGEL, S. *Nonparametric statistics.* McGraw-Hill, New York, **1956,** 312 p.

STERMAN, M. B. and CLEMENTE, C. D. Forebrain inhibitory mechanisms: sleep patterns induced by basal forebrain stimulation in the behaving cat. *Exp. Neurol.*, **1962,** *6*: 103–117.

OLFACTORY AND HORMONAL INFLUENCES ON THE BASAL FORE-BRAIN OF THE MALE RAT

DONALD W. PFAFF AND CARL PFAFFMANN

INTRODUCTION

Steroid sex hormones apparently act on the brain, affecting the control of pituitary gonadotropic hormones and the execution of mating behavior[9,18,25]. The preoptic region and surrounding structures in the basal forebrain may mediate these sex hormone effects. Lesions[9,18,19], implantation of small amounts of steroid hormone[25] and electrical stimulation[10,47] in this region all have been shown to affect pituitary gonadotropic function or mating behavior. Moreover, the amount and time course of uptake of radioactive estradiol and testosterone by cells in the preoptic region and other structures in the basal forebrain have a closer resemblance to uptake in known sex steroid target organs than does uptake in most other regions of the brain[35–37].

Some investigators have successfully used microelectrode recordings to study the effects of estrogens or progesterone on single or multiple unit activity[4,21,24]. The main object of the present study was to detect and describe some effects of testosterone on the electrical activity of the brain of the male rat. Primary attention was directed to the study of units in and around the preoptic region.

It was expected that testosterone might affect the 'resting activity' of units (activity between presentations of stimuli), the magnitude of response of units to stimuli, or both. Peripheral stimuli and changes in the internal environment which have been shown to affect firing by units in the preoptic region are noxious stimulation of the skin[31], changes in the temperature of the brain[32] and administration of serotonin, epinephrine[8] and anesthetics[31]. Although the effectiveness of odors in altering preoptic activity has not been tested, anatomical results indicate that an olfactory input to the preoptic region exists[39,46], and two reports of electrophysiological studies have included evidence of olfactory input to the lateral hypothalamus[4,41]. Therefore, a second object of the present study was to determine whether units in the preoptic region respond to olfactory stimulation, and particularly to see whether responses to odors could be influenced by administration of testosterone.

Recent reports on the effects of progesterone on the electrical activity of the brain have shown that it is desirable to include more than one site and type of recording in an experiment on hormone effects; particularly for determining how selectively the hormone acts in the brain[4,21]. In the present experiment, in addition to recording in the preoptic region, single units were recorded in the olfactory bulb and in the mesencephalic reticular formation. The electroencephalogram (EEG) was recorded as an index of activity in the cerebral cortex and was usually monitored simultaneously with microelectrode recording, to study the relations between the EEG and single unit activity. To test the suggestion that hormone effects on olfactory input could be mediated by changes in the access of odors to olfactory receptors[29], the rate of nasal air flow was determined before and after testosterone administration. Carotid blood pressure, body temperature and heart rate were measured, to estimate the generality of testosterone effects under the same conditions in which it affected single unit activity.

METHODS

Experiments were performed on male Sprague–Dawley rats obtained from Charles River Breeding Laboratories, and weighing between 200 and 250 g. The rats were castrated at least 2 weeks before being used, in order to reduce endogenous levels of testosterone. The rats were anesthetized with urethane (1.5 g/kg, i.p.) and were usually immobilized with gallamine triethiodide (Flaxedil, American Cyanamid Co., 50 mg/kg, i.p.). Before surgery atropine was administered (0.3 mg/kg, s.c.).

A routine tracheotomy was performed to permit artificial respiration (Rodent Respirator, Harvard Apparatus Co.). Air was drawn through the nose after tracheotomy by intermittent application of a vacuum to a polyethylene tube which reached into the back of the nose from the site of tracheotomy.

Recording and stimulating procedures

The head of the rat was stabilized in a stereotaxic instrument. After incision and retraction of the skin, the bone dorsal to the olfactory bulb or the appropriate cortical region was thinned by drilling. The deepest layer of bone and the dura were then removed carefully with forceps.

Single units were recorded with micropipettes filled with 3 *M* sodium chloride. Tip diameters were between 1 and 3 μ, and DC resistances were between 0.5 and 5 MΩ. The reference electrode was clipped to the retracted skin. The micropipette was positioned using a micromanipulator (La Précision Cinématographique), according to the stereotaxic atlas of König and Klippel[22], except for the olfactory bulb, for which an atlas was not required. Input from the micropipette was led to a Grass P6 preamplifier equipped with a cathode follower, and then to a Tektronix 502 oscilloscope and an audio monitor. Frequencies below 400 and above 10,000 c/sec were filtered out. Permanent records of spike discharges were made on magnetic tape (Magnecord model 1048) or on film (Grass Kymograph Camera). The frequency of spike discharges was quantitatively evaluated using an integrating circuit, or a spike frequency histogram generator equipped with a Schmitt trigger and a counting circuit. The outputs of these devices were displayed with an Esterline Angus penwriter or a Grass Model 7 Polygraph.

The electroencephalogram (EEG) was recorded from 2 screws set in the bone over the cortex, one in the parietal bone and the other in the frontal bone on the same side. Frequencies below 1 and above 75 c/sec were filtered out. Olfactory bulb wave activity was recorded either from two stainless steel wires (each 75 μ in diameter, insulated to the tip) one placed about 2 mm deep in the bulb and the other resting on the surface of the bulb, or from 2 screws set in the bone over the bulbs, one over the anterior region of one bulb and the other over the posterior region of the contralateral bulb. Frequencies below 3 and above 75 c/sec were filtered out. Blood pressure was monitored with a Statham P23AC strain gauge connected to one common carotid artery. The electrocardiogram was recorded from skin electrodes placed on the left side of the chest and at the base of the tail. The pressure in the polyethylene tube used to apply a vacuum to the back of the nose was recorded using a Statham P23AC strain gauge connected to the tube in the manner shown in Fig. 11A. The EEG, olfactory bulb waves, electrocardiogram and potentials from the Statham strain gauges were amplified and displayed using a Grass Model 7 Polygraph. Grass Model 7P3A preamplifiers were used with the polygraph, except for the output of the strain gauge, which required a Grass 7P1ADC preamplifier. Rectal temperature was monitored using an electronic thermometer (Tri-R Instruments, Jamaica, N.Y.).

Electrical stimulation of the ipsilateral olfactory bulb was delivered through bipolar wire electrodes, each 90 μ in diameter and insulated to within about 1 mm of the tip. The stimuli were square waves, 5–20 V, 0.1–0.8 msec duration, delivered 0.2–2/sec. During testing for effects of testosterone on unit responses to olfactory bulb shock, it was advantageous to use a combination of amplitude and duration of stimulation in the middle of the range of effective values.

Air, cleaned with a silica gel and activated charcoal, was passed by the nose of the rat at a rate measured with a flowmeter. A Sage infusion pump was used to add measured amounts of odor-saturated air from a syringe to the stream of cleaned air. In each experiment the concentrations of all the odor stimuli were the same, and were between 0.01 and 0.1 of saturation. In particular, conditions of olfactory stimulation were kept the same before and after administration of testosterone. Most odorants were the best grades available from a variety of chemical companies. Urine for the use as odorant was collected from female Sprague–Dawley rats, weighing 250–300 g, obtained from Charles River Breeding Laboratories. Estrous females were brought into a state of behavioral receptivity by subcutaneous injections of 0.2 mg estradiol benzoate in 0.2 ml sesame oil 48 h before the beginning of urine collection and 0.5 mg progesterone in 0.5 ml sesame oil at the beginning of urine collection. Other females had been ovariectomized at least 6 weeks before urine collection and received only injections of sesame oil. Urine was collected over a 24-h period in standard metabolism cages. It was used when fresh or after storage in a frozen state for 24 h.

Testosterone and control injections

Almost all testosterone injections were intraperitoneal and contained between 600 and 1000 μg of testosterone propionate. A few injections were intracarotid and contained about 500 μg of testosterone propionate. The vehicles used were 30–50 μl of propylene glycol or ethanol. Injecting ethanol or propylene glycol alone in these volumes usually had no effect on unit firing or EEG. Occasionally, a slight depression of single unit activity, increased synchronization of the EEG or slight depression of electrophysiological responses to sensory stimuli occurred, beginning within 1 or 2 min and lasting no longer than 6–8 min after injection.

In 12 experiments, testosterone propionate was applied directly to the preoptic area by cannula. The tip of a 12 mm length of 20-gauge stainless steel hypodermic tubing was positioned in the preoptic region using stereotaxic procedures. This cannula was angled into the preoptic region through a hole drilled in a more anterior position on the skull, to allow room for directing the micropipette into the same part of the preoptic region. A 10 mm length of 27-gauge stainless steel tubing connected to PE10 polyethylene tubing was inserted into the 20-gauge cannula and was used to flush the cannula with 30 μl of physiological saline, which sometimes held cholesterol or testosterone suspensions. The 27-gauge insert fitted loosely in the cannula, and the saline was flushed slowly through the cannula with a Sage infusion pump so that cells in the preoptic area could be exposed to testosterone or cholesterol without appreciable pressure changes in the region of the pipette. During each experiment control records were taken, and then the effects of filling the cannula with physiological saline, or with cholesterol suspended in saline (4 μg/μl), or with testosterone suspended in saline (4 μg/μl) were measured. Filling the intracranial cannula with 30 μl of the control substances (physiological saline or cholesterol suspension) usually had no effect on the activity of the units. Occasionally, the size of the spike was affected briefly or the resting activity increased for 1 or 2 min. Responses to olfactory bulb shock or to odors were not affected by the control substances.

Histological and statistical procedures

The bottom of each electrode track was marked by a lesion at the tip of the pipette (50 μA DC, for 50 sec) or a dye according to the method of Thomas and Wilson[44]. After the experiment the brain was fixed in 10% formalin. Serial sections 50 μ thick were cut and stained with Weil or cresyl violet, permitting confirmation of electrode position.

Electrophysiological records were examined for effects of testosterone on the magnitude of responses to electrical or sensory stimuli and on the level of activity between presentation of stimuli (the 'resting activity'). Average resting activity and average response magnitudes were calculated from the quantitative measures provided by the integrated circuit or spike counting circuit or from photographs of the spike activity. In the case of testosterone effects on responses to olfactory bulb shock, average response magnitudes and standard deviations were calculated for blocks of 40 shocks presented every few minutes.

Statistical tests were performed to determine the reliability of the differences between proportions of single unit samples which displayed certain characteristics. Differences between proportions involving more than 30 units were tested with a standard parametric test (ref. 12, p. 208). Differences between proportions involving smaller numbers of units were tested using the Fisher exact probability test[43]. Two aspects of selection of units and data probably had a bearing on the results: (a) units selected for tests of testosterone effects tended to have large amplitude spikes, so that they could be held long enough to complete the experiment, and stable firing rates, so that effects of testosterone could be detected; (b) negative results from testing units for responses to peripheral stimuli have not been included unless other units in the same preparation proved to be responsive.

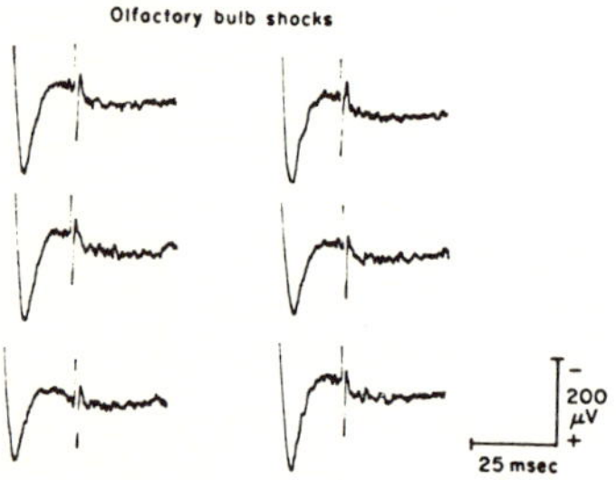

Fig. 1. Responses of a single unit in the preoptic area to 6 successive electric shocks of the ipsilateral olfactory bulb (11 V, 0.3 msec, 1/sec). Latency of response is 19 msec. Unit showed no resting activity.

TABLE I

EFFECTS OF ODORS AND OTHER STIMULI ON SINGLE UNIT ACTIVITY IN THE PREOPTIC AREA, MESENCEPHALIC RETICULAR FORMATION AND OLFACTORY BULB

Stimulus	*No. of units tested*	*No. of units responding*	*Response direction*		
			Excitatory	*Inhibitory*	*Mixed*
Preoptic area					
Olfactory bulb shock	44	25	24	1	—
Odors	117	88	56	21	11
Pain	54	32	23	9	—
Light	12	1	1	—	—
Sound	7	0	—	—	—
Mesencephalic reticular formation					
Odors	24	15	10	—	5
Pain	24	16	13	3	—
Olfactory bulb					
Odors	41	39	28	5	6

RESULTS

Olfactory input to the preoptic area

Responses to electrical stimulation of the olfactory bulb were recorded from 25 of 44 units tested in and around the preoptic region (Fig. 1; Table I). The median response latency was 20 msec, and latencies ranged from 10 to 76 msec. Units located anterior to the anterior commissure responded with a median latency of 15 msec, which was significantly shorter than the 26 msec median latency recorded from units under or behind the anterior commissure ($P < 0.02$) (Fig. 2).

Responses to odors were recorded in 88 out of 117 units (76%) in and around the preoptic region (Figs. 2 and 3). A significantly smaller percentage of units (59%) responded to painful tail, foot or nose pinches ($P < 0.05$). Some units responded only to odors, and other units responded both to odors and pain (Table II).

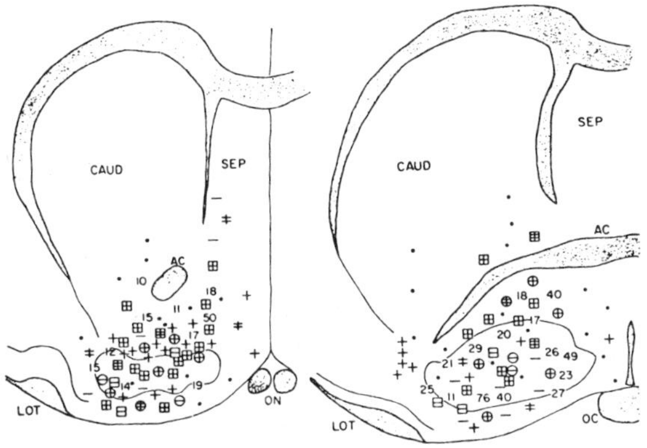

Fig. 2. Frontal sections showing units in and around the preoptic region which responded to olfactory stimulation. Medial forebrain bundle is drawn schematically. Numbers give the location and show the response latencies (msec) of units which responded to olfactory bulb shock. Other symbols denote units which responded to odors: +, unit excited by odors; −, unit inhibited by odors; ±, unit excited by some odors, inhibited by others; ●, unit unresponsive to odors and pain; ○, unit which responded to odors but not to pain; □, unit which responded to odors and to pain. CAUD, caudate nucleus; SEP, septum; AC, anterior commissure; LOT, lateral olfactory tract; ON, optic nerves, OC, optic chiasm.

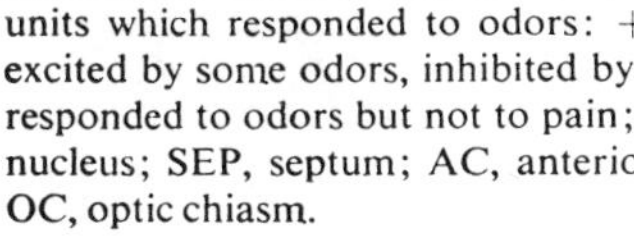

Fig. 3. Response of a single unit in the preoptic area (medial forebrain bundle) to the odor of urine from an estrous female rat (odor concentration, 1% of saturation).

TABLE II

MODALITY SPECIFICITY OF SINGLE UNIT RESPONSES TO ODORS AND PAIN

Brain region	*Total number of units tested**	*Responses*			
		Odor-specific	*Pain-specific*	*Both odor and pain*	*Neither odor nor pain*
Preoptic area	54	16 (30%)	0 (0%)	32 (59%)	6 (11%)
Mesencephalic reticular formation	24	1 (4%)	2 (8%)	14 (59%)	7 (29%)

* For both odor and pain responses.

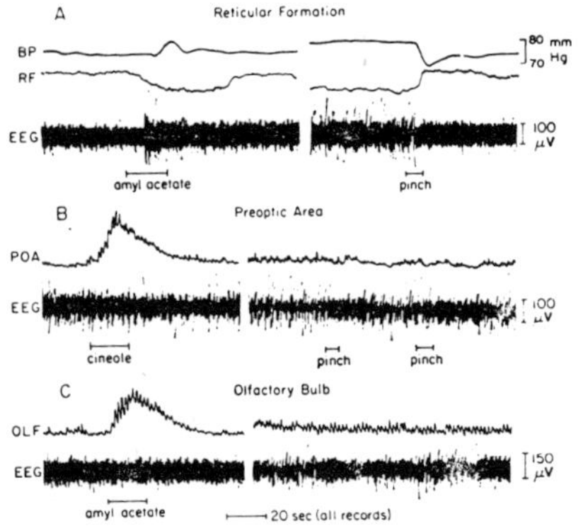

Fig. 4. Simultaneous recording of EEG and unit activity. A, Responses in the EEG, the integrated activity of a mesencephalic reticular formation single unit (RF) and the carotid blood pressure (BP) to the odor of amyl acetate and to a tail pinch. B, Response to the odor of cineole shown in the integrated activity of a preoptic area single unit (POA) without any response in the EEG; and responses to tail pinches in the EEG without responses in the preoptic unit. C, Dissociation of olfactory bulb unit integrated activity (OLF) from EEG activity.

In 9 experiments, single units which responded to odors were held during bilateral transection of the olfactory bulbs. Responses to odors, but not to pinches, were abolished by olfactory bulb transection, and must therefore have been mediated by the olfactory bulb rather than by the trigeminal innervation of the nasal mucosa. Ipsilateral olfactory bulb transection, alone, was usually sufficient to abolish responses to odors.

Units which responded to odors were distributed diffusely throughout the preoptic areas whether or not they responded to pain (Fig. 2).

64% of the odor-responsive units, showed only excitatory responses, 24% showed only inhibitory responses, and 12% were excited by some odors and inhibited by others. Among the odor responses from units in the dorsal part of the preoptic region only 12% were inhibitory, whereas 47% of the responses from the more ventrally located units were inhibitory ($P < 0.005$) (Fig. 2). Also, the percentage of inhibitory responses from units in the anterior preoptic region, in front of the anterior commissure (23%), was significantly smaller than that from units under or in back of the anterior commissure (52%) ($P < 0.02$). For the preoptic area, taken as a whole, the proportion of responses which were inhibitory was significantly greater than in the olfactory bulb ($P < 0.005$).

Responses to odors by midbrain units and EEG

Responses to odors and to pain were recorded from units in the mesencephalic reticular formation (Fig. 4A; Tables I and II). All of the mesencephalic units tested were located in the lateral reticular formation, directly lateral to the central gray and just ventral to the deep layers of the pretectal area or superior colliculus.

Responses to odors were detected frequently in the EEG in 28 preparations, and in the blood pressure in 8 preparations (Fig. 4A). Virtually, all EEG responses to pinches were desynchronizations (Fig. 4A), but EEG responses to odors included many synchronizations as well as desynchronization.

Single unit activity was often recorded simultaneously with EEG, to determine the degree of association between changes of firing rate in units and widespread changes of electrical activity in the cortex. Single unit firing rates and EEG activity changed as a result of sensory stimulation and during 'spontaneous' changes in resting activity. (Testosterone-induced changes are discussed in a later section.) A significantly higher proportion of midbrain reticular formation units than preoptic area units ($P < 0.01$) or olfactory bulb units ($P < 0.05$) showed consistent changes of firing rates at the same times that the EEG changed state (Table III; Fig. 4). Most reticular formation units increased in firing rates when the EEG became more desynchronized ($P < 0.01$), whereas units in the preoptic area and olfactory bulb which changed firing rates during EEG changes were more evenly split into groups which increased and decreased.

TABLE III

CHANGES IN FIRING RATES OF SINGLE UNITS DURING EEG DESYNCHRONIZATION

Type of change of firing rate upon EEG desynchronization	*Location of single units*					
	Midbrain ret. form.		*Preoptic area*		*Olfactory bulb*	
	No.	*(%)*	*No.*	*(%)*	*No.*	*(%)*
Increase	14	(64)	6	(24)	3	(21)
Decrease	4	(18)	3	(12)	4	(29)
No consistent change	4	(18)	16	(64)	7	(50)
Total number	22		25		14	

Effects of testosterone

Preoptic area

Intracerebral application. In 12 experiments the effect of testosterone on the firing of single units in the preoptic area was tested. Testosterone suspended in 30 μl physiological saline was introduced through a cannula, which extended into the preoptic region 0.5–1 mm anterior to the recording micropipette. In 9 experiments the olfactory bulbs were bilaterally transected anterior to stimulating electrodes so that the olfactory bulb could be activated in isolation from peripheral receptor changes. In 3 other experiments the bulbs were left intact so that responses to odors as well as shock could be determined.

Filling the intracranial cannula with 30 μl of the testosterone suspension affected the resting activity of preoptic units and their responses to olfactory bulb shock and odors (Table IV; Fig. 5). Changes in unit activity began within 5–15 min and lasted until 25–50 min after testosterone administration. Responses to olfactory bulb shock were increased between 30 and 180% by testosterone administration (Fig. 5). Control administration of saline or cholesterol did not significantly influence unit activity. Histological examination showed that units which were affected by direct application of testosterone to the brain were located throughout the preoptic area (Fig. 6A). The cannula tips were found to be located 0.5–1 mm anterior and sometimes medial to the site of the micropipette.

Systemic injections. Following intraperitoneal injections of testosterone, reliable changes occurred in single unit activity in the preoptic area (Table IV). The effects began within 5–15 min and lasted until 40–85 min after the injection. Effects of testosterone on the resting activity of preoptic units occurred in a total of 15 of the 28 experiments (Fig. 7B), including 10 increases, and 5 decreases. Units which had increased resting firing rates after testosterone injections were located more ventrally in the preoptic area than units which decreased or did not change ($P < 0.01$) (Fig. 6B).

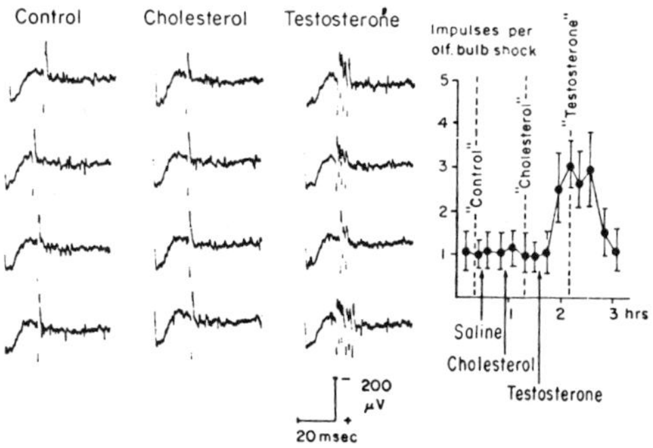

Fig. 5. Effect of direct testosterone application by cannula to the preoptic area on single unit responses to electrical stimulation of the olfactory bulb. The unit had no resting discharge. The graph shows that the average number of spikes per response increased after testosterone application, but not after cholesterol or saline (average ± standard deviation plotted). Dotted vertical lines in the graph show the times in the experiment from which the records on the left were chosen.

TABLE IV

EFFECTS OF TESTOSTERONE ON ELECTRICAL ACTIVITY OF THE BRAIN, AND OTHER MEASURES

Type of recording	*Spontaneous activity*				*Responses**				
	No. of experiments	*No. of effects*	*Type of effects*		*No. of experiments*	*No. of effects*	*Type of effects Response magnitude*		*Response direction reversals*
			Increases	*Decreases*			*Increases*	*Decreases*	
Preoptic area single units									
Intracerebral application	12	6	5	1	12	10	10	—	—**
					3	2	2	—	—
Systemic injection	28	15	10	5	28	18	12	—	6
Olfactory bulb									
Single units	18	7	5	2	8	12	8	3	1
Wave activity	10	6	6	—	10	5	3	2	—
Reticular formation									
Single units	14	5	1	4	14	7	5	2	—
EEG	26	10	7 (synchr)	3 (desynchr)	26	13	11	2	—
Nasal air flow	14	8	7	1	—	—	—	—	—
Blood pressure	8	1	1	—	—	—	—	—	—
Body temperature	29	2	2	—	—	—	—	—	—
Heart rate	24	0	—	—	—	—	—	—	—

* Unless otherwise noted, stimuli were various odors and painful pinches. Partial specificity of response change is described in text.
** Stimuli were electrical shocks to the olfactory bulb.

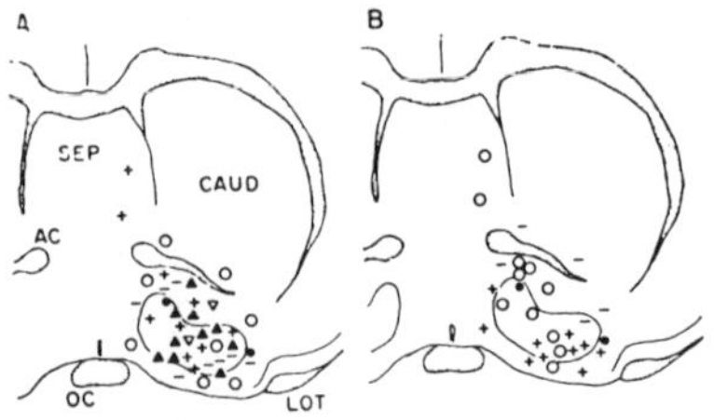

Fig. 6. Frontal sections showing locations of single units in and around the preoptic area which were influenced by testosterone administration. Anatomical abbreviations as in Fig. 2. A, Influence of testosterone on single unit responses to olfactory input. ▲, units influenced by direct application of testosterone to preoptic area (▽, units not influenced). Other symbols denote units tested with systemic testosterone injections; +, more spikes/response after testosterone; −, fewer spikes/response; ○, no change in response, but resting activity changed; ●, no change in response or resting activity. B, Influences of systemic testosterone injections on resting discharge of same units as shown in A: +, increase after testosterone; −, decrease after testosterone; ○, no change, but responses were changed; ●, no change in responses or resting activity.

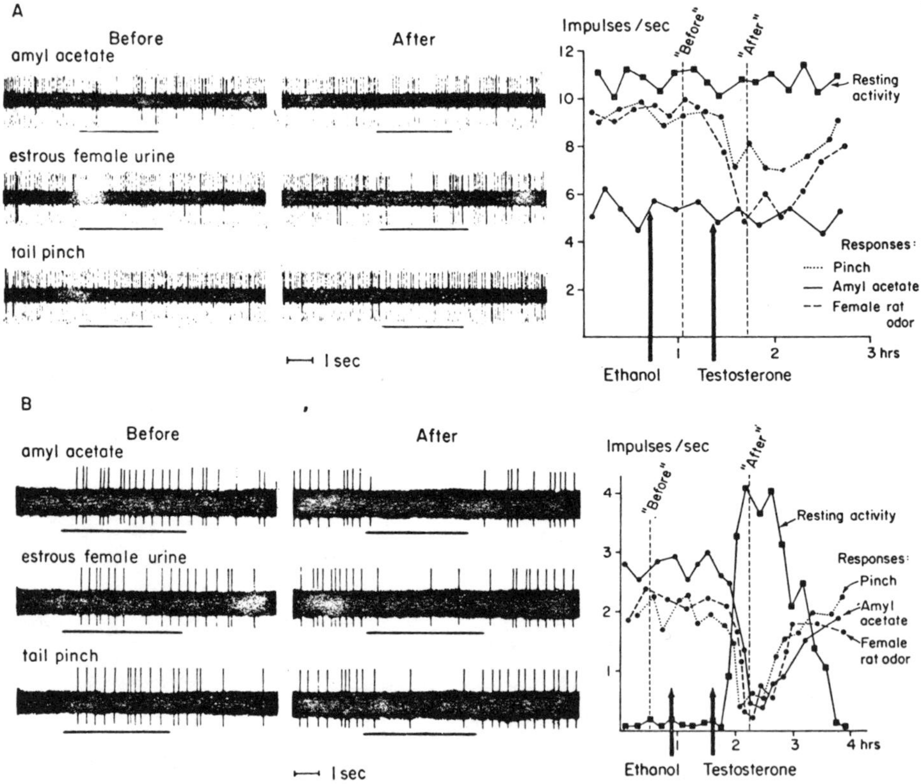

Fig. 7. Effects of intraperitoneal testosterone injections on the electrical activity of units in the preoptic area. The records on the left were selected from times in the experiments shown in the graphs by dotted vertical lines. Testosterone and ethanol (control) injections are indicated by arrows. A, Inhibitory responses to estrous female urine odor and to painful pinches were increased after testosterone injection (*i.e.* fewer spikes/sec during response), while resting activity and responses to amyl acetate odor were not affected. B, After testosterone injection, single unit resting activity increased, and responses to all 3 stimuli changed from excitations to inhibitions.

Twelve preoptic units showed reliably greater changes of activity in response to stimulation after testosterone injection (Fig. 7A), some showing larger inhibitions and others showing larger excitations. Six preoptic units showed reversals in response direction after testosterone injections (Fig. 7B); three showing reversals from excitation to inhibition, and the other three showing the opposite change. Units showing larger response magnitudes after testosterone were not located in consistently different regions of the preoptic area from units showing reversal of response directionality. However, units with testosterone-induced changes toward fewer spikes per response were usually located in more ventral positions than units with changes toward more spikes per response, and units whose responses were not changed at all were usually located outside the medial forebrain bundle (Fig. 6A). Changes in responses to odors were always at least as large as changes in responses to pain. Among the odors, there was a tendency toward larger changes in response to the female urine odors than to the non-urine odors (Fig. 7A).

Olfactory bulb

Unit activity. Following intraperitoneal injections of testosterone, single unit activity in the olfactory bulb changed reliably in 12 of 18 experiments, beginning within 10–15 min and lasting until 40–80 min after injection (Table IV). The predominant type of response change was an increase in magnitude of weak responses (Figs. 8A and B). Most of the enhanced responses were excitations, but some were inhibitions. In 3 experiments which included a large range of odor concentrations, the negatively accelerated stimulus-response curve found by prior investigators, was observed[28,30,45] and the magnitude of the testosterone effect on responses to odors appeared dependent upon the initial level of response (Fig. 8C). An experiment which used a large range of rates of nasal air flow yielded a similar effect; namely enhancement of responses by testosterone occurred with a low rate of nasal air flow but not with a high rate. Testosterone-induced changes in responses to odors were at least as large as changes in responses to pain. Changes after testosterone tended to be larger for the female urine odors than for non-urine odors.

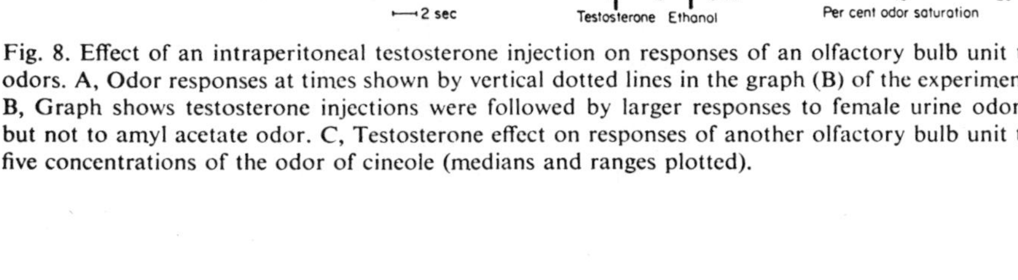

Fig. 8. Effect of an intraperitoneal testosterone injection on responses of an olfactory bulb unit to odors. A, Odor responses at times shown by vertical dotted lines in the graph (B) of the experiment. B, Graph shows testosterone injections were followed by larger responses to female urine odors, but not to amyl acetate odor. C, Testosterone effect on responses of another olfactory bulb unit to five concentrations of the odor of cineole (medians and ranges plotted).

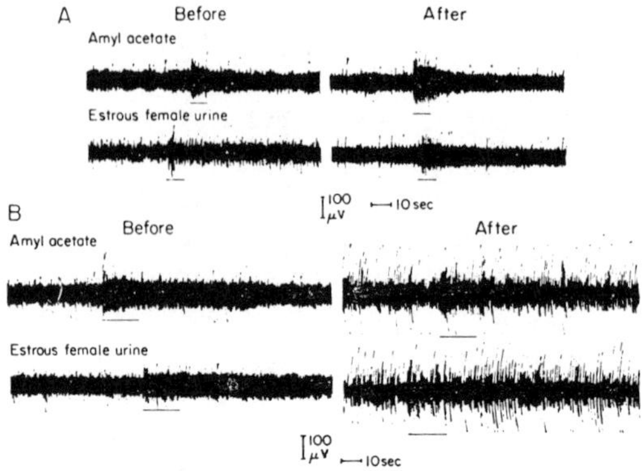

Fig. 9. Testosterone effects on olfactory bulb wave activity. 'Before' records are representative of control periods. 'After' records show the maximum testosterone effect. A, An experiment in which testosterone injection was not followed by resting activity change. B, Another experiment, in which testosterone was followed by a large increase of resting activity which obscured responses to odors.

Histological examination of the electrode tracks in the olfactory bulb showed that 8 of the 12 units affected by testosterone were in the mitral cell layer and that the other four were in the external plexiform layer.

Wave activity. After intraperitoneal injections of testosterone, changes in olfactory bulb wave activity occurred in 8 of 10 experiments, beginning within 5–15 min and lasting until 45–70 min after injection (Table IV). Changes after testosterone in spontaneous wave activity were always toward larger amplitude olfactory bulb waves (Fig. 9B). The type of response change after testosterone was related to the resting activity change. If the resting activity did not change, responses to odors were larger after testosterone than before (Fig. 9A). In the 2 experiments which showed large increases in the amplitude of the resting activity, responses to odors after testosterone injection appeared to be masked by the resting activity (Fig. 9B).

Mesencephalic reticular formation

Effects of testosterone injection were detected in the electrical activity of units in the mesencephalic reticular formation, appearing within 8–20 min and lasting until 50–80 min following injection (Table III). The electrode tracks from these experiments were located in the lateral reticular formation directly lateral to the central gray and just below the deep layers of the pretectal area or the superior colliculus. Changes in responses to painful stimuli were at least as large as changes in responses to olfactory input, in contrast to the results from preoptic area units.

EEG

Effects of testosterone injections on the EEG were detected, beginning within 5–15 min and lasting until 40–90 min following testosterone injection (Table IV; Fig. 10). Seven of the 10 effects on resting activity were in the direction of a more synchronized record (increased high-voltage low-frequency activity) and 3 records became more desynchronized after testosterone injections. EEG responses to stim-

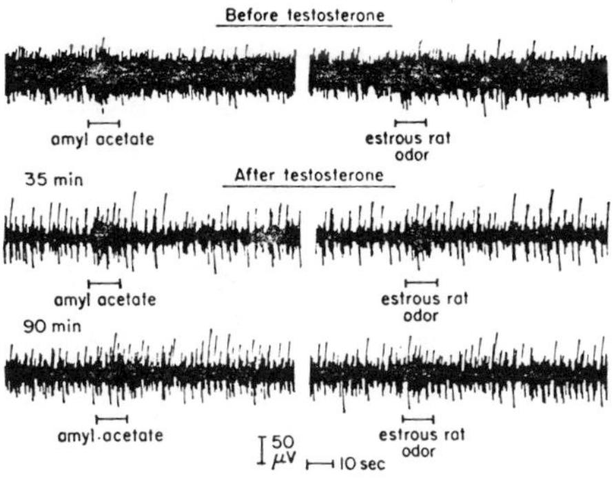

Fig. 10. Testosterone effect on the EEG. 'Before' records are representative of control periods. 'After' records show testosterone effect at its peak (35 min) and during recovery (90 min).

TABLE V

NUMBER OF EXPERIMENTS IN WHICH TESTOSTERONE EFFECTS OCCURRED IN THE EEG RESTING RECORD AND IN SINGLE UNIT RESTING ACTIVITY IN THE MIDBRAIN RETICULAR FORMATION AND THE PREOPTIC AREA

Testosterone effect on EEG	*Testosterone effects on unit activity*			
	Mesencephalic ret. form.		*Preoptic area*	
	Present	*Absent*	*Present*	*Absent*
Present	4	1	1	4
Absent	1	8	2	5
	$P < 0.05$		$P > 0.1$	

ulation after testosterone were larger than before, except when obscured by increased resting activity. Simultaneous EEG and single unit recording showed that the appearance of testosterone effects in EEG resting activity was associated with changes in unit activity in the midbrain reticular formation ($P < 0.05$) but not in the preoptic area ($P > 0.1$) (Table V). Increased EEG synchronization was associated with decreased reticular formation activity.

Nasal air flow and other measures

The rate of air flow through the nose before and after testosterone injections was determined indirectly by the pressure changes in the vacuum line to the nasopharynx by which air was drawn through the nose (Fig. 11A). Calibration with a flowmeter showed that increased pressure (because of greater constriction of air passageways) was associated with lower rate of air flow (Fig. 11B). Adrenalin sprayed into the external nares decreased the pressure pulses, presumably by widening the air passageway and facilitating air flow. Histamine spray had the opposite effect.

In 7 of 14 experiments, testosterone injections produced a 12–50% decrease in the magnitude of pressure pulses (Figs. 11C and D; Table IV). Changes began to appear within 5–15 min and lasted until 50–90 min after testosterone injection. It can be inferred that whenever testosterone injections affected nasal air flow, air

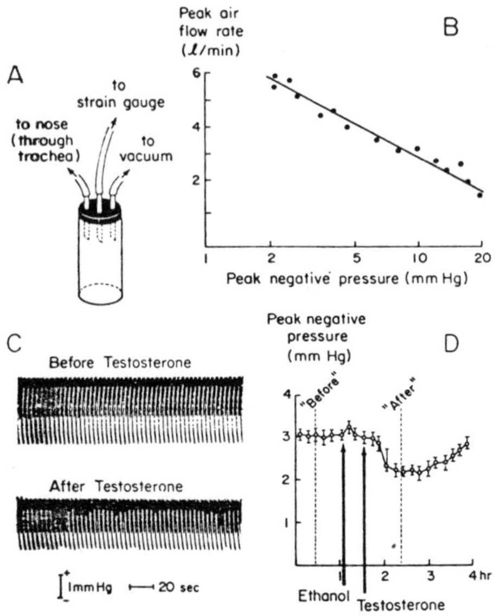

Fig. 11. Testosterone effect on nasal air flow rate. A, Scale drawing of connection between strain gauge and tubing used for applying vacuum to the back of the nose. B, Calibration curve showing relation between peak negative pressures (measured by the strain gauge) and peak rates of air flow (measured by a flowmeter). C, Polygraph records of the strain gauge output during intermittent vacuum applications ('artificial sniffs'). Records selected from times in the experiment shown in graph (D) by vertical dotted lines. D, Graph of an experiment showing testosterone effect on nasal pressures during artificial sniffs, and thus on nasal air flow (average ± standard deviation).

flow increased. Although such changes could play a role in some of the electrophysiological effects of testosterone, they cannot account for all of them, because testosterone effects on olfactory bulb activity were recorded in experiments where nasal air flow was not affected by testosterone injections.

Testosterone effects on electrophysiological measures were also observed in experiments in which heart rate, rectal temperature or blood pressure were simultaneously monitored and did not change. Thus, it is not likely that the electrophysiological effects were secondary to cardiovascular or temperature changes. In fact, testosterone effects on blood pressure, rectal temperature or heart rate were rarely seen (Table IV).

DISCUSSION

One aim of the present investigation was to search for cells in basal forebrain structures which responded to olfactory input. Having found a large number of cells in the preoptic area which responded to odors, it was necessary to show that the input causing the responses was truly olfactory. One alternative—that the input causing odor responses came from the trigeminal innervation of the nasal mucosa—seems unlikely because (a) olfactory bulb ablation abolished responses to odors, (b) many cells responded with short latencies to electrical shock applied directly to the olfactory bulb, and (c) some cells which responded to odor did not respond to somatosensory stimuli such as tail, foot or nose pinches. A second alternative was that responses to odors by cells in the preoptic area are part of some generalized electrophysiological response such as an arousal response caused by any novel stimulus. As such, preoptic area responses should be associated with responses to odors in the EEG[16,21] or the cardiovascular system[5,11]. However, responses to odors by many units in the preoptic area were seen without changes in the EEG, blood pressure or heart rate. Moreover, preoptic area responses often occurred with shorter latency and lower thresholds than EEG or blood pressure responses to odors. In general, firing rates of units in the preoptic area and olfactory bulb were not related as closely to the state of the EEG as was firing of units in the mesencephalic reticular formation. Finally, movement artifacts from arousal were impossible during these experiments because the rats were immobilized with Flaxedil and artificially respirated.

The main object of the present investigation was to find cells in the brain whose electrical activity was influenced by testosterone. The results provide direct proof that such cells exist, at least in the preoptic region, since direct application of testosterone to this region changed the activity of units there. The changes in unit activity were due to the direct action of testosterone in the preoptic region, rather than to indirect mechanisms, because the few minutes before the onset of the testosterone effect would allow time only for (a) entry into the brain of only part of the cannula's contents, which included considerably less testosterone than that required for effects following systemic injections, and (b) for diffusion considerably less than a millimeter from the cannula tip[27].

Some specific alternatives to the interpretation that testosterone influences cells in the preoptic area directly are that testosterone might affect respiratory movements, passage of air through the nose, blood pressure, heart rate, body temperature or the EEG, and that changes in these functions might be reflected, secondarily, by changes in preoptic area activity. The effectiveness of direct preoptic application of testosterone provides evidence that these indirect mechanisms are not necessary for testosterone effects in the basal forebrain. In addition, changes in respiratory and other movements were prevented by the use of Flaxedil, artificial respiration, and a vacuum line for 'artificial sniffing' of constant strength. Changes in the resistance to air flow through the nose did occur in some cases (*cf.* ref. 45), but in other instances electrical activity changed after testosterone while nasal air flow did not change. Moreover, nasal air flow was not a factor in experiments where the olfactory system was stimulated by shocks to the proximal positions of transected olfactory bulbs. Changes in blood pressure, heart rate and body temperature after testosterone injections were rarely seen, even in experiments where neuronal activity did change. The EEG usually showed some change after testosterone injections, but preoptic area effects were not correlated with EEG changes.

The generalized effects of testosterone resemble the diffuse electrophysiological effects of progesterone injections[21]. However, the present results also show that there are direct testosterone effects on the basal forebrain. These, together with the more generalized effects, could contribute to the overall effect of testosterone on the brain.

Direct testosterone application primarily caused an increase in the resting activity and an increased response to olfactory input by preoptic units. Intraperitoneal injections were followed by more diverse changes: either increases or decreases of resting activity by preoptic and olfactory bulb units, and, although most of the response changes were increases, there were also several reversals of response direction. It seems difficult to apply a unitary interpretation to all of these results, such as 'testosterone enhancement of olfactory input to the brain'.

After systemic injection, testosterone is taken up by cells throughout the brain of the male rat (ref. 35; McEwen and Pfaff, in preparation), and so could act at other sites in addition to the microelectrode recording site. Thus the change recorded from a nerve cell after testosterone injection could be due to testosterone acting directly on that cell plus testosterone action on other parts of the brain, transmitted to the recording site along anatomical pathways. Indeed, reversal in the direction of single unit responses to odors, resembling that after testosterone injection, can also be caused by electrical stimulation of the reticular formation[26]. Other effects of reticular formation stimulation and of behavioral arousal on olfactory activity have also been reported[1,3,15,20,34]. Anatomical pathways from the reticular formation to the preoptic area have been described in degeneration[17,33] and histochemical studies[2,14,42]. These studies show fibers running in the medial forebrain bundle from the mesencephalic tegmentum to the preoptic area, diagonal band of Broca and the olfactory tubercle. In turn, fibers going to the olfactory bulb from basal forebrain structures have been described[7,39].

In the male rat brain therefore, there may at least be two different types of testosterone action, each associated with different characteristics of testosterone uptake. First, the direct physiological action of testosterone in the basal forebrain, as recorded after direct application through a cannula, may have the specific effect of enhancing olfactory input to the rest of the brain. It is in this brain region that cells show high level, prolonged uptake of radioactive testosterone from the bloodstream (refs. 35–37; McEwen and Pfaff, in preparation). This region also shows significant differences between responses to odors from receptive and non-receptive female rats[38], and other functions concerned with reproduction (see Introduction). On the other hand, testosterone in other brain regions, including the reticular formation, might affect 'non-specific' behavioral arousal or locomotor activity[40]. These other brain regions show relatively low-level, short-lasting testosterone uptake.

The electrophysiological effects of intraperitoneal testosterone injections observed in these experiments began within a few minutes after the time of injection and started to disappear between 0.5 and 1.5 h after injection. This time course parallels that of [^{3}H]testosterone levels in the blood after intraperitoneal injection (McEwen and Pfaff, in preparation) and is closer to that of the early biochemical effects of testosterone on the prostate gland, seminal vesicles and liver, which occur within 2 h[13,23], than to the time course of behavioral actions of testosterone, which take days to appear (ref. 6; Pfaff, in preparation). To detect electrophysiological changes which follow the same time course as the behavioral effects of testosterone will require recording from chronically prepared, unanesthetized animals.

This investigation did not include independent confirmation that the hormone reaching the brain after intraperitoneal testosterone injections was still in the form of testosterone rather than a metabolite. However, direct intracerebral applications of pure testosterone were effective, and it has also been shown in other studies that a high percentage of the radioactivity found in the brains of male rats after intraperitoneal injections of [^{3}H]testosterone is still in the form of testosterone (McEwen and Pfaff, in preparation). The question of what effects other androgens, estrogens or other steroid hormones would have on the same preoptic units remains for further study.

SUMMARY

1. Single units in the medial forebrain bundle and elsewhere in the preoptic area of anesthetized male rats responded to electrical shocks of the olfactory bulb and to odors. The odor responses were mediated by the olfactory bulb. Inhibitory responses were recorded more often in the preoptic area than in the olfactory bulb and were mainly recorded from units located in more ventral and posterior parts of the basal forebrain than units with excitatory responses.

2. Responses to odors were recorded from single units in the mesencephalic reticular formation, and in the EEG.

3. Changes in firing rates of units in the mesencephalic reticular formation were more closely associated with changes in the EEG than firing rates of units in the preoptic area or olfactory bulb.

4. Administration of testosterone directly into the preoptic area or by systemic injection influenced the electrical activity of preoptic units. Direct preoptic administration increased the magnitude of single unit responses to electrical shock of the olfactory bulb and to odors. Systemic administration had more complex effects, including increases in response magnitude and reversals of response direction.

5. Testosterone effects were also detected in single unit recording in the olfactory bulb and the mesencephalic reticular formation, in olfactory bulb wave activity and in the EEG.

ACKNOWLEDGEMENTS

This work was supported by NSF grant GB-4198, an NSF postdoctoral fellowship (D.P.) and by the Population Council.

The authors wish to thank Dr. Christiana Leonard for her helpful suggestions during the preparation of this manuscript.

REFERENCES

1 ADRIAN, E. D., The electrical activity of the mammalian olfactory bulb, *Electroenceph. clin. Neurophysiol.*, 2 (1950) 377–388.

2 ANDEN, N.-E., DAHLSTROM, A., FUXE, K., LARSSON, K., OLSON, L., AND UNGERSTEDT, U., Ascending monoamine neurons to the telencephalon and diencephalon, *Acta physiol. scand.*, 67 (1966) 313–326.

3 ARDUINI, A., AND MORUZZI, G., Sensory and thalamic synchronization in the olfactory bulb, *Electroenceph. clin. Neurophysiol.*, 5 (1953) 235–242.

4 BARRACLOUGH, C., AND CROSS, B., Unit activity in the hypothalamus of the cyclic female rat: Effect of genital stimuli and progesterone, *J. Endocr.*, 26 (1963) 339–359.

5 BAUST, W., AND NIEMCZYK, H., Studies of the adrenalin-sensitive component of the mesencephalic reticular formation, *J. Neurophysiol.*, 26 (1963) 692–704.

6 BEACH, F. A., AND HOLZ-TUCKER, M., Effects of different concentrations of androgen upon sexual behavior in castrated male rats, *J. comp. physiol. Psychol.*, 42 (1949) 433–453.

7 CRAGG, B. G., Centrifugal fibres to the retina and olfactory bulb, and composition of the supraoptic commissures in the rabbit, *Exp. Neurol.*, 5 (1962) 406–427.

8 CUNNINGHAM, D., STOLWIJK, J., MURAKAMI, N., AND HARDY, J., Responses of neurons in the preoptic area to temperature, serotonin and epinephrine, *Amer. J. Physiol.*, 213 (1967) 1570–1581.

9 DONOVAN, B. T., Regulation of the secretion of follicle-stimulating hormone. In G. W. HARRIS AND B. T. DONOVAN (Eds.), *The Pituitary Gland, Vol. 2*, Univ. Calif. Press, Berkeley, Calif., 1966, pp. 49–98.

10 EVERETT, J. W., Neural control of reproductive functions of the adenohypophysis, *Physiol. Rev.*, 44 (1964) 373–431.

11 FRAZIER, D. T., TAQUINI, C., BOYARSKY, L., AND WILSON, M., Hypothalamic unit response to increases in arterial blood pressure, *Proc. Soc. exp. Biol. (N.Y.)*, 120 (1965) 450–454.

12 FREUND, J. E., *Modern Elementary Statistics*, Prentice–Hall, Englewood Cliffs, N. J., 1952, pp. 208–209.

13 FUJII, T., AND VILLEE, C., Effect of testosterone on ribonucleic acid metabolism in the prostate, seminal vesicle, liver and thymus of immature rats, *Endocrinology*, 82 (1968) 463–467.

14 FUXE, K., Distribution of monoamine nerve terminals in the central nervous system, *Acta physiol. scand.*, 64, Suppl. 247 (1965).

15 GAULT, F., AND COUSTAN, D. R., Nasal air flow and rhinencephalic activity, *Electroenceph. clin. Neurophysiol.*, 18 (1965) 617–624.

16 GOODMAN, S., AND MANN, P., Reticular and thalamic multiple unit activity during wakefulness, sleep and anesthesia, *Exp. Neurol.*, 19 (1967) 11–24.

17 GUILLERY, R. W., Afferent fibres to the dorso-medial thalamic nucleus in the cat, *J. Anat. (Lond.)*, 93 (1959) 403–418.

18 HARRIS, G. W., AND CAMPBELL, H. J., Regulation of the secretion of luteinizing hormone and ovulation. In G. W. HARRIS AND B. T. DONOVAN (Eds.), *The Pituitary Gland, Vol. 2*, Univ. Calif. Press, Berkeley, Calif., 1966, pp. 99–165.

19 HEIMER, L., AND LARSSON, K., Impairment of mating behavior in male rats following lesions in the preoptic-anterior hypothalamic continuum, *Brain Research*, 3 (1966–1967) 248–263.

20 HERNÁNDEZ-PEÓN, R., LAVIN, A., ALCOCER-CUARON, C., AND MARCELIN, J., Electrical activity of the olfactory bulb during wakefulness and sleep, *Electroenceph. clin. Neurophysiol.*, 12 (1960) 41–58.

21 KOMISARUK, B. R., MCDONALD, P. G., WHITMOYER, D. I., AND SAWYER, C. H., Effects of progesterone and sensory stimulation of EEG and neuronal activity in the rat, *Exp. Neurol.*, 19 (1967) 494–507.

22 KÖNIG, J. F., AND KLIPPEL, R. A., *The Rat Brain*, Williams and Wilkins, Baltimore, Md., 1963.

23 LIAO, S., LEININGER, K. R., SAGHER, D., AND BARTON, R. W., Rapid effect of testosterone on ribonucleic acid polymerase activity of rat ventral prostate, *Endocrinology*, 77 (1965) 763–765.

24 LINCOLN, D., AND CROSS, B., Effect of oestrogen on the responsiveness of neurones in the hypothalamus, septum and preoptic area of rats with light-induced persistent oestrus, *J. Endocr.*, 37 (1967) 191–203.

25 LISK, R. D., Sexual behavior; hormonal control. In L. MARTINI AND W. GANONG (Eds.), *Neuroendocrinology, Vol. 2*, Academic Press, New York, 1967, pp. 197–239.

26 MANCIA, M., GREEN, J. D., AND VON BAUMGARTEN, R., Reticular control of single neurons in the olfactory bulb, *Arch. ital. Biol.*, 100 (1962) 463–475.

27 MICHAEL, R. P., An investigation of the sensitivity of neurological areas to hormonal stimulation. In S. S. KETY AND J. ELKES (Eds.), *Regional Neurochemistry*, Pergamon, Oxford, 1961, pp. 465–472.

28 MOULTON, D. G., Studies in olfactory acuity. III. Relative detectability of *n*-aliphatic acetates by the rat, *Quart. J. exp. Psychol.*, 12 (1960) 203–213.
29 MOULTON, D. G., AND BEIDLER, L. M., Structure and function in the peripheral olfactory system, *Physiol. Rev.*, 47 (1967) 1–52.
30 MOZELL, M. M., Electrophysiology of the olfactory bulb, *J. Neurophysiol.*, 21 (1958) 183–196.
31 MURAKAMI, N., STOLWIJK, J., AND HARDY, J. D., Responses of preoptic neurons to anesthetics and peripheral stimulation, *Amer. J. Physiol.*, 213 (1967) 1015–1024.
32 NAKAYAMA, T., HAMMEL, H., HARDY, T., AND EISENMAN, J., Thermal stimulation of electrical activity of single units of the preoptic region, *Amer. J. Physiol.*, 204 (1963) 1122–1126.
33 NAUTA, W. J. H., AND KUYPERS, H., Some ascending pathways in the brainstem reticular formation. In H. H. JASPER (Ed.), *Reticular Formation of the Brain*, Little, Brown, Boston, 1958, pp. 3–30.
34 PAGANO, R., The effects of central stimulation and nasal air flow on induced activity of olfactory structures, *Electroenceph. clin. Neurophysiol.*, 21 (1966) 269–277.
35 PFAFF, D. W., Uptake of testosterone-H^3 and estradiol-H^3 by the male and female rat brain An autoradiographic study, *Science*, 161 (1968) 1355–1356.
36 PFAFF, D. W., Uptake of estradiol-17β-H^3 in the female rat brain. An autoradiographic study, *Endocrinology*, 82 (1968) 1149–1155.
37 PFAFF, D. W., Autoradiographic localization of heterologous sex hormones in the rat brain, *Experientia (Basel)*, 24 (1968) 958–959.
38 PFAFF, D. W., AND PFAFFMANN, C., Behavioral and electrophysiological responses of male rats to female rat urine odors. In C. PFAFFMANN (Ed.), *Olfaction and Taste*, Rockefeller Univ. Press, New York, 1969, in press.
39 POWELL, T. P. S., COWAN, W. M., AND RAISMAN, G., The central olfactory connexions, *J. Anat. (Lond.)*, 99 (1965) 791–813.
40 REED, J. D., Spontaneous activity of animals, *Psychol. Bull.*, 44 (1947) 393–412.
41 SCOTT, J., AND PFAFFMANN, C., Olfactory input to the hypothalamus: electrophysiological evidence, *Science*, 158 (1967) 1592–1594.
42 SHUTE, C., AND LEWIS, P., The ascending cholinergic reticular system; neocortical, olfactory and subcortical projections, *Brain*, 90 (1967) 497–520.
43 SIEGEL, S., *Nonparametric Statistics*, McGraw-Hill, New York, 1956, pp. 96–104.
44 THOMAS, R. C., AND WILSON, V. J., Precise localization of Renshaw cells with a new marking technique, *Nature (Lond.)*, 206 (1965) 211–213.
45 TUCKER, D., Physical variables in the olfactory stimulation process, *J. gen. Physiol.*, 46 (1963) 453–490.
46 VALVERDE, F., *Studies on the Piriform Lobe*, Harvard Univ. Press, Cambridge, 1965.
47 VAUGHAN, E., AND FISHER, A. E., Male sexual behavior induced by intracranial electrical stimulation, *Science*, 137 (1962) 758–759.

Diurnal Variation in the Effects of Progesterone on Multiple Unit Activity in the Rat Hypothalamus

EI TERASAWA AND CHARLES H. SAWYER [1]

A study has been made of the effects of progesterone on multiple unit activity (MUA) in the hypothalamus of ovariectomized estrogen-primed rats maintained under light-controlled conditions (14 hr light, 10 hr dark). With large microelectrodes (25 μ), recordings were made of integrated MUA in the arcuate nucleus-median eminence (ME) and the preoptic region of proestrous rats (nucleated vaginal smears) under light urethane anesthesia. Cortical EEG, EKG, and respiration were also monitored. Injection of progesterone (2.5 mg sc in oil) induced a "sleepy" EEG within an hour, regardless of time of administration. However, afternoon (14:30) injections induced a depression in ME multiunit activity followed by several hours of elevated activity starting around 17:00, while injections at 11:00 evoked a rise in activity preceding the phases of depression and secondary elevation (a triphasic effect). In natural proestrus progesterone at 11:00 activates release of pituitary ovulating hormone ("advances the critical period"), and the initial elevation in multiunit activity may represent a neural correlate of this process. The secondary rise in activity occurs at about the time of onset of behavioral estrus. Anterior deafferentation of the hypothalamus eliminates the diurnal variation in responsiveness to progesterone, and injection of the steroid is followed by a slow rise in multiunit activity regardless of time of day.

Introduction

For many years endocrinologists have recognized that the ovarian steroid hormone progesterone may either facilitate or inhibit ovulation, a process controlled by the central nervous system (CNS) even in "spontaneously ovulating" species (10, 13, 24, 29). In a rat with a 5-day estrous cycle, injection of progesterone early on the third day of diestrus advances ovulation 24 hr (12, 14), whereas an afternoon injection on the second

[1] The work was supported in part by grants from the National Institutes of Health (NB 01162) and the Ford Foundation. Present address of Dr. Terasawa: Department of Physiology, Yokohama University, School of Medicine, Yokohama, Japan. The authors gratefully acknowledge the assistance of David Whitmoyer (electronics), Virginia Hoover (surgery), Arlene Koithan and Beverly Bedard (histology), Keiko Akutagawa (drawings), Rudolph Sabbot (photography) and Elise Bozzo (bibliography).

day of diestrus in a 4-day cycle delays for 24 hr the release in an ovulatory surge of pituitary gonadotrophin. Recently, several investigators (7, 8, 25, 28, 34) have shown that administering the steroid on the morning of proestrus activates the release of pituitary ovulating hormone(s) prior to the afternoon "critical period" when release would ordinarily occur. This "advancement of the critical period" can be blocked with drugs such as atropine and pentobarbital, and the CNS is obviously involved.

Many investigators have looked for electrophysiological correlates of the actions of progesterone. Kawakami and Sawyer (21) described biphasic changes in brain thresholds in the rabbit associated with progesterone's facilitation-inhibition effects in that species. Studying the unit firing of lateral hypothalamic neurons in the female rat under urethane anesthesia, Barraclough and Cross (3) reported that intravenous progesterone in propylene glycol inhibited the excitatory effect of vaginal stimulation. They considered this a specific effect on hypothalamic neurons but they did not monitor electrical activity in other parts of the brain. When Ramirez, Beyer, Komisaruk and their associates (5, 23, 27) repeated their experiment and simultaneously recorded the cortical EEG, they found that changes in hypothalamic unit firing rate and responsiveness to peripheral stimuli paralleled EEG changes, suggesting that both were reflections of the anesthetic effects of progesterone on a urethane background and therefore not specific. However, Haller and Barraclough (19) and Terasawa and Sawyer (31) reported that urethane given on the morning of proestrus did not block ovulation, and Haller and Barraclough (19) found that the anesthetic did not block progesterone's advancing ovulation. Later, with electrochemical stimulation of the preoptic area, Terasawa and Sawyer (32) observed an elevation of multiple unit activity (MUA) in the arcuate nucleus-median eminence region independent of cortical EEG changes but correlated with activation of the release of pituitary ovulating hormone. In view of these findings, the present experiments were undertaken to look for progesterone-induced changes in the firing patterns of hypothalamic neurons which might be related to activation and inhibition of adenohypophyseal function.

Materials and Methods

Eighty-one mature Sprague-Dawley ovariectomized rats weighing 250–350 g were maintained in a light-controlled (14 hr light, 10 hr dark) air conditioned room. Two to 4 weeks after ovariectomy 58 of them were treated for 2 days with estrogen (5 μg estradiol benzoate, sc, at 16:00–18:00 daily) to produce a state of artificial proestrus on the day of electrical recording. On the morning of this third day nucleated vaginal smears confirmed the proestrous condition.

Surgery and recording were conducted under light urethane 120 mg/ 100 g body wt) anesthesia. A polyethylene cannula was inserted into the trachea to expedite breathing in the stereotaxic frame. The head was oriented according to the atlas of Albe-Fessard, Stutinsky, and Liboudan (1). To avoid the use of intravenous propylene glycol, progesterone (1.25–5.0 mg) was injected subcutaneously in 0.1 ml sesame oil. Control injections were made of the sesame oil vehicle alone. Stainless steel screws were fixed over the frontal cortex for EEG recording. Two "macro-micro" electrodes, made from No. 00 stainless steel insect pins insulated with Epoxylite to their 20–40 μ tips, were inserted into the hypothalamus independently by hydraulic micromanipulators.

Multiple unit activity (MUA) was amplified with a solid state preamplifier, displayed, and photographed on a Tektonix 565 oscilloscope screen, integrated, and the integrated level recorded with an Offner type R Dynograph for periods up to 18 hr by methods described earlier (33). EEG, EKG, and respiration were also monitored. Integrated MUA levels before and after treatment with progesterone were compared during periods of EEG synchrony characteristic of sleep.

Hypothalamic "deafferentations" were made with the Halasz knife (18) 2 to 8 weeks prior to recording. The axis of the knife was centered at $A = 6.0$, and a complete rotation ("complete deafferentation") isolated a cylinder of 1.5 mm radius and 3.8 mm height. Anterior and posterior deafferentations were achieved with appropriate half-circle rotations of the knife. Recording sites were marked with the Prussian blue reaction and their locations and the degree of deafferentation ascertained histologically (33).

Results

Correlations Between Sleep-Wakefulness Changes in the Cortical EEG and Local Subcortical Alterations in Multiple Unit Activity. Before a study could be made of specific effects of progesterone on the firing of subcortical neurons, it was desirable to know whether these neurons reacted independently of overall changes in the cortical EEG. To this end a survey was made of 277 cases in which the EEG was monitored while changes were recorded in the level of integrated MUA of subcortical neurons. Some of these records were taken during the course of an earlier study (33). The types of correlations were divided into three classes: (a) type A, in which elevations in MUA were related to EEG desynchrony (arousal) and depressions to a synchronized pattern of cortical EEG (sleep); (b) type S, in which elevations in MUA were related to EEG synchrony and depressions to desynchrony; and (c) type N, in which no correlation could be seen between changes in MUA and cortical EEG.

Most of the data are summarized in Table I. Good type A correlations between multiple units and sleep-wakefulness EEG patterns were seen in the thalamus, reticular formation, and central gray matter, lateral and posterior hypothalamic regions, retrochiasmatic region, and paraventricular and ventromedial hypothalamic nuclei. Type S correlations were common in the hippocampus and amygdala, especially the cortical nucleus of the amygdala. A large number of cases (53 out of 76) of independent multiple units were encountered in the arcuate nucleus-median eminence (ARC-ME) region (type N). Only eight cases in the ARC-ME showed strong correlations with EEG sleep-wakefulness, of which six were type A and two, type S. Other areas with a high (>40%) percentage of cases of independent MUA include the tract of the diagonal band, the medial preoptic area, the optic chiasma or tract, the dorsomedial nucleus of the hypothalamus, and the medial nucleus of the amygdala.

Multiple unit records taken from the arcuate nucleus or median eminence showed relatively uniform neuronal activity when compared with the diversity of unit amplitudes registered from other parts of the brain (Fig. 1). In view of the uniform "size" of units in the ARC-ME, changes in the level of integrated MUA in this region were attributable to alterations in firing rate of the neurons. Comments on the effects of progesterone in Fig. 1 and the effects of deafferentation in Table 1 will be made below.

Effects of Progesterone on the Cortical EEG. A clear view of the effects of subcutaneous injections of progesterone on the EEG was somewhat difficult to obtain because of the relatively slow absorption of the steroid from its oil vehicle, the concurrent effects of urethane anesthesia, the long time course of these "acute" recording experiments, and the occasional irreversible influence of asphyxia resulting from a temporarily plugged tracheal cannula (30).

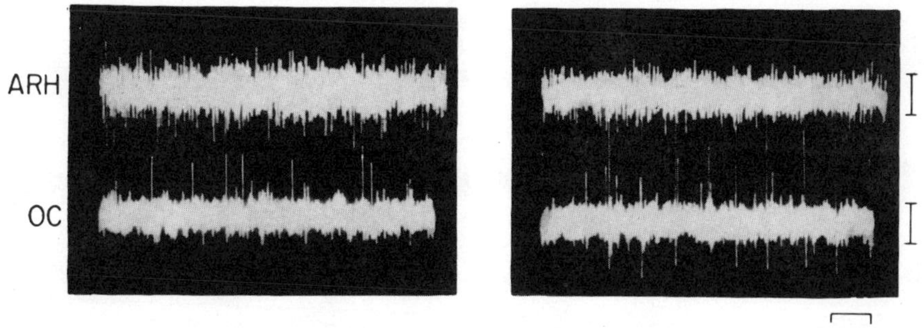

FIG. 1. Oscilloscopic records of multiple unit activity in the arcuate nucleus (ARH) and optic chiasm (OC) before (left) and after (right) a late-afternoon injection of progesterone. Note the reduced activity in ARH after progesterone. The record was taken from rat No. 15 in Table 2. Calibration marks: 20 msec; 20 μv.

However, a consistent pattern of effects emerged from the many experiments, and the influences of progesterone on the EEG proved to be independent of the time of day at which the steroid was administered (Fig. 2). Within 30–40 min of the subcutaneous injection prolonged spindle bursts appeared and continued for several hours. After about 5 hr the long spindle bursts were interspersed with short bursts of the type commonly seen during pentobarbital anesthesia. The mixture of long and short spindle bursts persisted for about 12-15 hr, giving way at that time to a phase of EEG arousal and small spindles which continued to the end of the experiment. Occasionally, the initial phase of the progesterone effect consisted of barbiturate-like short spindle bursts rather than the long lasting spindles. In most of these progesterone experiments the ovariectomized rats were primed with estrogen. In the absence of estrogen the EEG effects of progesterone differed only very slightly if at all from those described above. Perhaps, in the absence of estrogen, the length and amplitude of the long spindle bursts were somewhat diminished, but the duration of the progesterone effect was, if anything, prolonged.

Effects of Progesterone on Multiple Unit Activity in the Intact Hypothalamus. In contrast to the uniform sleeplike effects of progesterone on the cortical EEG throughout the day of artificial proestrus, diurnal variations in responsiveness to the steroid were observed in the integrated multiple unit record of the arcuate nucleus-median eminence. The results

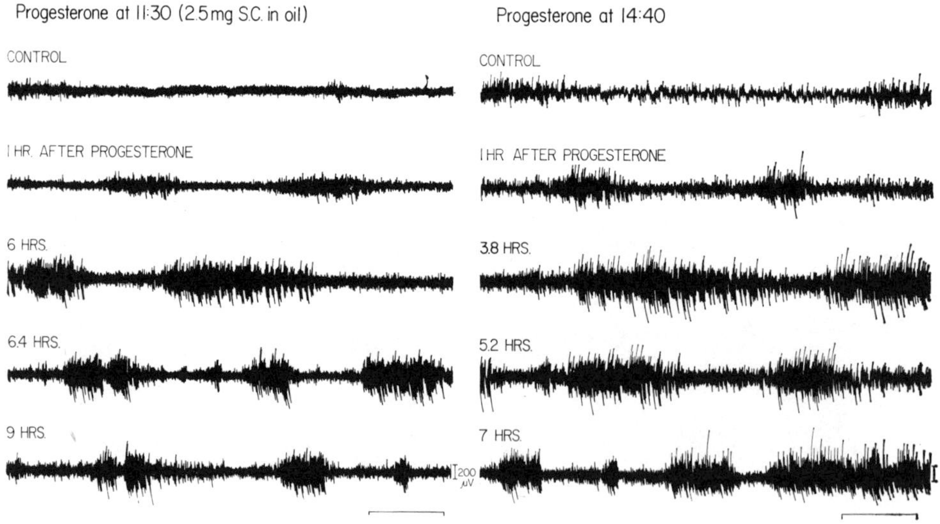

FIG. 2. Effects on the cortical EEG in two rats (no. 147, left; no. 123, right) induced by injecting progesterone at different hours of the day of "artificial proestrus." A sleeplike synchronous EEG with spindles resulted from administering the steroid regardless of the time of day. Calibration marks: 1 min; 200 μv.

TABLE 1

CORRELATION BETWEEN ELEVATION OF INTEGRATED MULTIPLE UNIT ACTIVITY (MUA) AND EEG SLEEP-WAKEFULNESS CHANGES

		Type of correlation					
		EEG-Dependent					
MUA Electrode site	Total No. rats	MUA elevation with EEG arousal cases[a]	%	MUA elevation with EEG sleep cases[a]	%	MUA change independent of EEG cases	%
Tract of diagonal band	14	8	57	0	0	6	43
Lateral preoptic area	3	1+(1)	67	0	0	1	33
Medial preoptic area	34	10+(6)	47	0	0	18	53
Suprachiasmatic nucleus	4	(3)	75	0	0	1	25
Anterior hypothalamic area	5	2+(1)	60	0	0	2	40
Paraventricular nucleus	9	5+(1)	67	0	0	3	33
Retrochiasmatic area	9	7	78	1	11	1	11
Optic chiasma or tract	8	1+(1)	25	0	0	6	75
Arcuate nucleus (ARC) and/or median eminence (ME)	76	6+(14)	26	2+(1)	4	53	70
Ventromedial nucleus (VMH)	6	3+(1)	67	0	0	2	33
Area between ARC + VMH	12	8	67	(1)	8	3	25
Dorsomedial nucleus (DMH)	7	3	43	0	0	4	57
Lateral hypothalamic area	9	5+(1)	67	0	0	3	33
Posterior hypothalamus and premamillary area	4	4	100	0	0	0	0
Thalamus and zona incerta	13	11	84	(1)	8	1	8
Internal capsule, putamen and globus pallidus	12	8	67	0	0	4	33
Reticular formation and central gray	5	4+(1)	100	0	0	0	0
Hippocampus	5	1	20	3	60	1	[illegible]
Amygdala-medial nucleus	5	0	0	2	40	3	60
Amygdala-cortical nucleus	6	1	17	4+(1)	83	0	0
ARC-ME, completely deafferented	10	0	0	0	0	10	100
ARC-ME, incompletely deafferented	9	1+(2)	33	0	0	6	67
ARC-ME, posteriorly deafferented	2	0	0	0	0	2	100
ARC-ME, anteriorly deafferented	6	(2)	33	0	0	4	67

[a] Numbers in parentheses represent relatively weak changes.

are summarized in Table 2 and illustrated in Fig. 3. The integrated MUA records from the ARC-ME of rats No. 147 and 123 in Fig. 3A and B were taken simultaneously with the EEG tracings from these same rats, shown in Fig. 2A and B, respectively.

Animals receiving the progesterone in the morning (9:44-13:00) showed a triphasic response in six out of nine cases (Fig. 3A, Table 2). There was an initial rise in integrated MUA (latency, 24–48 min; latency to peak, 30 min–2 hr; recovery time, 1hr–3.4 hr), a secondary depression (latency, 1.2–3.4 hr; latency to lowest point, 3.6–5.1 hr; recovery time 5–7.2 hr, and a tertiary elevation (latency, 5–7 hr); latency to peak, 7–10 hr; recovery time, 8.2–11.4 hr). The other three animals showed biphasic responses, lacking the initial peak in MUA but including depression and elevation phases covering the same time courses as phases II and III of the triphasic responses (Table 2).

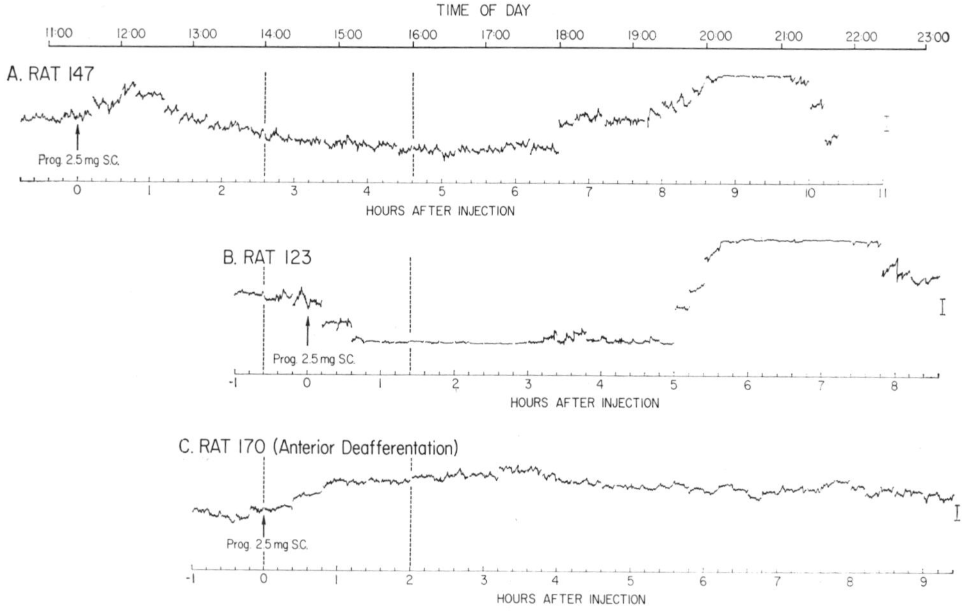

FIG. 3. Effects of morning and afternoon injections of progesterone on integrated multiple unit activity in the arcuate nucleus-median eminence of the rats whose EEG samples were shown in Fig. 2. A. Note the rise, fall, and secondary rise in integrated MUA following the morning injection (rat 147); and B, the biphasic fall and rise induced by the afternoon injection (rat 123). The 14:00–16:00 "critical period" is marked with vertical dotted lines. C, shows the slow rise in MUA in the anteriorly deafferented hypothalamus following progesterone treatment. Calibration marks: 100 mv.

TABLE 2

TIME RELATIONSHIPS OF THE SEQUENTIAL PHASES OF MULTIPLE UNIT ACTIVITY IN THE MEDIAN EMINENCE FOLLOWING TREATMENT WITH PROGESTERONE AT DIFFERENT HOURS OF THE DAY OF "PROESTRUS"

Rat no.	Progesterone injection sc in oil		Elapsed time in hr after progesterone treatment								
			Phase I: Elevation			Phase II: Depression			Phase III: Elevation		
	Time	Dosage (mg)	Latency	Latency to peak	Recovery time	Latency	Latency to lowest point	Recovery time	Latency	Latency to peak	Recovery time
122	13:00	2.5	0.4	1.2	1.4	1.4	3.6	5.0	5.0	7.0	11.0
147	11:22	2.5	0.4	0.8	1.6	1.4	5.1	6.8	7.0	9.4	10.2
149	10:20	1.25	0.8	2.0	3.4	3.4	4.4	5.2	5.2	6.9	8.2
155	10:05	1.25	0.4	1.5	2.6	2.8	4.1	5.2	5.2	6.4	8.4
163	10:29	2.5	0.6	1.0	1.6	1.6	5.0	6.0	6.0	10.0	11.4
166	10:34	1.25	0.4	0.6	1.0	1.2	4.0	7.2	7.2	9.8	11.4
157	9:44	1.25	—	—	—	2.8	5.2	5.8	5.8	6.6	8.2
150	10:10	1.25	—	—	—	1.6	3.1	4.8	4.8	>6.0	>6.4
159	10:26	2.5	—	—	—	2.6	3.4	5.0	5.4	7.5	8.6
123	14:45	2.5	—	—	—	0.4	2.6	5.4	5.4	6.6	12.0
125	14:45	2.5	—	—	—	0.8	2.8	5.0	5.0	6.8	7.6
102	16:00	2.5	—	—	—	1.2	3.4	6.4	6.4	7.4	>8.0
126	18:25	2.5	—	—	—	0.4	2.7	4.2	4.2	4.8	10.4
121	15:00	2.5	—	—	—	0.8	4.2	5.4	5.4	6.4	8.0
139	13:06	2.5	—	—	—	0.2	3.2	4.2	4.2	5.2	>7.0
114	13:12	2.5	—	—	—	0.6	3.0	5.2	—	—	—
115	16:08	2.5	—	—	—	1.0	5.2	7.6	—	—	—
101	15:11	2.5	—	—	—	—	—	—	3.4	5.7	10.4
130	14:50	2.5	—	—	—	—	—	—	3.4	7.6	10.2

Rats injected with progesterone in the afternoon (13:06–18:25) generally gave a biphasic response: they lacked the initial rise in MUA seen in animals treated in the morning but showed the phases of depression and subsequent elevation. Two out of ten rats gave only the phase of depression and two others, only the late rise in MUA. The time courses of these responses can be seen in Fig. 3B and Table 2. Figure 1 shows the oscilloscopic picture of depression of multiple units following the afternoon injection of progesterone. The latency of the depression phase was much shorter than that which followed the morning injection (in which a rising phase was interspersed), but the recovery time from the drop in MUA and the whole time course of the later elevated phase were similar to those which followed the morning injection of progesterone.

Twelve ovariectomized rats which had not been primed with estrogen were injected with progesterone (2.5–5 mg sc) in the afternoon (14:00–19:00). In six of them the ARC-ME multiple unit level showed a monophasic rise of long latency (2.8–3.2 hr); latency to peak, 3.8–6.1 hr; and recovery time too late to be determined, generally > 10 hr. In four others the delayed rise in MUA was preceded by a slight drop in activity which reached its lowest point between 2.6–5.6 hr after progesterone administration. The other two showed only the slight depression in MUA with no subsequent rise above the control level.

Effects in Other Regions of the Brain. Among 15 ovariectomized estrogen-primed rats with electrodes in the medial preoptic area or the diagonal band there were four different patterns of response to progesterone injected in the morning of artificial proestrus. Five of these animals showed a monophasic elevation in multiple units with a latency of 1–3.2 hr, a latency to peak of 3.6 hr, and a recovery time of 5.8–9.4 hr. Four of the rats gave a biphasic response with initial depression, and two showed a triphasic response with initial elevation as in the ARC-ME. The other four rats appeared unaffected by the steroid. Fourteen similar rats were injected with progesterone in the afternoon; only three of these showed any effect of the steroid, one a biphasic response and the other two cases an increase in MUA. Without estrogen priming, 16 rats with electrodes in the medial preoptic area or diagonal band, injected with progesterone in the morning or afternoon, failed to show any response attributable to the steroid.

Even with estrogen priming, several rats with electrodes in the lateral hypothalamic region, dorsomedial hypothalamic nucleus, central gray matter, reticular formation, and zona incerta showed little if any change in MUA following treatment with progesterone either in the morning or afternoon.

Effects of Progesterone after deafferentation of the Hypothalamus. The results are summarized in Table 3 and illustrated in Figs. 3C and 4. Although the number of rats was small the effects of deafferentation on the responses to treatment with progesterone were quite constant. Either anterior deafferentation (Fig. 3C) or complete deafferentation (Fig. 4) nullified the biphasic effect of an afternoon injection of progesterone on multiple units in the ARC-ME and replaced it with a gradual rise in activity, a monophasic response with a long recovery time. In the medial preoptic area, rostral to the region of deafferentation but anatomically very close to it, the response to progesterone after the operation was gen-

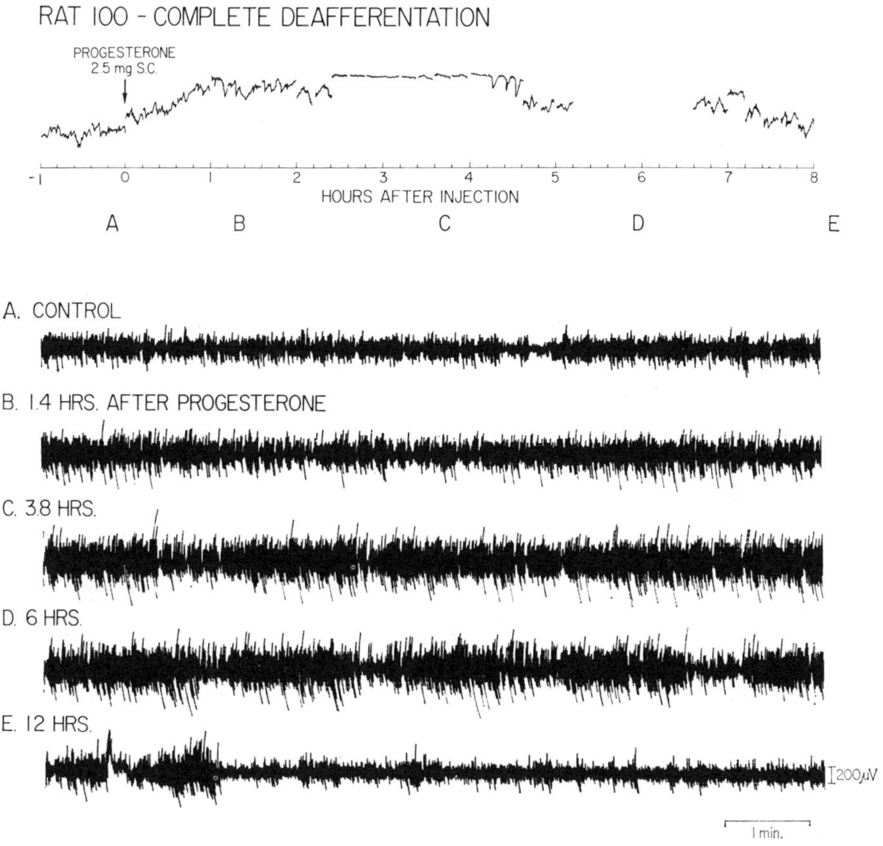

FIG. 4. Effects of progesterone on integrated multiple unit activity in the completely deafferented hypothalamus of rat No. 100. Progesterone was injected at 16:53 (Table 3). EEG samples (A-E), extracted from the record at intervals, show the synchronized high-amplitude response to the steroid. Calibration marks: 1 min; 200 μv.

TABLE 3

TIME RELATIONSHIPS OF PHASES OF MULTIPLE UNIT ACTIVITY (MUA) IN THE MEDIAN EMINENCE AND MEDIAL PREOPTIC AREA FOLLOWING PROGESTERONE TREATMENT IN HYPOTHALAMICALLY-DEAFFERENTED RATS

				Elapsed time in hr after progesterone treatment								
		Progesterone injection sc in oil		Arcuate nucleus-median eminence			Medial preoptic area					
				Elevated MUA			Depressed MUA			Elevated MUA		
Rat no.	Type of deafferentation	Time	Dosage (mg)	Latency	Latency to peak	Recovery time	Latency	Latency to lowest point	Recovery time	Latency	Latency to peak	Recovery time
94	Anterior	23:03	2.5	1.2	4.8	>5.0	0.2	1.2	3.2	—	—	—
96	Anterior	16:22	2.5	3.4	6.4	8.4						
98	Anterior	18:04	1.0	1.0	5.8	>7.0	0.2	0.4	2.4	2.4	5.6	>7.0
99	Complete	14:46	1.0				0.4	2.4	4.2	4.2	5.0	>9.4
100	Complete	16:53	2.5	0.2	3.4	7.6	0.4	3.2	4.4	4.4	9.6	17.0
105	Complete	13:40	2.5	1.6	9.4	13.0	0.6	1.8	3.2	3.2	5.8	8.0
168	Anterior	13:18	1.25	4.2	5.4	6.8						
169	Anterior	13:21	2.5	2.6	6.2	>8.0						
170	Anterior	13:47	2.5	0.6	3.6	11.0						

erally a biphasic one with initial depression (Table 3). There were no morning injections in this series.

Deafferentation did not appreciably affect the response of the cortical EEG to progesterone (Fig. 4). The prolonged sleep-like effect occurred with return to a partially aroused state after 12 hr or more. Although deafferented multiple units were almost completely independent of sleep-wakefulness EEG changes (Table I), the multiple unit tracings (Fig. 3C, Fig. 4) were extracted from records during periods of EEG synchronization or sleep, just as they were in experiments on intact brains.

Discussion

The "triphasic" effect of the morning injection of progesterone on hypothalamic MUA in the estrogen primed ovariectomized rat resembles in many ways the "biphasic" effect on brain thresholds described by Kawakami and Sawyer (21) in the estrogen-primed ovariectomized rabbit. The latter was, however, not affected by the diurnal factors controlling the response in the rat. The first phase, considered facilitatory in the rat because it resembled the response to ovulation-inducing preoptic stimulation (32), corresponded to the initial lowering of thresholds of EEG arousal and EEG afterreaction in the rabbit. The second phase of depressed activity in the rat corresponds to the period of elevated thresholds in the rabbit during which it is difficult to stimulate ovulation in the intact rabbit. The third phase (secondary elevation of MUA) in the rat has its counterpart in "estrous rebound" lowering of thresholds in the rabbit. The functional significance of the secondary rise in MUA in the rat is unknown, but one may speculate that it is related to the onset of estrous behavior, which occurs at that time in natural proestrus. In both the rat and rabbit these characteristic responses represent a synergistic effect of progesterone with estrogen; in the absence of estrogen the response to progesterone is commonly a monophasic slow rise in MUA (rat) or a monophasic elevation in threshold of EEG afterreaction (rabbit).

Our demonstration of progesterone-induced specific changes in hypothalamic MUA, independent of the steroid's effect on cortical EEG, might be considered as confirmation of earlier proposals (3, 9) that such specific changes do occur. However, our hypothalamic electrodes were in the arcuate nucleus-median eminence region in which the unit activity is largely of the "N" type, independent of sleep-wakefulness, whereas the earlier recordings of the Cambridge group (3) were in the lateral hypothalamus in which the unit activity is more commonly of the "A" type, facilitated during arousal. The results of Ramirez *et al.* (27), in which units were recorded in VMH, more closely resembled effects in the lateral hypothalamus, and the influences of progesterone in VMH units were not specific but parallel to changes in cortical EEG. In the absence of an EEG control one is not justified in claiming that single neurons respond specifically. Our new results do, nevertheless, confirm the later findings of Haller and Barraclough (19) that urethane permits the stimulatory effects of progesterone. Interestingly, the sleep-inducing effects of progesterone, which we observed in confirmation of many earlier investigators (2, 20, 22, 23), were relatively independent of the time of day and even independent of the hypothalamus: they occurred in the rat with a completely deafferented hypothalamus.

The induction by progesterone of "specific" changes in MUA in the arcuate nucleus-median eminence of the intact brain does not in itself mean that the so-called progesterone "receptors" necessarily lie in the basal hypothalamus. The slow changes in the completely deafferented hypothalamus following progesterone treatment do suggest that the steroid exerts a direct action on neurons in this area. Progesterone implants in the VMH-arcuate region by Döcke and Dörner (11) indicated to them that progesterone facilitates ovulation by lowering basal hypothalamic thresholds to cyclic neural stimuli arriving from the medial preoptic-anterior hypothalamic regions, and our results are not inconsistent with that hypothesis. Progesterone implantation experiments in Davidson's laboratory (10) suggest that the inhibitory feedback effect of the steroid is also exerted at the level of the median eminence. However, the fact that the medial preoptic area (MPO) shows biphasic changes in MUA when they are absent from the hypothalamus following anterior deafferentation suggests that receptors responsible for those changes lie rostral to the hypothalamus, possibly in the preoptic region itself or in some rhinencephalic area. The diurnal nature of the triphasic response suggests that progesterone may directly influence neurons related to the timing mechanism for pituitary activation. No attempt was made to deafferent the preoptic area, as was achieved in a few animals by Halász (18). A preoptic locus of progesterone receptors would be consistent with the proposal of Barraclough, Yrarrazaval, and Hatton (4) that the medial preoptic-suprachiasmatic region is essential for induction of ovulation by progesterone.

Our results show that under conditions in which progesterone stimulates the release of pituitary ovulating hormone prior to the critical period of proestrus, as in the experiments of Zeilmaker (34), Naller, Antunes-Rodrigues, and McCann (25), Brown-Grant (7), Redmond (28), and Caligaris, Astrada, and Taleisnik (8), it triggers or facilitates a phase of elevated MUA in arcuate nucleus neurons which is completed before the onset of the critical period. Odell and Swerdloff (26) have shown that in estrogen-primed ovariectomized or postmenopausal women progesterone stimulates a sharp peak in gonadotrophin secretion. However, there is doubt as to whether progesterone parallels estrogen secretion in anticipating gonadotrophin release in the natural cycles of either women or rats. Feder, Resko, and Goy (16) and Goldman *et al.* (17) have reported rises in progestins in arterial blood and ovarian venous effluent, respectively, in rats on the morning of proestrus, but in a later paper Feder *et al.* (15) could find little evidence of progesterone secretion prior to the critical period. Further work will be needed to determine what role, if any, endogenous progesterone plays in triggering the release of an ovulatory surge of gonadotrophin in either species.

Our results reveal a diurnal fluctuation in the responsiveness of MUA in the arcuate nucleus-median eminence region to subcutaneous injections of progesterone. These changes correlate with hypothalamo-pituitary activation and inhibition by progesterone. Our deafferentation results indicate that extrahypothalamic influences are responsible for the diurnal changes in responsiveness. Whether this is attributable to extrahypothalamic location of progesterone "receptors" or to other factors remains for future investigation.

References

1. Albe-Fessard, D., F. Stutinsky, and S. Liboudan. 1966. "Atlas Stéréotaxique du Diencéphale du Rat Blanc." Editions CNRS, Paris.
2. Arai, Y., M. Hiroi, J. Mitra, and R. A. Gorski. 1967. Influence of intravenous progesterone administration on the cortical electroencephalogram of the female rat. *Neuroendocrinology* **2** : 275–282.
3. Barraclough, C. A., and B. A. Cross. 1963. Unit activity in the hypothalamus of the cyclic female rat: effect of genital stimuli and progesterone. *J. Endocrinol.* **26** : 339–359.
4. Barraclough, C. A., S. Yrarrazaval, and R. Hatton. 1964. A possible hypothalamic site of action of progesterone in the facilitation of ovulation in the rat. *Endocrinology* **75** : 838–845.
5. Beyer, C., V. D. Ramirez, D. I. Whitmoyer. and C. H. Sawyer. 1967. Effects of hormones on the electrical activity of the brain in the rat and rabbit. *Exp. Neurol* **18** : 313–326.
6. Beyer, C., and C. H. Sawyer. 1969. Hypothalamic unit activity related to control of the pituitary gland, pp. 255–287. *In* "Frontiers in Neuroendocrinology, 1969", W. F. Ganong and L. Martini [eds.]. Oxford University Press, New York.
7. Brown-Grant, K. 1967. The effects of a single injection of progesterone on the oestrous cycle, thyroid gland activity and uterus-plasma concentration ratio for radio-iodide in the rat. *J. Physiol. London* **190** : 101-121.
8. Caligaris, L., J. J. Astrada, and S. Taleisnik. 1968. Stimulating and inhibiting effects of progesterone on the release of luteinizing hormone. *Acta Endocrinol.* **59** : 177–185.
9. Cross. B. A., and I. A. Silver. 1966. Electrophysiological studies on the hypothalamus. *Brit. Med. Bull.* **22** : 254–260.
10 Davidson, J. M. 1969. Feedback control of gonadotropin sceretion, pp. 343–388. *In* "Frontiers in Neuroendocrinology, 1969", W. F. Ganong and L. Martini [eds.]. Oxford University Press, New York.

11. Döcke, F., and G. Dörner. 1969. A possible mechanism by which progesterone facilitates ovulation in the rat. *Neuroendocrinology* **4**: 139–149.

12. Everett, J. W. 1948. Progesterone and estrogen in the experimental control of ovulation time and other features of the estrous cycle in the rat. *Endocrinology* **43**: 389–405.

13. Everett, J. W. 1969. Neuroendocrine aspects of mammalian reproduction. *An. Rev. Physiol.* **31**: 383–416.

14. Everett, J. W., and C. H. Sawyer. 1949. A neural timing factor in the mechanism by which progesterone advances ovulation in the cyclic rat. *Endocrinology* **45**: 581–595.

15. Feder, H. H., K. Brown-Grant, C. S. Corker, and D. Exley. 1969. Systemic plasma progesterone levels during the pro-oestrous critical period. *J. Endocrinol.* **43**: xxix.

16. Feder, H. H., J. A. Resko, and R. W. Goy. 1968. Progesterone levels in the arterial plasma of pre-ovulatory and ovariectomized rats. *J. Endocrinol.* **41**: 563–569.

17. Goldman, B. D., I. A. Kamberi, P. K. Siiteri, and J. C. Porter. 1969. Temporal relationship of progestin secretion, LH release and ovulation in rats *Endocrinology* **85**: 1137–1143.

18. Halász, B. 1969. The endocrine effects of isolation of the hypothalamus from the rest of the brain, pp. 307–342. *In* "Frontiers in Neuroendocrinology, 1969," W. F. Ganong and L. Martini [eds.]. Oxford University Press, New York.

19. Haller, E. W., and C. A. Barraclough. 1968. Hypothalamic regulation of ovulation: effects of urethane and progesterone. *Proc. Soc. Exp. Biol. Med.* **129**: 291–295.

20. Heuser, G.. G. M. Ling, and M. Kluver. 1967. Sleep induction by progesterone in the preoptic area in cats. *Electroencephalogr. Clin. Neurophysiol.* **22**: 122–127.

21. Kawakami, M., and C. H. Sawyer. 1959. Neuroendocrine correlates of changes in brain activity thresholds by sex steroids and pituitary hormones. *Endocrinology* **65**: 652–668.

22. Kobayashi, T., T. Kobayashi, S. Takezawa, K. Oshima, and H. Kawamura. 1962. Electrophysiological studies on the feed-back mechanism of progesterone. *Endocrinol. Jap.* **9**: 302–320.

23. Komisaruk, B. R., P. G. McDonald, D. I. Whitmoyer, and C. H. Sawyer. 1967. Effects of progesterone and sensory stimulation on EEG and neuronal activity in the rat. *Exp. Neurol.* **19**: 494–507.

24. Lisk, R. D. 1969. Progesterone: role in limitation of ovulation and sex behavior in mammals. *Trans. N.Y. Acad. Sci.* **31**: 593–601.

25. Nallar, R. J. Antunes-Rodrigues, and S. M. McCann. 1966. Effect of progesterone on the level of plasma luteinizing hormone (LH) in normal female rats. *Endocrinology* **79**: 907–911.

26. Odell, W. D., and R. S. Swerdloff. 1968. Progestogen-induced luteinizing and follicle-stimulating hormone surge in postmenopausal women: a simulated ovulatory peak. *Proc. Nat. Acad. Sci. U.S.* **61**: 529–536.

27. Ramirez, V. D., B. R. Komisaruk, D. I. Whitmoyer, and C. H. Sawyer. 1967. Effects of hormones and vaginal stimulation on the EEG and hypothalamic units in rats. *Amer. J. Physiol.* **212**: 1376–1384.

28. Redmond, W. C. 1968. Ovulatory response to brain stimulation or exogenous luteinizing hormone in progesterone-treated rats. *Endocrinology* **83**: 1013–1022.

29. SAWYER, C. H. 1969. Regulatory mechanisms of secretion of gonadotrophic hormones, pp. 389–430. *In* "The Hypothalamus", W. Haymaker, E. Anderson, and W. J. H. Nauta [eds.]. Thomas, Springfield, Illinois.
30. SAWYER, C. H., M. KAWAKAMI, B. MEYERSON, D. I. WHITMOYER, and J. J. LILLEY. 1968. Effects of ACTH, dexamethasone and asphyxia on electrical activity of the rat hypothalamus. *Brain Res.* **10**: 213–226.
31. TERASAWA, E., and C. H. SAWYER. 1968. Effects of luteinizing hormone (LH) on multiple unit activity in the rat hypothalamus. *Fed. Proc.* **27**: 269.
32. TERASAWA, E.. and C. H. SAWYER. 1969. Changes in electrical activity in the rat hypothalamus related to electrochemical stimulation of adenohypophyseal function. *Endocrinology* **85**: 143–149.
33. TERASAWA, E., D. I. WHITMOYER, and C. H. SAWYER. 1969. Effects of luteinizing hormone on multiple-unit activity in the rat hypothalamus. *Amer. J. Physiol.* **217**: 1119–1126.
34. ZEILMAKER, G. H. 1966. The biphasic effect of progesterone on ovulation in the rat. *Acta Endocrinol.* **51**: 461–468.

EFFECTS OF TESTOSTERONE INFUSIONS UPON EEGs OF NORMAL MALE ADULTS[1]

W. VOGEL, D. M. BROVERMAN, E. L. KLAIBER,

G. ABRAHAM AND F. L. CONE

Previous work (Vogel *et al.* 1968, 1969) reported relationships of EEG indices to the Automatization Cognitive Style, which is defined as greater or lesser ability to perform repetitive tasks than expected from the individual's general level of intellectual performance (Broverman 1964). Male Strong Automatizers (subjects with relatively greater abilities to perform repetitive tasks) had slower alpha frequencies while performing a repetitive mental task (serial subtraction problems) than Weak Automatizers. Strong Automatizers also show more evidence of testosterone stimulation than Weak Automatizers (Broverman *et al.* 1964; Klaiber *et al.* 1967).

The present report describes an experimental attempt to manipulate the EEG and behavioral phenomena previously found to be associated with the Automatization Cognitive Style, through the acute peripheral administration of testosterone to normal adult males.

The association of automatized behaviors with slow alpha frequencies is conceptualized in the following manner. Normally, the alpha rhythm (8–12 c/sec) is predominant during states of waking rest and is replaced by the beta rhythm (18–30 c/sec) during mental activity. However, during the performance of a repetitive task, the alpha rhythm gradually returns as the task becomes mastered, or automatized. Darrow (1947) has argued that, in such instances, alpha represents "an inhibitory process involving the discharge of subcortical and sympathetic impulses back into the cortex, thereby moderating or terminating the cortical excitation". This "termination of cortical excitation" is closely associated with the "automation" or "habituation" of learned behaviors, with a subsequent shift from "cortical to subcortical control" over behavior, according to Darrow (1957). We accept Darrow's argument, but would expand his theory to take account of individual differences in alpha frequency: the slower the alpha frequency during mental performances, the more it ought to be associated with automatized behaviors (Vogel *et al.* 1968).

---

[1] The data included in this paper were presented at the 7th International Congress of EEG and Clinical Neurophysiology, San Diego, 1969, and at the meetings of the Eastern Psychological Association, Atlantic City, 1970.

Darrow's (1947) formulation suggests that alpha rhythms during mental performances are sympathetic, or adrenergic, in origin. Earlier we indicated that the effects of testosterone upon many behaviors of both humans and animals are similar to those of pharmacological agents known to enhance central adrenergic functioning (Broverman *et al.* 1968). Both adrenergic stimulants and testosterone tend to increase proficiency in performances of automatized tasks (Broverman *et al.* 1968; Klaiber *et al.* 1971). Thus, we hypothesize that testosterone acts centrally as an adrenergic stimulant. Accordingly, infusions of testosterone should experimentally induce the slower alpha frequencies during mental performances such as have been observed in subjects who appear to differ naturally in androgen stimulation, *i.e.*, Strong as contrasted with Weak Automatizers (Klaiber *et al.* 1967; Vogel *et al.* 1968).

Subjects. Sixty-seven normal 21-year-old male college students were paid for their participation in the study.

PROCEDURE

Morning (*a.m. session.*)Continuous intravenous infusions of 10% ethanol and normal saline were started for all subjects as previously described (Klaiber *et al.* 1971). The material was infused at 1.91 ml/min using a Harvard infusion pump. The 10% ethanol and normal saline solution was utilized so that testosterone could be added to the solution later in the experiment. Testosterone is highly soluble in ethanol but only weakly soluble in aqueous solutions. To control for physiological factors, all subjects were told that they were receiving infusions of testosterone. After 2 h, EEG recordings under both rest and mental performance were obtained. The mental performance consisted of serial subtractions in which 17 was subtracted from 981, and from each successive remainder for a 3 min period.

Afternoon (*p.m.*) *session.* Immediately thereafter, in forty of the sixty-seven subjects, the infusion solution was changed, without the subjects' knowledge, to provide testosterone 0.8 mg/h, which is double the rate of testosterone reported for normal adult males (Levin *et al.* 1967). After 4 h, a second set of EEG recordings and mental performances was obtained.

Procedures run on the remaining twenty-seven control subjects were identical to the above, except that no testosterone was infused; rather, the saline-ethanol solution was continued throughout the 6 h infusion period. The total amount of alcohol infused into each of the sixty-seven subjects was 68.76 ml, or approximately 2.4 oz.

To control for psychological factors, all subjects were told that they were receiving infusions of testosterone. Except for the attending physician who supervised the infusion procedure, none of the personnel who were associated with the study and who were responsible for giving and scoring the EEG and mental performance data was aware of which subjects were receiving testosterone.

The EEG data were obtained on a Grass model 5D

polygraph, with Grass model 5P5E pre-amplifiers and Grass 5P5 amplifiers. The time constant was 0.2 sec. The sensitivity used was 30 μV/cm pen deflection. Grass EC2 electrode cream was applied under Grass E5 gold disc electrodes. The EEG data used for this report were obtained from one pair of occipital electrodes with each electrode placed 3 cm above the inion and 2 cm from the midline.

Not all sixty-seven subjects were included in the EEG analysis. Only fifty-two subjects produced sufficient alpha to proceed with the analysis, *i.e.*, five or more 1 sec periods of uninterrupted alpha during the 3 min serial subtraction task for both the *a.m.* and *p.m.* examination periods. Average alpha frequency for these fifty-two subjects was assessed by determining (to the nearest full cycle) the frequencies of the waves for each second in which alpha was uninterruptedly evident during each 3 min serial subtraction period, and then averaging the frequencies for that person for that period. Each record was scored independently by the senior author and by an experienced EEG technician. Inter-rater reliability for alpha frequency was better than 0.90 and intra-rater reliability was 0.95. Disagreements were resolved by later consultation between the scorers.

Since we wished to assess the effect of testosterone on alpha frequency, experimental and control subjects were matched for average *a.m.* alpha frequency to within ± 0.4 c/sec. This procedure eliminated six subjects, so that we were left with twenty-three experimental and twenty-three control subjects.

Blood samples for assays of plasma testosterone concentrations, by the method of Riondel *et al.* (1963) were drawn from twenty-three of the experimental subjects, and from twenty of the control subjects. This procedure was introduced after the experiment had started; hence, three subjects in the control group were not included.

TABLE I

Effects of testosterone *vs.* saline infusion on mean number of problems correct.

	a.m.	*p.m.*	Change, *p.m.–a.m.**
Testosterone (N=23)	38.9	35.9	−3.0
Saline (N=23)	39.3	31.0	−8.3

* Change, *p.m.–a.m.*, testosterone *vs.* saline groups, $F = 4.58$, $P < 0.05$.

RESULTS

For all forty-six subjects in the combined experimental and control groups, mental performance declined from *a.m.* to *p.m.* in terms of number of subtraction problems performed correctly in 3 min. However, as shown in Table I, the experimental subjects showed significantly less deterioration in performance than did the control subjects ($F = 4.58$; $P < 0.05$).

For all forty-six subjects combined, alpha frequency during mental performances showed no significant change from *a.m.* to *p.m.* However, as shown in Table II, the alpha frequencies of the experimental subjects were slower in the afternoon than in the morning, whereas the reverse occurred in the control subjects. The trends of alpha frequency in the experimental and control subjects are significantly different ($F = 5.58$; $P < 0.05$). Thus the infusion of testosterone appeared to exert a slowing influence upon alpha frequencies.

The slowing of alpha frequency in the experimental subjects was presumably due to the influence of the infused testosterone. The reason for the acceleration of alpha frequency in the control subjects may relate to changes in their plasma testosterone concentrations as reported below.

Relationship of post-infusion plasma testosterone concentration (PTC) to alpha frequency in control subjects. The PTCs of the control subjects declined 21% ($P < 0.002$) from morning to afternoon. The decline could have been due either to the stress of the infusion procedures (Levin *et al.* 1967), or to diurnal factors (Resko and Eik-Nes 1966). However, those control subjects who maintained relatively high post-infusion PTCs showed, like the experimental subjects, a decrease in alpha frequency; subjects with the lowest post-infusion PTCs showed a marked acceleration in alpha frequency. The difference in change in alpha frequency between the 2 groups

TABLE II

Effects of testosterone *vs.* saline infusion on mean alpha frequency.

	a.m.	*p.m.*	Change, *p.m.–a.m.**
Testosterone (N=23)	9.75	9.52	−0.23
Saline (N=23)	9.72	10.00	+0.28

* Change, *p.m.–a.m.*, testosterone *vs.* saline groups, $F = 5.58$, $P < 0.05$. The mean number of seconds of alpha on which the *a.m.* and *p.m.* alpha frequency scores were based were: testosterone group, 17.5 and 23.7; saline group 18.5 and 22.5, group differences not significant by F test.

of subjects was statistically significant (F = 4.68; $P < 0.05$). This observation was based on eight control subjects with above median post-infusion PTCs who could be matched on *a.m.* alpha frequency ±0.4 c/sec to eight control subjects with below median post-infusion PTCs (see Table III). Thus, those control subjects who were best able to maintain their plasma testosterone concentrations did not show the accelerated alpha frequency found in control subjects who had marked drops in post-infusion PTCs.

Relationship of post-infusion plasma testosterone concentration (PTC) to alpha frequency in experimental subjects. Not unexpectedly, the experimental subjects being infused with testosterone showed a significant ($P < 0.001$) rise to post-infusion PTCs. However, considerable variation in the extent of the rise occurred. Eleven subjects averaged a 15% rise, whereas twelve other subjects had an average increase of 143%. The reason for such differences in the post-infusion PTCs are unknown. Such differences could be explained by variations in metabolic clearance or production rates of testosterone, by differences in liver enzyme activities, or by variations in the extent to which the circulating testosterone was rendered physiologically inactive via binding to specific testosterone-binding protein molecules (August *et al.* 1969). Consideration of other factors, however, led to the conclusion that the most likely of these possibilities was reduced metabolic clearance due to excessive binding of testosterone (Klaiber *et al.* 1971), based on the fact that the infused testosterone failed to suppress plasma gonadotrophin levels

TABLE III

The relationship of alpha frequency to post-infusion plasma testosterone concentrations in control subjects.

Concentration	Mean alpha frequency		
	a.m.	*p.m.*	Change, *p.m.–a.m.**
Hi-testosterone (N = 8) (0.51 to 0.92 μg/100 ml)	9.78	9.61	−0.17
Low testosterone (N = 8) (0.27 to 0.50 μg/100 ml)	9.63	10.20	+0.57

* Change, *p.m.–a.m.* high *vs.* low testosterone groups, F = 4.68, $P < 0.05$. The mean number of seconds of alpha on which the *a.m.* and *p.m.* alpha frequency scores were based were: "hi" group, 17.0 and 22.5; "low" group, 19.5 and 21.5, group differences not significant by F test.

in the subjects with the higher post-infusion PTCs, but did in subjects with lower post-infusion PTCs. Thus, high levels of post-infusion PTC seem to reflect a relative physiological inactivity of testosterone. It is worthy of note, therefore, that the experimental subjects with the relatively high post-infusion PTCs actually showed, like the control subjects, an *increase* in alpha frequency. The tendency of infused testosterone to lead to slowing of alpha frequency was largely limited to those experimental subjects who had relatively low post-infusion PTCs, *i.e.*, those subjects who were better able to utilize the infused testosterone. The difference in changes in alpha frequency in the two groups is statistically significant ($F = 6.03$; $P < 0.05$). This observation was based on ten experimental subjects with above median post-infusion PTC who could be matched on *a.m.* alpha frequency ± 0.4 c/sec to ten experimental subjects with below median post-infusion PTC (see Table IV).

DISCUSSION

The effects of testosterone vs. saline infusion on alpha frequency. Our hypothesis that the infusion of testosterone would induce a slowing of alpha frequencies is confirmed. The infused testosterone also induced a heightened proficiency in performances of a repetitive mental task.

Moreover, changes in alpha frequency were also significantly related to changes in plasma testosterone concentration (PTC). Control subjects with the greatest drops in PTC

TABLE IV

The relationship of alpha frequency to post-infusion plasma testosterone concentrations in experimental subjects.

Concentration	Mean alpha frequency		
	a.m.	*p.m.*	Change, *p.m.–a.m.**
Hi-testosterone (N=10) (0.92 to 2.96 μg/100 ml)	10.02	10.14	+0.12
Low testosterone (N=10) (0.51 to 0.88 μg/100 ml)	10.24	9.76	−0.48

* Change, *p.m.–a.m.*, high *vs.* low testosterone groups. $F = 6.03$, $P < 0.05$. The mean number of seconds of alpha in which the *a.m.* and *p.m.* alpha frequency scores were based were: "hi" group, 18.0 and 21.5; "low" group, 18.0 and 23.9; group differences not significant by F test.

showed the greatest increment in alpha frequency. Faster alpha frequencies were also found in experimental subjects who appeared least able to clear the infused testosterone metabolically.

Adrenergic stimulants, such as amphetamine, are known to have a positive effect on performances of repetitive mental tasks (Broverman *et al.* 1968). We have shown previously that chronic injections of testosterone affected EEG alpha driving responses to photic stimulation in a manner similar to adrenergic stimulants (Stenn *et al.*, in preparation). Taken together, these findings suggest to us that testosterone may achieve its behavioral and EEG effects through a facilitatory effect upon the central adrenergic system.

The Automatization Cognitive Style (a measure of proficiency at the performance of repetitive mental tasks) has been found related to a wide variety of behavioral and physiological characteristics in addition to those previously cited, *e.g.*, rate of physical maturation and physical development (Broverman *et al.* 1964); distractability (Broverman 1960); learning ability and resistance to mental fatigue (Broverman *et al.* 1966); occupational efficiency (Broverman 1964); and EEG resistance to photic stimulation (Vogel *et al.* 1969). The current findings have relevance to this body of work. Specifically, we would suggest that the subcortical adrenergic regulating mechanism postulated by Darrow (1947, 1957) which we believe to be reflected by slow alpha frequencies during mental performances, may be a significant contributory factor to the various behavioral traits associated with Strong and Weak Automatizers. This mechanism, in turn, appears to be sensitive to and manipulatable by testosterone, a gonadal steroid hormone.

SUMMARY

Continuous intravenous infusions of 10% ethanol and normal saline were started in each of forty-six normal young adult males. After 2 h, the infusion material was changed to include testosterone at the rate of 0.8 mg/h for four hours in twenty-three subjects, while infusion of saline-ethanol was continued in the remaining twenty-three control subjects. Simultaneous EEGs and mental performance data (serial subtraction problems) were obtained before and after the point at which the infusion material was changed. The subjects receiving testosterone solved more problems correctly ($P < 0.05$) and evidenced slower alpha frequencies ($P < 0.05$) than those subjects receiving saline. High as contrasted with low post-infusion testosterone levels in the control group were associated with slow alpha frequencies. However, very high as contrasted with lower post-infusion levels in the testosterone-infused group were associated with fast alpha frequencies. This latter finding is possibly attributable to the fact that very high testosterone levels may reflect reduced metabolic clearance due to excessive protein binding of testosterone. Such binding would result in reduced physiological activity of testosterone, *e.g.*, a lessened effect upon the

EEG. Our results confirm the hypothesis that testosterone, acting through the central nervous system, affects cognitive and EEG events in normal persons.

REFERENCES

August, G. P., Thachuk, M. and Grumback, M. M. Plasma testosterone-binding affinity and testosterone in umbilical cord plasma, late pregnancy, prepubertal children and adults. *J. clin. Endocr.*, **1969,** *29*: 891–899.

Broverman, D. M. Dimensions of cognitive style. *J. Personality*, **1960,** *28*: 167–185.

Broverman, D. M. Generality and behavioral correlates of cognitive styles. *J. cons. Psychol.*, **1964,** *28*: 487–500.

Broverman, D. M., Broverman, I. K. and Klaiber, E. L. Ability to automatize and automatization cognitive style: a validation study. *Percept. Motor Skills*, **1966,** *23*: 419–437.

Broverman, D. M., Broverman, I. K., Vogel, W., Palmer, R. D. and Klaiber, E. L. The automatization cognitive style and physical development. *Child Develop.*, **1964,** *35*: 1343–1359.

Broverman, D. M., Klaiber, E. L., Kobayashi, Y. and Vogel, W. Roles of activation and inhibition in sex differences in cognitive abilities. *Psychol. Rev.*, **1968,** *75*: 23–50.

Darrow, C. W. Psychological and psychophysiological significance of the EEG. *Psychol. Rev.*, **1947,** *54*: 157–168.

Darrow, C. W. Electroencephalographic "blocking" and "adaptation". *Science*, **1957,** *126*: 74–75.

Klaiber, E. L., Broverman, D. M. and Kobayashi, Y. The automatization cognitive style, androgens, and monoamine oxidase. *Psychopharmacologia (Berl.)*, **1967,** *11*: 320–336.

Klaiber, E. L., Broverman, D. M., Vogel, W., Abraham, G. E. and Cone, F. L. Effects of infused testosterone on mental performances and I.C.S.H. *J. clin. Endocr.*, **1971,** *32*: 341–349.

Levin, J., Lloyd, C. W., Lobotsky, J. and Friedrich, E. H. The effect of epinephrine on testosterone production. *Acta endocr. (Kbh.)*, **1967,** *55*: 184–192.

Resko, J. A. and Eik-Nes, K. B. Diurnal testosterone levels in peripheral plasma of human male subjects. *J. clin. Endocr.*, **1966,** *26*: 573–576.

Riondel, A., Tait, J. F., Gut, M., Tait, S. A. S., Joachim, E. and Liddle, B. Estimation of testosterone in human peripheral blood using S^{35} thiosemicarbazide. *J. clin. Endocr.*, **1963,** *23*: 620–628.

Vogel, W., Broverman, D. M. and Klaiber, E. L. EEG and mental abilities. *Electroenceph. clin. Neurophysiol.*, **1968,** *24*: 166–175.

Vogel, W., Broverman, D. M., Klaiber, E. L. and Kun, K. J. EEG response to photic stimulation as a function of cognitive style. *Electroenceph. clin. Neurophysiol.*, **1969,** *27*: 186–190.

The Gonad-Brain Relationship: Effects of Female Sex Hormones on Electroshock Convulsions in the Rat

DOROTHY E. WOOLLEY† AND PAOLA S. TIMIRAS

ABSTRACT. The effects of ovariectomy and ovarian hormones on brain excitability were investigated in rats by measuring: (a) minimal electroshock seizure threshold, and (b) maximal electroshock seizure pattern. Increased excitability or greater convulsive reactivity is indicated by a decreased threshold and by alterations in the duration of the tonic and clonic components of a maximal seizure, i.e., shortening of tonic flexion and/or lengthening of tonic extension. These procedures and treatments were studied: (a) ovariectomy, before and after puberty, with or without hormonal replacement therapy; (b) administration of estradiol and progesterone, alone or in combination, in intact, castrated or hypophysectomized male or female rats; and (c) administration of testosterone and methylandrostenediol to compare the central nervous effects of male and female sex steroids. Body and organ weights were measured and compared with the changes in convulsability. The main results were: (a) *Ovariectomy.* After sexual maturation intact females demonstrated greater convulsability than rats ovariectomized *before* puberty. This was shown by lower seizure thresholds and shorter tonic flexor phases in intact rats as compared with castrated females. However, when ovariectomy was performed *after* puberty, difference in convulsability was not observed even 3 weeks after operation. (b) *Sex steroids.* Administration of estradiol to intact mature males and to ovariectomized immature and mature females markedly lowered seizure thresholds. This excitatory action of estradiol was apparent 2 to 7 days after treatment was started, and continued for the duration of treatment; it occurred at doses from 500 μg to 4 μg/100 g body weight/day and was proportional to the dose administered. Similar effects of estradiol in hypophysectomized rats demonstrated that the convulsant action of the hormone was *not* mediated through the pituitary trophic hormones. Progesterone (500 μg/100 g body weight/day) rapidly and significantly raised the seizure threshold in female rats but had no immediate effect in males. This anticonvulsant action in females was transient and was replaced after 20 days of treatment by a moderate convulsant effect in both males and females. Testosterone and methylandrostenediol (500 μg/100 g body weight/day)

THE RELATIONSHIP between gonadal activity and brain function has long been recognized as a dual one. The numerous studies concerned with the effects exerted by the nervous system via the hypothalamic-hypophyseal axis on the development and function of the gonads have been reviewed recently by Harris (1). Other studies have investigated the second aspect of the relationship, namely, the influence exerted by gonadal hormones on the activity of the nervous system. Several observations have indicated that sex hormones participate in the regulation not only of mating behavior but also of various types of adaptive behavior such as running activity (2–4), aggressiveness (5), dominance pattern (6), and perhaps maze-learning ability (7). The behavioral data have led Beach (8, 9) to formulate the hypothesis that the sex steroids must alter thresholds within the nervous system. The influence of the gonadal hormones on the central nervous system was further demonstrated by their ability to produce general anesthesia (10, 11), to elevate the convulsive threshold (12), and to inhibit brain respiration (13). A relation between sex hormones and brain excitability was also suggested by clinical studies, reviewed by Logothetis *et al.*

Supported by a grant (S-60-14) from the Committee for Research in Problems of Sex of the National Academy of Sciences.

† This work is part of a thesis submitted by the senior author in partial fulfillment of the requirements for the degree of Doctor of Philosophy in Physiology. It was performed during the tenure of a USPHS predoctoral fellowship.

significantly lowered seizure threshold after 9 to 20 days of injections in intact adult male rats; however, this fall in threshold was less marked than that produced by estradiol. Thus estradiol appeared to have a more marked central excitatory action than progesterone, testosterone or methylandrostenediol. In addition, progesterone exhibited both an anticonvulsant and a convulsant action in female rats. It is concluded that sex steroids are capable of altering thresholds and convulsive patterns in the brain and thus play a basic role in aspects of central nervous system physiology other than those exclusively concerned with sexual functions.

---

(14), in epileptic females in whom it was possible to correlate incidence and severity of seizures with phases of ovarian activity.

A direct approach to the study of the relationship between gonadal function and brain activity thresholds was that taken by Kawakami and Sawyer (15) who studied the effects of sex steroids "on sex behavior and pituitary function" in correlation with "changes in thresholds of two opposing cerebral systems: the 'EEG arousal threshold' involving the brainstem reticular formation (I), and the 'EEG after-reaction threshold' involving the rhinencephalon and hypothalamus (II)." According to these authors "changes in I are more closely related to sexual behavior, whereas alterations in II are correlated with pituitary thresholds for the release of ovulating hormone." And they conconcluded "that both the facilitatory and inhibitory effects of sex steroids" on I and II "are mediated by means of altered thresholds of cerebral activity." That the sex steroids alter brain thresholds is also suggested by data from our laboratory which showed that threshold and pattern of electroshock convulsions differ significantly in adult male and female rats of the same age and strain (16) and that this difference may be attributed to the type and level of circulating sex steroids (17, 18).

Because of the practical importance of the sex steroids in some neurological diseases and the frequent use of these hormones in therapy, we pursued further the experimental study of the gonad-brain relationship. Our objective in this investigation was to study the effects of ovarian hormones on brain excitability in rats. The following conditions and treatments were considered: (a) ovariectomy, before and after puberty, with and without replacement therapy; (b) administration of estradiol and progesterone, alone or in combination, in intact, castrated or hypophysectomized male or female rats. Data from one experiment with male sex steroids are also presented to compare the central nervous effects of male and female hormones. In all experiments, brain excitability was assessed by measuring the threshold and pattern of electroshock convulsions, a method used routinely in several laboratories in investigations of the same type (19, 20). In addition, body and organ weights were measured to compare the well-known metabolic and endocrine actions of the sex steroids with their lesser-known effects on brain thresholds.

Materials and Methods

Animals. The Long-Evans strain of rats was used. Water and a standard rat diet in pellets were available *ad libitum* to all animals. Hypophysectomized rats received in addition 60% glucose and moistened mash. Animal quarters were illuminated by artificial light only, automatically controlled to produce 12 hours of light and 12 hours of darkness. Hypophysectomies were performed by the parapharyngeal approach and ovariectomies through 2 separate costo-lumbar incisions. All operations were checked for completeness at autopsy.

Body weights were recorded at start and end of each experiment and at least once a week during the experimental period. *Organs* were dissected immediately after sacrifice and weighed fresh. When immature females were studied, each animal was checked daily for the appearance of vaginal opening; the time of opening was considered as an indication of puberty and sexual maturation.

Vaginal smears were performed periodically in adolescent and mature females to determine whether or not the vaginal estrous cycle was normal or had been altered by the hormonal treatment and experimental conditions.

Sex steroids. These sex steroids were subcutaneously injected: estradiol dipropionate, progesterone, testosterone propionate, and methylandrostenediol (MAD). Each steroid was dissolved in Mazola oil[1] so that the quantity to be injected each day was contained in 0.1 ml. Because of its low solubility

[1] Certain vegetable oils have been found to possess estrogen-like activity when injected subcutaneously in immature female mice (21). However, in the present experiments, the oil vehicle (Mazola) alone did not seem to alter the electroshock threshold or to present any indication of estrogenic activity.

TABLE 1. Experimental arrangements and procedures

	Sex and sexual maturity at start of experiment	Surgical procedure	Hormones,* μg/100 g body weight/day				Duration of treatment or experiment in days	Convulsive parameters tested
			Estradiol	Progesterone	Testosterone	Methylandrostenediol		
			Experiment 1					
1	Immature females	Sham-operation	—	—	—	—	50	—
2		Ovariectomy	—	—	—	—		—
3		Sham-operation	—	—	—	—		EST†, MES†
4		Ovariectomy	—	—	—	—		EST, MES
			Experiment 2					
1	Immature females	—	—	—	—	—	102	EST, MES
2		Ovariectomy	—	—	—	—		EST, MES
3		Ovariectomy	0.1–4.0	—	—	—		EST, MES
4		Ovariectomy	—	250–375	—	—		EST, MES
			Experiment 3					
1	Mature females	—	—	—	—	—	24	EST
2		Ovariectomy	—	—	—	—		EST
3		Ovariectomy	10	—	—	—		EST
4		Ovariectomy	10	500	—	—		EST
5		Ovariectomy	—	500	—	—		EST
			Experiment 4					
1	Mature males	—	—	—	—	—	20	—
2		—	500	—	—	—		—
3		—	500	500	—	—		—
4		—	—	500	—	—		—
5		—	—	—	500	—		—
6		—	—	—	—	500		—
7		—	—	—	—	—		EST
8		—	500	—	—	—		EST
9		—	500	500	—	—		EST
10		—	—	500	—	—		EST
11		—	—	—	500	—		EST
12		—	—	—	—	500		EST
			Experiment 5					
1	Mature males	—	—	—	—	—	20	EST
2		—	10	—	—	—		EST
3		—	50	—	—	—		EST
4		—	200	—	—	—		EST
5		—	500	—	—	—		EST
			Experiment 6					
1	Mature females	—	—	—	—	—	24	EST
2		Hypophysectomy	10	—	—	—		EST

* All hormones were dissolved or suspended in oil and injected subcutaneously. Control animals were injected subcutaneously with the oil vehicle.

† For explanation of abbreviations, see text.

in oil, MAD was injected as a suspension.

Electroshock techniques. The apparatus and techniques employed have been described in detail elsewhere (22). Only the general aspects of these procedures will be presented here.

Minimal electroshock seizure threshold (EST) test. The EST is defined as the minimal amount of 60 cps. current in milliamperes (ma.) delivered through corneal electrodes for 0.2 seconds, which results in a barely detectable clonic convulsion of the ears, jaws, and forepaws. This convulsion lasts for only a few seconds and is not associated with loss of equilibrium.

Maximal electroshock seizure (MES) pattern. The MES is elicited by the same techniques outlined above for the EST but with a stimulus of 150 ma., which is 5 to 6 times stronger than the current used for the threshold determinations (the threshold current is usually 20 to 30 ma. for adult rats). This supramaximal stimulus produces a generalized tonic-clonic convulsion characterized by a constant progression of events as follows: tonic hindleg flexion, tonic hindleg extension, and intermittent whole-body and limb clonus. The duration of each of these phases of the maximal convulsion constitutes the *MES pattern.* The phases are timed in seconds by automatic timers connected to the stimulator.

General Plan of Experiments

The experimental arrangements and procedures are summarized in Table 1.

In Experiment 1, 40 immature female rats were divided into 4 equal groups (Table 1). Ovariectomies and sham-operations were performed when the animals were 30 days of age and had an average body weight of 60 g. The experiment was terminated when the animals had reached 80 days of age. In Experiment 2, 40 immature female rats were divided into 4 equal groups (Table 1). Ovariectomy was performed at 30 days of age when the animals had an average body weight of 60 g. All rats were sacrificed at 132 days of age and the uterus, hypophysis, adrenals, and thymus were weighed at autopsy. Estradiol was injected in the following daily doses per 100 g body weight: 1st week, 0.10 μg; next 12 days, 0.15 μg; next 16 days, 0.25 μg; for the remainder of the experiment, 4 μg. Progesterone was injected in the following daily doses per 100 g body weight: 1st 9 days, 250 μg; next 27 days, 285 μg; for the remainder of the experiment, 375 μg. Doses were gradually increased in order to induce vaginal opening and/or to obtain changes in electroshock threshold.

In Experiments 1 and 2, EST was measured 3 times a week throughout the experimental period. MES pattern was determined in Experiment 1 at 44 and 64 days of age and in Experiment 2 at 53, 74, 107, and 132 days of age. In Experiment 3, 30 young adult female rats were divided into 5 equal groups (Table 1). Ovariectomy was performed when the animals had reached an average body weight of 220 g. Hormonal injections were started 1 week after ovariectomy. The daily doses of estradiol and progesterone, either singly or in combination, and the duration of the treatment are given in Table 1. At autopsy the uterus and the adrenals were weighed. In all animals EST was measured 1 to 3 times a week, 1 week before ovariectomy, and then throughout the experimental period. In Experiment 4, 132 male rats with an average initial body weight of 220 g were divided into 2 major groups: the animals of the 1st group served as unshocked controls and those of the 2nd group were electroshocked at regular intervals. Each major group was further divided into 6 subgroups of 11 animals each, according to the steroid injected (Table 1). Seminal vesicles, levator ani, hypophysis, adrenals, and thymus were weighed at autopsy. In Experiment 5, 30 male rats with an average initial body weight of 250 g were divided into 5 equal groups (Table 1). The rats of 4 groups were injected daily with 4 doses of estradiol for 20 days (Table 1). All animals underwent electroshock. At autopsy the weight of the seminal vesicles was recorded. In Experiments 4 and 5, EST was determined in the appropriate groups 3 times a week for 2 weeks before the start of the injections and then for the duration of the study. In Experiment 6, 20 female rats with an average body weight of 140 g were hypophysectomized and divided into 2 equal groups (Table 1). Uterus and adrenals were weighed at autopsy. The EST was measured in all animals 3 times a week for 2 weeks before the start of the hormonal treatment and then for the duration of the experiment.

Results

As stated above, convulsive reactivity was quantitated by measuring both minimal electroshock seizure threshold

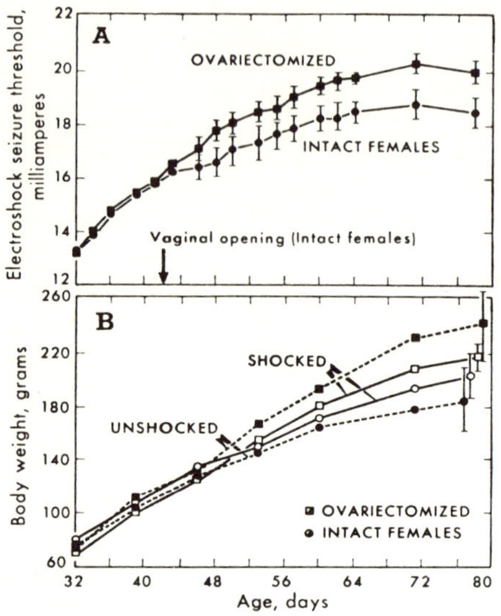

FIG. 1. Electroshock seizure thresholds (A) and body weights (B) of intact and ovariectomized rats. Vertical bracketed lines represent 95% confidence intervals of the means. Ovariectomies and sham-operations were performed at 30 days of age. Vaginal opening had occurred in all intact females at 42 days of age.

and maximal electroshock seizure pattern. Increased convulsive reactivity is indicated by a decreased threshold, a shorter duration of the tonic flexion or a longer duration of the tonic extension during a maximal seizure. Convulsive reactivity or convulsability, as determined by these methods, is believed by several authors (19, 23, 24) to measure a type of neural excitability. Therefore, brain excitability and convulsability, as measured by electroshock techniques, are often considered synonymous. The interchangeable use of these terms is permissible provided the parameters employed are adequately defined.

Effects of ovariectomy on electroshock convulsions

In view of our previous observations that brain convulsive reactivity is greater in adult female rats than in males of the same age and strain (16), it was considered of interest to study the influence of ovariectomy and replacement therapy on convulsability. The effects of ovariectomy performed before and after sexual maturation were compared.

a. Ovariectomy in immature rats (Experiment 1). Intact females after sexual maturation demonstrated greater convulsability than animals of the same age ovariectomized before puberty. The seizure thresholds were markedly lower in mature intact females than in the ovariectomized. The difference in thresholds between the two groups became statistically significant (*t*-test and 95% confidence limits) six days after vaginal opening had occurred in all intact females and remained significant for the duration of the experiment (Fig. 1A).

Both intact and ovariectomized rats demonstrated the progressive rise in

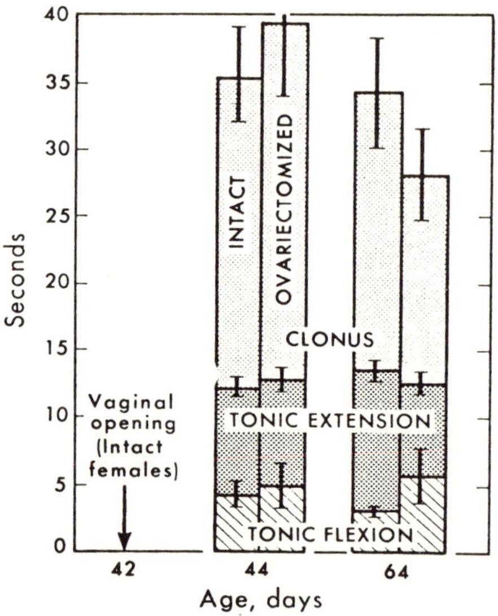

FIG. 2. Phases of the maximal electroshock seizure pattern of intact and ovariectomized rats. Vertical bracketed lines represent 95% confidence intervals of the means for each phase.

threshold shown to be associated with increasing age after 30 days of age (25). A similar characteristic rise occurred in all our experiments. This diminishing convulsive reactivity with age has been observed in rats (25–27) and mice (28), and evidence has been presented that the general decline in nervous system responsivity is due to aging, rather than to weight increase (25, 28, 29).

The greater convulsability of the mature intact females, as compared with the prepuberally ovariectomized adults, is also demonstrated by the differences in the maximal seizure patterns of the two groups. At 64 days of age intact females have a shorter tonic flexion and a longer tonic extension than ovariectomized rats (Fig. 2). It is to be noted that there was a delay between the time of vaginal opening and the onset of the changes in convulsability both in seizure thresholds and maximal seizures.

It is interesting that repeated electroshock did not interfere with the regularity of the estrous cycle as measured by vaginal smears. This is in agreement with our previous findings (18).

The final body weights of ths shocked and unshocked intact females were lower than those of the ovariectomized animals (Fig. 1 B). Electroshock alone did not significantly modify the rate of body growth in either intact or ovariectomized rats. It is to be pointed out that the shocked intact and the ovariectomized groups differed significantly in convulsability but not in body weight.

b. Ovariectomy with replacement therapy in immature females (Experiment 2). As in Experiment 1, intact mature females had lower thresholds and consequently greater convulsability than rats ovariectomized before puberty (Fig. 3 A).

Estradiol was administered at four dose levels to ovariectomized rats for 100 days (Fig. 3). The initial doses (0.10,

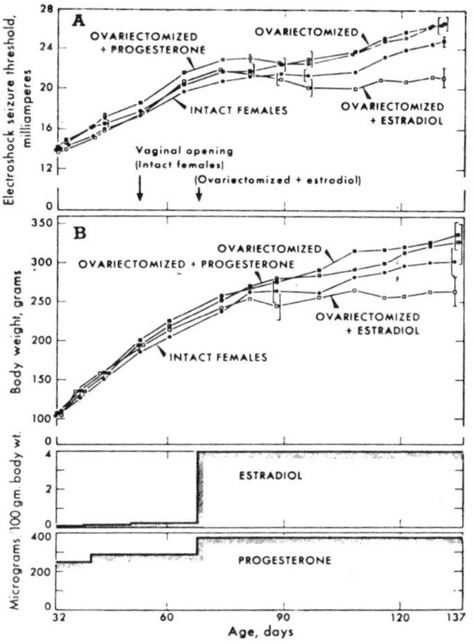

FIG. 3. Electroshock seizure thresholds (A) and body weights (B) of intact and ovariectomized rats with and without hormone therapy. Daily doses of hormones are shown at the bottom of the graph. Vertical bracketed lines represent 95% confidence intervals of the means.

0.15, and 0.25 μg/100 g body weight) did not significantly change the threshold and were not sufficient to prevent a two-week delay in the appearance of vaginal opening as compared with intact controls. After the dose was increased to 4.0 μg thresholds of estradiol-treated rats fell below those of the controls. By the end of the treatment period, threshold values of the injected animals were 20% and 15% lower than those of the ovariectomized and intact rats, respectively (Fig. 3 A). It appears then that the minimal effective daily dose of estradiol on the electroshock threshold lies between 0.25 and 4.0 μg/100 g body weight.

Progesterone lowered brain excitability as shown by a rise in the threshold above that of intact and ovariectomized

Table 2. Organ weights of intact and ovariectomized rats with or without replacement therapy

Treatment or procedure	No. of rats	Uterus, mg	Pituitary, mg	Adrenals, mg	Thymus, mg
None (intact controls)	10	440* ±54	11.5 ±0.4	87.4 ±5.0	237 ±26
Ovariectomized †	9	31 +3 (<.01) ‡	13.1 ±0.7 (<.01)	59.2 ±4.5 (<.01)	386 ±28 (<.01)
Ovariectomized + estradiol §	9	319 ±11 (<.01)	25.3 ±2.2 (<.01)	80.0 ±6.6	117 ±19 (<.01)
Ovariectomized + progesterone §	6	51 ±1 (<.01)	13.5 ±0.6 (<.02)	49.0 ±5.6 (<.01)	390 ±59 (<.05)

* Mean ± standard error.
† Ovariectomy was performed at 30 days of age.
‡ Figures in parentheses are P values based on the *t*-test for significance of differences between means of intact females and experimental groups.
§ For hormone doses see text and Figure 2.

controls from 44 to 81 days of age. After 81 days the thresholds of progesterone-injected rats were similar to those of the ovariectomized controls despite the continued daily administration of the hormone.

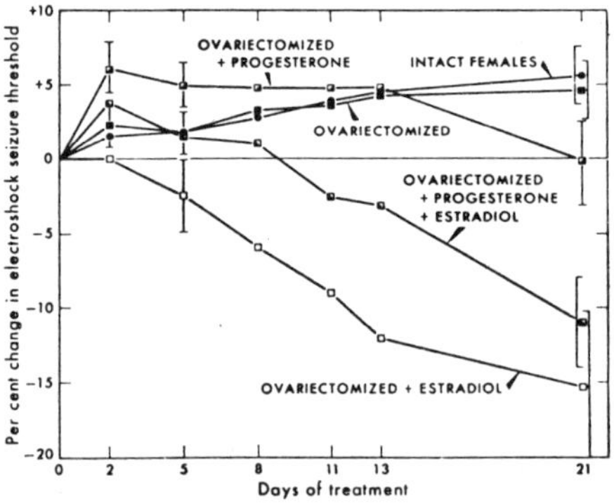

Fig. 4. Per cent changes in electroshock seizure thresholds in intact and ovariectomized rats with and without hormone therapy. Percent changes in thresholds are calculated in terms of pretreatment values. See text for doses. Ovariectomy was performed after sexual maturation had occurred. Vertical bracketed lines are 95% confidence intervals of the means.

Changes in the maximal seizure pattern were similar to those observed in previous experiments. Ovariectomy decreased convulsability as in Experiment 1 (Fig. 2). Administration of estradiol and progesterone shortened tonic flexions and lengthened tonic extension, thus reverting to normal the pattern altered by castration. These convulsant effects of the two hormones have already been described (17).

Body weights were similar in all groups except in that receiving estradiol (Fig. 3 B). In the latter, final body weights were lower than those of the other three groups. Whereas this difference in body weights became statistically significant only near the end of the experiment, the changes in threshold appeared earlier during the treatment with estradiol or progesterone.

Estradiol decreased thymus weight, increased pituitary weight, prevented the postcastration decrease in adrenal weight, but failed to restore completely the uterus weight. Progesterone did not alter the postcastration picture (Table 2).

c. Ovariectomy with replacement therapy in mature rats (Experiment 3). Ovariectomy in the adult female did not alter the seizure threshold (Fig. 4). This finding contrasts with the results reported above (Experiments 1 and 2) in which ovariectomy before sexual maturation resulted in a decreased convulsability.

The thresholds of ovariectomized rats receiving estradiol were lower than pretreatment values for this group as well as for values of control rats (Fig. 4). The difference between estradiol-injected and control groups was statistically significant by the fifth day of treatment and the final thresholds of injected rats were 20% below those of the controls. Thus estradiol had the same excitatory action in all ovariectomized rats regardless of the time of castration (Figs. 3, 4).

Progesterone significantly increased the threshold of ovariectomized above control values only during the first week of injections. Continued treatment tended to lower the threshold (Fig. 4). The administration of progesterone with estradiol to castrates delayed the fall in threshold produced by estradiol alone (Fig. 4). As in Experiment 2, the final body weights of the estradiol-injected rats were lower than those of the intact and ovariectomized controls (Table 3). In ovariectomized animals, estradiol, progesterone and the combined treatment increased the weight of the uterus to normal or above; adrenal weights did not differ significantly from intact control values.

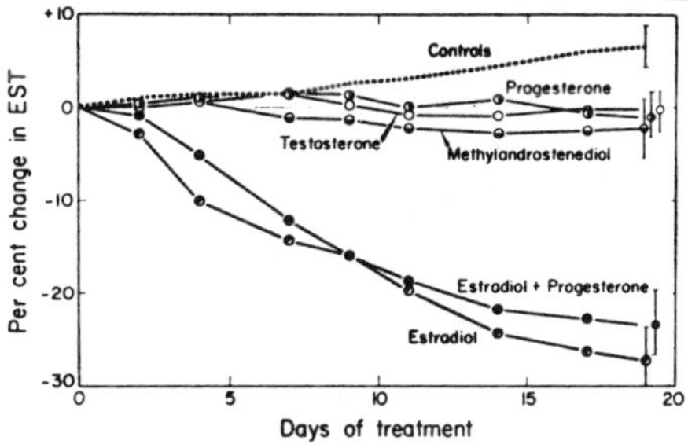

FIG. 5. Comparison of effects of male and female sex steroids on the electroshock seizure threshold (EST) in intact adult male rats. Thresholds are expressed as per cent changes of pretreatment values. Vertical bracketed lines are 95% confidence intervals of the means.

TABLE 3. Effects of estradiol and progesterone administration for 24 days on body and organ weights of adult ovariectomized or hypophysectomized female rats

Surgical procedure and daily doses of steroids per 100 g body weight	No. of rats	Body weight, g		Organ weights, mg	
		Initial	Final	Uterus	Adrenals
Intact controls	6	238 ±12*	271 ±15	475 ±64	70.8 ±5.8
		Ovariectomy†			
Controls	6	243 ±13	290 ±15	83 ±7	60.5 ±7.2
Estradiol, 10 μg	6	235 ±10	244 ±13 (<.01)‡	759 ±116 (<.01)	71.0 ±4.6
Estradiol, 10 μg + progesterone, 500 mg	6	242 ±11	259 ±14	676 ±125 (<.01)	73.7 ±10.9
Progesterone, 500 mg	6	235 ±12	265 ±14	476 ±68 (<.01)	77.5 ±6.4
		Hypophysectomy§			
Controls	7	135 ±2	140 ±4	60 ±4	10.6 ±0.6
Estradiol, 10 μg	7	137 ±3	128 ±7	393 ±41 (<.01)	13.3 ±0.9 (<.05)

* Mean ±standard error.

† Ovariectomy was performed 1 week before beginning of injections.

‡ Figures in parentheses are P values based on the *t*-test for significance of differences between means of hormone injected groups and appropriate controls.

§ Hypophysectomy was performed 3 weeks before beginning of injections.

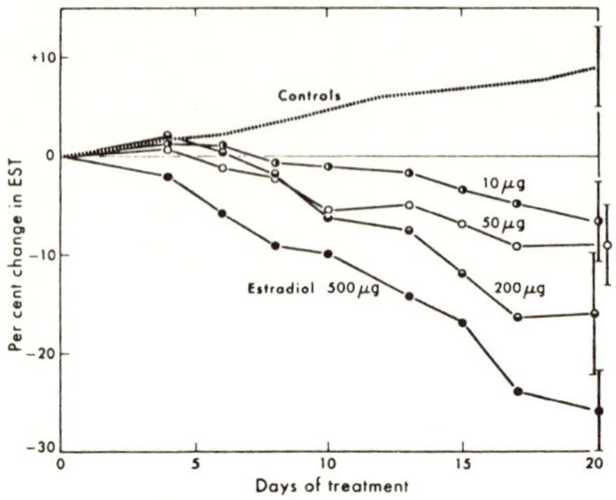

FIG. 6. Comparison of effects of 4 daily doses of estradiol on electroshock seizure thresholds (EST) in intact adult male rats. Thresholds are expressed as per cent changes of pretreatment values. Vertical bracketed lines are 95% confidence intervals of the final means.

Effects of sex steroids on electroshock convulsions in intact adult male rats

a. Estradiol, progesterone, estradiol plus progesterone, testosterone and methylandrostenediol (MAD) (Experiment 4). The thresholds of the estradiol-injected male rats decreased rapidly and were significantly lower than those of the controls two days after the start of the injections (Fig. 5). The addition of progesterone to estradiol delayed the initial fall in the threshold but after one week of the combined treatment there were no significant differences between the two groups; final thresholds were 27% and 23% below pretreatment values in the estrogen-injected and estrogen plus progesterone injected rats, respectively.

Progesterone, testosterone, and MAD did not modify the thresholds significantly during the first nine to 11 days of treatment; thereafter they significantly lowered the thresholds below control values.

Body and organs weights in corresponding shocked and unshocked groups were similar (Table 4). Final body weights of animals receiving estradiol alone or combined with progesterone were lower than control values.

The weights of the seminal vesicles and levator ani were significantly increased by testosterone, whereas MAD had no effect on the weight of the seminal vesicles and reduced that of the levator ani. Atrophy of these organs was produced by estradiol alone or in combination with progesterone; progesterone alone produced only a moderate involution of these organs.

Pituitary and adrenal hypertrophy were observed in all animals receiving estradiol. Progesterone alone did not affect these organs. Testosterone reduced pituitary weight to a greater extent than MAD did; neither affected adrenal weight. Thymus involution was produced by all steroids except progesterone.

b. Four doses of estradiol (Experiment 5). After 20 days of estradiol injections the mean electroshock thresholds of all experimental groups were significantly lower than pretreatment and control thresholds (Fig. 6). The decreases in

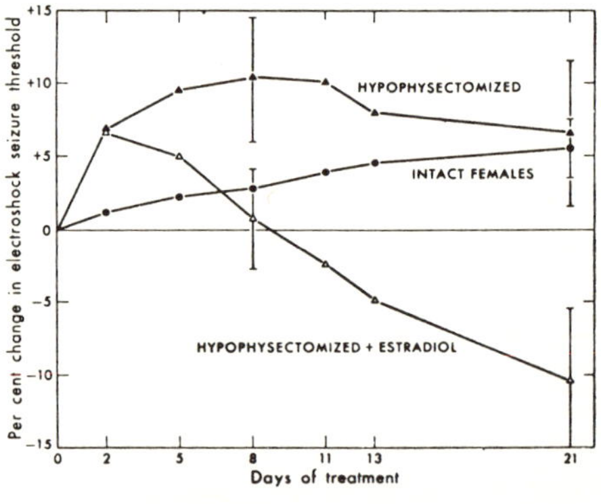

FIG. 7. Effects of estradiol on electroshock seizure thresholds of hypophysectomized female rats. The thresholds are expressed as per cent changes of pretreatment values. Vertical bracketed lines are 95% confidence intervals of the means.

threshold were proportional to the dose of estradiol.

In addition to lowering the electroshock threshold, estradiol injections also decreased body and seminal vesicle weights (Table 5). The atrophy of the seminal vesicles and the catabolic action of estradiol, as shown by the loss in body weight, were near maximal at the lowest dose level (Fig. 6). This suggests that the excitatory action of estradiol on the brain of the adult rat occurs at a higher

TABLE 4. Effects of administration of sex steroids for 20 days on body and organ weights of male unshocked and shocked rats

Injection* groups	No. of rats	Body weight, g		% change	Organ weights, mg				
		Initial	Final		Seminal vesicles	Levator ani	Pituitary	Adrenals	Thymus
				Unshocked Groups					
Oil vehicle (controls)	11	222† ±2	298 ±4	+34	722 ±32	217 ±12	9.6 ±0.4	49.0 ±1.0	339 ±29
Estradiol dipropionate	11	228 ±3	192 ±4	−16	81 ±5 (<.01)‡	65 ±7 (<.01)	15.0 ±0.8 (<.01)	79.9 ±5.2 (<.01)	106 ±12 (<.01)
Estradiol+progesterone	11	223 ±3	190 ±4	−15	96 ±8 (<.01)	63 ±5 (<.01)	15.5 ±0.6 (<.01)	65.9 ±4.5 (<.01)	91 ±13 (<.01)
Progesterone	10	221 ±4	290 ±10	+31	580 ±33 (<.01)	182 ±11	10.8 ±0.4	52.1 ±1.7	332 ±31
Testosterone propionate	11	223 ±2	275 ±5	+23	1,873 ±224 (<.01)	308 ±9 (<.01)	7.2 ±0.3 (<.01)	47.8 ±1.5	116 ±10 (<.01)
Methylandrostenediol	11	213 ±3	262 ±5	+23	637 ±40	173 ±9 (<.01)	8.4 ±0.5 (<.05)	48.6 ±2.0	252 ±22 (<.05)
				Shocked Groups					
Oil vehicle (controls)	10	229 ±3	288 ±5	+26	708 ±52	204 ±11	10.9 ±0.5	49.7 ±2.0	298 ±19
Estradiol dipropionate	11	222 ±3	195 ±5	−12	88 ±4 (<.01)	74 ±6 (<.01)	14.4 ±0.6 (<.01)	63.7 ±1.3	110 ±10 (<.01)
Estradiol+progesterone	10	215 ±5	190 ±5	−12	100 ±4 (<.01)	74 ±9 (<.01)	14.7 ±0.4 (<.01)	78.2 ±8.7 (<.01)	85 ±9 (<.01)
Progesterone	9	214 ±3	270 ±5	+26	582 ±56	172 ±11 (<.05)	10.8 ±0.7	46.1 ±2.3	297 ±21
Testosterone propionate	11	224 ±2	257 ±5	±13	2,215 ±79 (<.01)	305 ±13 (<.01)	8.7 ±0.3 (<.01)	50.4 ±2.9	100 ±14 (<.01)
Methylandrostenediol	10	217 ±5	265 ±7	+22	686 ±51	195 ±11	10.9 ±0.7	58.3 ±4.0	230 ±20 (<.05)

* One mg of each steroid was injected subcutaneously daily.

† Mean ± standard error.

‡ Figures in parentheses are P values based on the *t*-test for significance of differences between means of organ weights of control and hormone-injected groups.

TABLE 5. Effects of administration of 4 dose levels of estradiol for 20 days on body and seminal vesicle weights of rats

Daily doses of estradiol (μg/100 g body weight)	No. of rats	Body weight, g		Seminal vesicles, mg
		Initial	Final	
0 (controls)	6	269 ±18*	327 ±20	1,011 ±77
10	6	257 ±15	239 ±9 (<.01)†	147 ±3 (<.01)
50	6	263 ±12	236 ±13 (<.01)	148 ±6 (<.01)
200	6	265 ±8	241 ±11 (<.01)	158 ±10 (<.01)
500	6	263 ±12	243 ±12 (<.01)	126 ±8 (<.01)

* Mean ±standard error.
† Figures in parentheses are P values based on the *t*-test for significance of differences between means of control and estradiol-injected rats.

dose level than the inhibitory effects on the secondary sex organs and body weight.

Effects of estradiol and progesterone on electroshock convulsions in hypophysectomized female rats (Experiment 6)

The rise in threshold of the hypophysectomized controls at the beginning of the experimental period, i.e., three weeks postoperation, agrees with Woodbury's observation of the threshold-raising effects of hypophysectomy (19).

A daily dose of 10 μg estradiol produced a significant fall in the thresholds of hypophysectomized rats (Fig. 7) of a similar magnitude as that observed in ovariectomized animals (Fig. 4). Thus estradiol has an excitatory action even in the absence of the pituitary. Body weights of the hypophysectomized rats were not significantly influenced by the hormonal treatment (Table 3). Estradiol tended to correct the posthypophysectomy atrophy of the uterus. Although the adrenal weights of all hypophysectomized rats were below those of the intact controls, estradiol slightly increased adrenal weights above those of the hypophysectomized controls in accord with previous observations (30).

Discussion

The present work demonstrates that physiological levels of the ovarian hormones influence convulsive reactivity in the rat. Thus, intact mature females have lower electroshock seizure thresholds and a more convulsant type of seizure pattern than rats of the same age ovariectomized before puberty. The fact that estrogens are the principal ovarian hormones in the mature cycling rat (31, 32) suggests that this difference in convulsability is due to the action of estrogens; the present results of estradiol administration support this view. Progesterone would be expected to have little influence on convulsability in the cycling female, because the rat lacks a spontaneous luteal phase and has a minimal secretion of progesterone (31, 32).

Previous work from this and other laboratories has shown that sexually mature female rats and mice display greater convulsive reactivity than males of the same age and strain (16, 28). The data presented in this study provide evidence that these demonstrated sex differences in convulsability are due, at least in part, to the high levels of estradiol in the female and to the convulsant action of this estrogen.

Ovariectomy performed before sexual maturation impairs the normal development of brain excitability; consequently prepuberally castrated adult females have a lower convulsability than intact ones. In contrast ovariectomy performed after puberty does not alter convulsability during the first month after castration (Fig. 4) or may even increase it after two months (33). These findings that the effects of ovariectomy on brain excitability depend on the age at which the operation is performed and the time after castration recall the well-known fact that the effect of ovariectomy on adrenal cortical weight, and perhaps on adrenal corticoid production, depends both on the age at which the animal is ovariectomized as well as the postcastration time at which the adrenals are examined (34). Perhaps further elucidation of the estradiol-adrenocortical interrelation will help explain the age-dependent effects of ovariectomy on convulsability.

The administration of estradiol in daily doses ranging from 500 μg down to 4 μg per 100 g body weight lowers seizure thresholds relative to those of uninjected controls; thus it is evident that the convulsant action occurs at physiological levels of the estrogen. This is further supported by data which indicate that the rhythmic variations in estrogen levels during the estrous cycle are accompanied by parallel variations in brain thresholds: convulsability is lowest during diestrus, higher during proestrus, and highest during estrus (18). Estradiol exerts its marked convulsant effect not only in female rats but also in males. Furthermore, the threshold-lowering action of estradiol for experimental seizures has also been observed in other animal species (guinea pig, dog) (35, 36).

The threshold-raising action of progesterone noted during the first week of hormone administration in female rats may be related to the high EEG arousal thresholds involving the brainstem reticular formation observed approximately 24 hours after progesterone injection in estrogen pretreated rabbits by Kawakami and Sawyer (15). These workers also observed a decreased EEG arousal threshold approximately five hours following progesterone administration. In our studies convulsive thresholds were not determined less than 24 hours after the start of injections and therefore a comparison of seizure and arousal thresholds during this period cannot be made.

Progesterone administration rapidly and significantly raises the seizures threshold in female rats, but causes no immediate effect in males. However, the anticonvulsant effect in females is transient, and after 20 days of treatment a mild convulsant effect is observed in both males and females. The anticonvulsant effect of progesterone in females may be explained by Yates' observation that homogenates from livers of adult female rats reduce ring A of Δ^4-3 ketosteroids (progesterone, testosterone, etc.) three to ten times faster than homogenates from males (37). Figdor (38) has reported that these reduced products have greater anesthetic potency, and probably also greater anticonvulsant potency, than the original compounds. The conversion of the anticonvulsant to a convulsant effect in females after prolonged administration of progesterone remains still unexplained. Further investigation of the metabolic conversion of the steroids might unfold the mechanisms involved.

In the present experiments progesterone exhibits a mild convulsant action in intact adult male rats. A similar action is observed also after testosterone and methylandrostenediol; however, the excitatory effect of these compounds is less marked than that of estradiol at the same dose level. The convulsant action of testosterone has been reported previously (10, 11), but not that of progesterone and methylandrostenediol.

Estradiol increases convulsability to approximately the same extent in hypophysectomized as in intact females. Thus the convulsant action of estradiol is exerted even in the absence of the pituitary trophic hormones and despite lower than normal levels of adrenal steroids. This finding is of importance because the pituitary and adrenal hypertrophy induced by estradiol in several of the present experiments suggested an increased ACTH and adrenocorticoid production. In turn, adrenocortical stimulation might have accounted for the convulsant action, because some adrenal steroids (cortisol and cortisone) increase convulsive reactivity (19).

The present results emphasize the convulsant actions of the sex steroids, especially estradiol, and may appear to be in conflict with the observations of previous investigators. Thus, progesterone and testosterone were among the steroids which produced anesthesia (10) and raised the threshold for electroshock seizures (12) in immature female rats. Estradiol showed neither anesthetic nor anticonvulsant activity in these acute experiments. However, it is to be pointed out that very high doses were required to produce anesthesia.

Our experimental findings on the effects of ovariectomy in reducing convulsability agree with clinical observations that (a) ovariectomy reduces epileptic seizures in humans; (b) seizures often begin, or pre-existing attacks recur or worsen, at the menarche; and (c) seizure incidence is significantly depressed at the menopause in some cases (see 14 for review). Furthermore, these experimental data support the contention of some clinicians that estrogens aggravate the epileptic condition and that the ovulatory and premenstrual exacerbation of seizures observed in some female epileptics may be due to high blood levels of estrogens during these phases of the menstrual cycle (14, 39). The increased convulsive reactivity produced by estradiol may be involved in the premenstrual tension syndrome first described by Frank (40). Frank himself believed that the underlying cause of the syndrome is a marked retention of estrogens in the blood during the premenstrual phase and he described several clinical cases in which this was found to be true. In rare instances epileptiform seizures during the syndrome were noted.

The lowered seizure thresholds produced by several of the sex steroids, especially estradiol, offer more direct evidence to substantiate Beach's hypothesis, prompted by a consideration of mating behavior studies, that the gonadal hormones must alter thresholds within the nervous system It is suggested that a parallelism can be drawn between convulsive thresholds and other indices of brain excitability, e.g., running activity and mating behavior. The capacity of the gonadal hormones, both male and female, to modify convulsability suggests that the sex hormones may play a basic role in aspects of central nervous system physiology other than those exclusively concerned with sexual functions.

Acknowledgments

The authors thank Dr. A. A. Renzi of Ciba Pharmaceutical Products Inc. for the gift of the hormones, Mr. A. J. Silva for technical assistance, and Dr. F. A. Beach for critical review of the manuscript.

References

1. Harris, G. W.: *1st Intern. Congr. Endocrinol.*, Copenhagen, Symp. Lect. 1960. p. 15.
2. Wang, G. H.: *Comp. Psychol. Mon.* **2** (Serial No. 6). 1923.
3. Richter, C. P. and C. G. Hartman: *Am. J. Physiol.* **108:** 136, 1934.
4. Young, W. C. and W. R. Fish: *Endocrinology* **36:** 181, 1945.

5. Kislak, J. W. and F. A. Beach: *Endocrinology* **56:** 684, 1955.
6. Clark, G. and H. G. Birch: *Psychosomat. Med.* **7:** 321, 1945.
7. Zuckerman, S.: Hormones, Psychology and Behavior and Steroid Hormone Administration. *Ciba Colloq. Endocrinol.* **3:** 34, 1952.
8. Beach, F. A.: *Hormones and Behavior.* Hoeber, New York, 1948.
9. Beach, F. A.: *Biological and Biochemical Bases of Behavior*, Harlow and Woolsey, ed. Univ. Wis. Press. 1958. p. 263.
10. Selye, H.: *Proc. Soc. Exper. Biol. & Med.* **46:** 116, 1941.
11. Heuser, G.: *Rev. Canad. Biol.* **17:** 229, 1958.
12. Spiegel, E. and H. Wycis: *J. Lab. & Clin. Med.* **30:** 947, 1945.
13. Gordan, G. S.: *Rec. Prog. Horm. Res.* **12:** 153, 1956.
14. Logothetis, J., R. Harner, F. Morrell and F. Torres: *Neurology* **9**(5): 352, 1959.
15. Kawakami, M. and C. M. Sawyer: *Endocrinology* **65:** 652, 1959.
16. Woolley, D. E., P. S. Timiras, M. R. Rosenzweig, D. Krech and E. L. Bennett: *Nature* **190:** 515, 1961.
17. Woolley, D. E., P. S. Timiras and D. M. Woodbury: *Proc. West. Pharm. Soc.* **3:** 11, 1960.
18. Woolley, D. E., P. S. Timiras, H. H. Srebnik and A. Silva: *Fed. Proc.* **20**(1): 198d. 1961.
19. Woodbury, D. M.: *Rec. Prog. Horm. Res.* **10:** 65, 1954.
20. Timiras, P. S. and D. M. Woodbury: *Endocrinology* **58:** 181, 1956.
21. Booth, A. N., E. M. Bickoff and G. O. Kohler: *Science* **131:** 1807, 1960.
22. Woodbury, L. A. and V. D. Davenport: *Arch. Int. Pharmacodyn.* **92**(1): 97, 1952.
23. Toman, J. E. P., E. A. Swinyard and L. S. Goodman: *J. Neurophysiol.* **9:** 231, 1946.
24. DeSalva, S. J., R. A. Evans, R. Stubbs and G. Bobalik: *Proc. Soc. Exper. Biol. and Med.* **99:** 658, 1958.
25. Gellhorn, E. and H. Ballin: *Proc. Soc. Exper. Biol. and Med.* **68:** 540, 1948.
26. Frölich, A. and I. A. Mirsky: *Arch. Neurol. and Psychiat.* **47:** 30, 1942.
27. Frölich, A.: *J. Mt. Sinai Hosp.* **19:** 4, 1952.
28. Clark, G. and D. S. Sarkaria: *J. Neuropathol. & Exper. Neurol.* **17:** 612, 1958.
29. DeSalva, S. J. and N. Ercoli: *Arch. Internat. Pharmacodyn.* **122:** 75, 1959.
30. Bourne, G. and S. Zuckerman: *J. Endocrinol.* **2:** 283, 1940.
31. Emmens, C. W. *Reproduction in Domestic Animals*, Vol. I, Cole and Cupps, ed. Academic Press, N. Y. 1959. p. 111.
32. Segal, S. J.: *Comparative Endocrinology*, Gorbman, ed. Wiley & Sons, N. Y. 1958. p. 553.
33. Vallecalle, E., A. Soto-Rivera, T. Garrido de Armas and A. Gonzalez Luque: *1st. Intern. Congr. Endocrinol.*, Copenhagen, Abs. of Communications. 1960. p. 99.
34. Tepperman, J., F. L. Engel and C. N. H. Long: *Endocrinology* **32:** 373, 1943.
35. Perrini, M.: *Folia Endocrinol.* **7:** 179, 1954.
36. Longo, V.: *Riv. di Pat. Nerv.* **57:** 432, 1941.
37. Yates, F. E., A. L. Herbst and J. Urquhart: *Endocrinology* **63:** 887, 1958.
38. Figdor, S. K., J. J. Kodet, B. M. Bloom, E. J. Agnello, S. Y. P'an and G. D. Laubach: *J. Pharmacol. & Exper. Therap.* **119:** 299, 1957.
39. Copelman, L. S.: *First Intern. Congr. Neurol. Sciences* **3:** 605, 1957.
40. Frank, R. T.: *Arch. Neurol. & Psychiat.* **26:** 1053, 1931.

AUTHOR INDEX

KEY-WORD TITLE INDEX